Realities of Nutrition

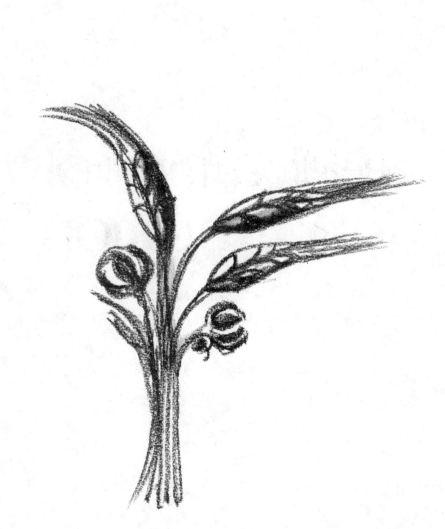

Realities of Nutrition

RONALD M. DEUTSCH

BULL PUBLISHING CO., P.O. Box 208, Palo Alto, CA 94302

Cover and Illustrations: Diana Dennington
Design: Joan Ingoldsby Brown

© Copyright 1976, Bull Publishing Co.

ISBN 0-915950-07-3
Library of Congress Catalog No. 76-23508
Printed in the United States of America

For

Diana and Kevin,

my family,

Who cheerfully surrendered

so many things

and so many days

to the making of this book.

BOOKS BY THE AUTHOR

In Nutrition
Realities of Nutrition
Nutrition Labeling (with the National Nutrition Consortium)
The *New* Nuts Among the Berries
The Family Guide to Better Food and Better Health

Psychology and Physiology
Pairing (with G. Bach)
Key to Feminine Response in Marriage

Fiction and Humor
The Grass Lovers
Is Europe Necessary?

BERKELEY SERIES IN NUTRITION

Food for Sport, Nathan J. Smith, M.D. (1976)

Realities of Nutrition, Ronald M. Deutsch (1976)

The Berkeley Series in Nutrition is a series of significant books about foods and nutrition, as they relate to the health and well being of people. It is our intent that all publications in this series will be carefully reviewed and evaluated before publication, to insure that the information is consistent with the current understanding of scientific research studies and practices in nutrition as it relates to the needs of humans.

Some books will provide an overview of the subject for the reader wanting reliable non-technical information. Others will be useful as college text books in non-major and major courses in nutrition. Still other books in the series are expected to contain specialized, technical information, for the professional in food and nutrition and related fields.

George M. Briggs, Ph.D.
Professor of Nutrition
Biochemist, Agriculture Experiment Station
University of California, Berkeley

Helen D. Ullrich, M.A., R.D.
Editor, Journal of NUTRITION EDUCATION
Lecturer in Nutrition
University of California, Berkeley
Editors

SOME PERSONAL WORDS

This book and I owe special gratitude to those people who reviewed and criticized the manuscript before it was put into its final form:

Dr. Roslyn Alfin-Slater
Dr. George Briggs
Dr. Alfred Harper
Dr. Paul Lachance
Dr. Gilbert Leveille
Margaret Phillips
Helen Ullrich

No one ever really wrote a book of this kind alone. Not only does it take other eyes to help keep facts clear and meaningful, but it takes other minds to help develop the perspectives which interpret those facts. Over the last few years, while this book was slowly taking shape, a number of people have contributed ideas, interpretations and examples from the literature of science, government, and commerce.

I owe thanks to such caring and informed people as Dr. Fredrick Stare, the

viii

inveterate teacher who always seems to have time to help; Dr. Philip White, who has patiently helped me to find the answers to awkward nutrition questions for at least 15 years; Dr. Mark Hegsted, who has extraordinary skill in detecting the smallest chink in the armor of any idea, and who has suggested a number of modifications for concepts which I have used here.

I am especially grateful also to: Beatrice Marks, who keeps me well informed about the realities of food production and marketing and the public's vision of nutrition; Dr. Paul Hopper, who has provided many insights into the labeling of food and into the food industry; Dr. Jean Mayer, who years ago taught me much about how to convey scientific realism in explaining the problems of obesity; Barbara Best, who has furnished me much of value about the consumer view; Dr. George York, who generously shares his broad knowledge of food-borne illness and of food science, and from whom I have pirated numbers of ideas about how to teach the real and imaginary hazards of foods; Dr. Fergus Clydesdale, who freely offers his acute understanding of the student mind and inquiry; Dr. Kristen McNutt, who has made valuable suggestions on how to communicate intricate technical data; Mildred Kaufman and Anita Owen, whose creative and realistic programs for the people (respectively) of Florida and Arizona have developed some very helpful practical concepts; and Dr. Richard Daniels, who with special acuity provides insights into the delicate relationship between industrial necessity and the public safety and health.

But beyond these (and many other) contributors of fact and philosophy, there are some special debts. One is to my wife, Diana, who has scoured the pages of the magazines and the shelves of the food markets to provide most of the examples of this kind used throughout the book. The other is to David Bull, who as an act of faith suggested that I write the book, who published it, who edited it, and who—no matter what the pressure—always accepted the simple explanation that, whatever the delay or the cost, it would make a better work.

With these thanks, however, I must add that any errors of fact, of understanding, or of presentation are solely mine.

R.M.D.
Laguna Beach, 1976

contents

ix

Realities of Nutrition

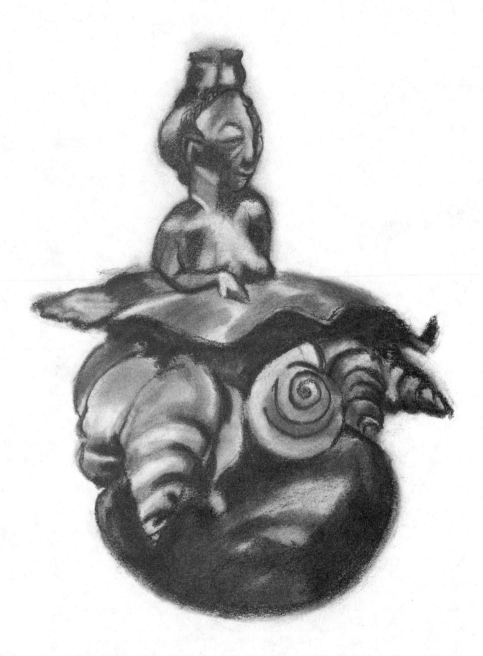

Food has been deeply involved in the myth and religion of virtually every culture. *Early Baluba Fetish. The Spirit of Fertility rising from a gourd and shells, symbolizing the food of land and sea. The Congo.*

chapter 1

THE PRICE OF ILLUSION

    While the nobles of ancient Rome banqueted on the choicest meats, and on game from every corner of their world, the fare of common folk consisted mostly of grain pastes, coarse breads, and millet porridges.[1] There was, however, one grim chance to break the dietary monotony. The stronger, nimbler slaves and criminals might be trained to become gladiators. During that training, and especially on the night before their trial on the Colosseum floor, they were given meat to make them strong.[2]

    Today's gladiators and their coaches still tend to agree, except of course that now they are much more "scientific," and refer to their training-table steak as *protein*. Recently, when Olympic athletes were interviewed, most said they needed to eat differently from other people.[3] Most commonly, they sought extra protein—some even saying that they couldn't get enough from food and had to take special protein pills and capsules.

1

Some Illusions and Realities of Protein

How realistic are these ideas in terms of what science knows? Contrary to popular belief, nutritionists find that heavy exercise requires little if any extra protein.[4] A running back and a desk clerk (of the same size) have about the same protein needs. Cross-country skiers used essentially the same amount of protein when they raced from 22 to 53 miles a day as they did while relaxing.[5]

But doesn't eating more protein make the body build more muscle? No. Increase of muscle is determined by ordinary growth, by heredity, or by exercise. What we eat merely supplies the materials for the increase; it doesn't *cause* it.[6]

When we do build more muscle, say, through exercise, don't we need extra protein to make it? We do need a little more, but the typical American diet already provides that extra amount.[7,8]

How Nutrition Illusions Can Be Costly

In recent years, there has been an astonishing boom of public interest in nutrition. (Not long ago, the world's most widely read magazine, *Reader's Digest,* found that nutrition had replaced sex as the biggest drawing card on the newsstands.[9]) Ironically, as we shall see, much of this popular interest is so misguided that it leads to deteriorating eating habits.

The protein illusions illustrate how this happens. There is, first of all, a penalty in dollars. Most protein sources, such as meats, are among our most expensive foods, so that when we try to add to a protein consumption which is already needlessly large, nutritionally we waste money. This may not be an important burden for the Dallas Cowboys or the U.S. Olympic Team, but it can be a critical nutrition factor for some people in our society.

For example, a number of athletes are persuaded to take protein supplements such as *Hi-Nrg.* The instructions for this product recommend that the buyer use one to four tablets a day. Four tablets cost about fifty cents. They contain, in total, roughly one-fourth of the protein in a single egg, a tiny fraction of our daily need, at a cost more than twenty times as great.

In a recent study of such supplements, the Federal Trade Commission (FTC) found that they were commonly recommended for the elderly, with such inducements as ". . . recommended as a dietary supplement for . . . aging persons," or, "Old folks, who have lost their taste for meat and eggs should consider them as a necessity for their diet."[10]

Since the elderly constitute one of our nutritionally compromised groups, and one reason for this is limited financial resources, let us see what the price of illusion may be for them. Using the FTC figures for costs, the day's protein allowance for an elderly man could be furnished by sirloin steak for less than eight percent of the cost of the supplement. Hamburger could do it for perhaps four percent, and nonfat dried milk for less than two percent.

However, there is more than an economic loss involved. For the reach for an emphasis on a diet high in protein can actually *un*balance our nutrition in some very destructive ways.

Protein is but a part of even "high-protein" foods. Even meat, the classic source, usually has less than a third of its calories in protein; most of its calories are in fats. So what many people believe to be a high protein diet usually proves to be a high fat diet. And we will see a number of reasons why high fat diets, which are typical American diets, are nutritionally undesirable.

One of the reasons why high fat diets are criticized by nutritionists is because fats are so much higher in calories than the other two major energy sources in foods, carbohydrates and proteins. (As we will discuss later, the ratio is approximately 9-4-4: A gram of fat provides approximately 9 calories, compared to about 4 for car-bohydrates and proteins.) So fats tend to drive other foods out of the diet, by taking up so much of our calorie budget. Some of the foods which are thus excluded, especially the carbohydrate-rich foods like grains, vegetables and fruits, are good sources of certain vitamins and minerals. When we lose those foods, we lose the vitamins and minerals which are found in them.

How good or bad is America's knowledge of nutrition? How many of us may be paying a high price in money, in health, or both for our lack of understanding about how food really furnishes the raw materials of life? Let us look at one recent study.[11]

How Real Is Our View of Nutrition?

Not long ago, a Federal agency sought to assess the nutritional thinking of a representative sample of the U.S. population. Here are some samples of the questions asked and the accuracy of the answers.

(1) *If people feel tired and run down, they probably need more vitamins and minerals.*

71 percent of the sample wrongly believed that this was true.

(We should note that, as is the case with all simplified questions, the most accurate answer to this one has its exceptions. For example, someone who suffered from iron deficiency might feel lacking in vigor. But the falsity of the statement lies in the implication that a deficiency of vitamins and minerals would be the *most likely* cause of weakness or fatigue. It would not.)

(2) *Older people need about the same amount of vitamins as young adults.*

67 percent of the sample said this idea was false, and were wrong. The needs of both groups are similar.

(3) *The chemicals added to our manufactured food take away much of its value for health.*

This was the most accurately answered question of the group. Only 48 percent of the responses were wrong.

(4) *Man-made vitamins are just as good as natural vitamins.*
Wrong answers were given by 65 percent.

(5) *Much of our food has been so processed and refined that it has lost its value for health.*
Wrong answers were given by 60 percent.

(6) *Chemical sprays that farmers use make our food a danger to health, even if they are used carefully.*
Wrong answers were given by 57 percent.

(7) *There is no difference in food value between food grown in poor, worn-out soil and food grown in rich soil.*

Wrong answers were given by 85 percent overall, and college graduates were wrong 88 percent of the time.

(8) *Many foods lose a lot of their value for health because they are shipped so far and stored so long.*
Wrong answers were given by 73 percent.

(9) *Food grown with chemical fertilizers is just as healthful as food grown with natural fertilizers.*
Wrong answers were given by 57 percent.

Statements numbered 2, 4, 7, and 9 are true. The rest are false. There are some exceptions to the truth or falsity of each of these questions. But there is a clear scientific basis for the "proper" answer to each—as will be apparent later.

On the average we can see that about two thirds of these Americans' answers to nutrition questions tended to be wrong. (Incidentally, college graduates' scores averaged only six percent better than those of the general population.) And when we come to more subtle nutrition problems, such as the evaluation of advertising claims, the practical balancing of the diet, or attempts to lose weight, the misconceptions are even more widely believed. Clearly, in the very real matter of food and health, a great majority of us are guided not by facts but by illusion.

Some of these illusions are ancient. From earliest time, man has made food and its mysteries a very basic part of his myth, his culture, and his religion.

THE SEARCH FOR NUTRITION MAGIC

In the oldest records of humanity, we find an awareness of a relationship between what we eat and what we are. We find in some form the idea that food supplies the energy of life, that food can become a part of us and can change us.[12, 13, 14, 15, 16]

For some facts of nutrition are obvious. It takes little science to learn that in general we feel good when we eat and bad when we go hungry. Mankind learned early that those who have plenty of food are likely to have less sickness. Indeed, the witch doctor and the scientist would probably agree on a basic definition of nutrition as—*the study of foods and their effects on the health, development, and performance of the individual.*

Up to a point, the study of foods by an early culture remains a very realistic business. For the first problem is to identify the potential sources of food, and to learn what is safely edible and what is dangerous. One finds truth by experiment.

For example, if a person finds that the blueberry is good and satisfying food, it may be tempting to try the lethal berries of the neighboring nightshade; but probably not a second time. It becomes important to know which mushroom is safe, which leaf, which root. Guessing in the world of food can easily go wrong. If one knows that the tuber of the potato is safe and nourishing, one would not have any way to guess that the leaves can be toxic. Or if one knows that the leaves of rhubarb are unsafe to eat, one might not guess that the stalks provide good food.

But even as such knowledge has accumulated, it has contributed little to a more basic understanding of how foods nurture. There is a magical quality to the relationship between food and life. Indeed, even for the modern scientist, nutrition is so close to the miracle of life itself that understanding often evokes a kind of awe. For nutrition is a kind of chemical witchery, in which we see such seeming commonplaces of the earth as the seeds of grasses, the leaves of plants, and the fruits of trees transformed into a human being.

Small wonder that primitive people endow foods with magical power and believe that qualities of the food may be transmitted to the eaters.[16,17]The people of the Aru and Buru Islands of the Pacific believed that a good way to become more nimble was to eat a dog. Certain American Indian braves believed that if they ate the genitals of the animals they hunted, they would become more potent.

In this light, we can see the logic of the Bakalai of Africa's Guinea Coast, who hold that each man has his own special taboo food, or *roondah*—and that if he dares to eat it, his wife will bear a child who resembles it. We can understand the thinking of those Moroccan tribesmen who, thinking the hyena to be stupid, believed that a woman who wanted to rebel against her husband had only to feed him a stew with a sauce made from hyena brains, and she would forever dominate the marriage.

Often such ideas are harmless. And sometimes they are confirmed repeatedly by the psychological effects of belief. Certain African tribes believe that to eat the flesh of the lion is to become brave and strong, but to dine on the hare means weakness and timidity. It does not take much imagination to see why the system seems to work, and what happened to the warrior who went into battle *believing* he would be weak and timid after eating rabbit. One can also understand why there have been those who would go hungry rather than risk the threat of the taboo.

The Frustrated Search of the Scientists

For well over 2,000 years nutrition has been viewed as a dominant force in medicine. Yet medical science has been slow to learn the realities of nutrition.

For centuries two schools of thought dominated medical teaching. In both, nutrition was seen to be at the foundation of health and disease.

One school was represented by Hippocrates, the famed physician of Greece's Golden Age, who is still regarded as the father of "modern" medicine. Aristotle reports Hippocrates' theory of disease, and his concern with the grosser physical qualities of foods, as follows:

"Either because of the quantity of things taken (eaten) or through their diversity or because the things taken happen to be strong and difficult of digestion, residues are thereby produced . . . And when the things that have been taken are of many kinds, they quarrel with one another in the belly, and . . . there is a change into residues . . . From the residues arise gases, which having arisen, bring on disease."[18]

This was typical of nutrition thinking for the next twenty centuries. There was also special emphasis on such attributes of food as its temperature, hardness, and color. For example, the Greek *Regimen in Health* gave this Hippocratic advice on eating in warm weather:

"In summer the barley-cake (a staple of the ancient Greek dietary) is to be soft, the drink diluted and copious, and the meats in all cases boiled. For one must use these in summer, that the body may be cold and soft."[18]

Rather close to the time of Hippocrates, in China of the sixth century B.C., another school of nutritional thinking arose, which is credited to Ho the Physician. He adapted to medicine the philosophic concept of two opposite yet mysteriously complementary forces as the core powers of the universe—*yin* and *yang*.

The *yin* is the female principle, typifying coolness and moistness. The *yang* is the male principle, standing for such qualities as warmth and expansion. These forces were seen to account for the occult characteristics of food, which supposedly influenced health by heightening the yin and yang of the body.

The Oriental idea entered the Arab world, and through it, the Greek. A thousand years ago it reached the medical school at Salerno, in Italy. By the time of the first Crusades—and partly because of them—the concept was brought into northern Europe. The Greek and Oriental nutrition traditions blended fairly well. For both related to the observable physical properties of foods. And whatever could not be explained in any other way could be attributed to the mystical balance or imbalance of yin and yang.

Nutrition science progressed little until the late 18th century, when the discoveries of oxygen and some of the first ideas of true chemistry at last began to open the way for understanding the life-giving qualities of food. Until that time (about 1780) all "civilized" people, despite their knowledge of astronomy, architecture, philosophy, and so forth, lived with a nutrition understanding which was really not a great deal different from that of the Aru or the Bakalai, the American Plains Indian, or the Australian aborigine. Nutrition as it would have been known to Columbus, Elizabeth the First, Sir Francis Drake, Isaac Newton, or young Benjamin Franklin is typified by this segment of a poem, the *Regimen sanitatis Salernitanum* (Health Regimen of Salerno), probably dating from the 1200s:

> "Peaches, apples, pears, milk, cheese, and salted meat,
> Deer, hare, goat and veal,
> These engender black bile and are enemies of the sick.
> Fresh eggs, red wines, fat broth,
> Together with fine pure flour, strengthen nature.
> Wheat, milk, young cheese,
> Testicles, pork, brain marrow,
> Sweet wine, food pleasant to the taste,
> Soft-boiled eggs, ripe figs, and fresh grapes,
> Nourish as well as make fat."[18]

Then, in the period 1780 to 1794, the French chemist Lavoisier showed that oxygen was taken into the body, and that it was used in a "burning" process which yielded heat. From these experiments came the first insights into food's work as fuel. In one famous line, Lavoisier forged the key to all true nutrition science—*"La vie est une fonction chimique."* (Life is a chemical function.)

From this basic work there developed the understanding that foods are merely the raw materials which provide the "chemicals" for the chemistry of life. But it took more than a century of work by thousands of scientists before we acquired more than the most superficial information about the composition of foods and how that composition affects our lives. Only in this century have we acquired any real understanding of food and nutrition.

Perhaps the newness of so much of our scientific understanding helps to account for the fact that so few people seem to accept fully the concept of nutrition as chemistry—and instead, would ascribe health values of foods to factors totally inconsistent with chemical science, and indeed not entirely unlike those ancient myths which we find so ridiculous.

The Power of Modern Nutrition Mythology

As an example of how we still value food myths, consider the wide belief in foods which are sold as "natural," and particularly our national adoption of "granolas" for breakfast cereals. These are simply mixtures of variously processed grains, with a little bit of dried fruit, nuts, and the like, and a good deal of sweetener. They are sold with an implication of greater health value, and by weight they cost twice as much or more than ordinary ready-to-eat cereals.

Granolas originated in Swiss and German spas about the beginning of the century, devised by "naturopaths" with little or no medical training. Fed to the wealthy guests who came to find health by drenching themselves inside and out with mineral waters, they were the core of some vegetarian "cures" which were popularized in this country by the likes of Dr. John Harvey Kellogg (inventor of the cereal flake).[19] More recently, enthusiasm for the granolas was revived by Gayelord Hauser and Adelle Davis, among others.

Scientifically, they have no special value. No matter how cleverly one mixes an ounce of grains, they are not likely to have extraordinary nutritional importance. The amount of fruit and nut in a serving has little significance for the diet. And the sweeteners (usually honey, or raw or brown sugar), which often constitute the second largest ingredient, have no practical health advantage over ordinary refined white sugar.

But Americans, concerned about better nutrition, and noting that the granolas are "natural," that they have no "additives" or white sugar, and generally seem homey and old-fashioned, have begun to buy them in quantity. At this writing, over 7 percent of the enormous ready-to-eat breakfast cereal market has been taken by granolas.[20]

How do these cereals compare to ordinary breakfast cereals? It depends on the cereal, of course, but many are relatively rich nutritionally. What are *not* added to granolas are the vitamins and minerals often added to ordinary cereals. The result is that the expensive granolas generally have about 70 to 90 percent less of key vitamins and minerals. Let us compare two kinds of cereals.

*Comparison of Nutrient Values of a Typical "Natural" cereal with a Popular Conventional cereal.		
	Quaker 100% Natural	**Cheerios**
Serving size	1 ounce (¼ cup)	1 ounce (1¼ cups)
Calories	120	110
Percentage of U.S. Recommended Daily Allowances		
Protein	2	6
Vitamin A	*	25
Vitamin c	*	25
Thiamin (B_1)	2	25
Riboflavin (B_2)	*	25
Niacin	2	25
Calcium	2	4
Iron	2	25
Vitamin D	*	10
Vitamin B_6	**	25
Vitamin B_{12}**	*	25

* *Contains less than 2% of U.S. RDA for this nutrient.*
***Value not given, but may be presumed low.*

From this tabulation one can see that a mother who seeks to improve her family's breakfast nutrition by turning to granolas spends more money, only to provide less nutritionally. For she has bought a generally mythological value (the word "natural" on the label), rather than a chemical one (the nutrients contained in the product). Myths can contribute to the quality of life, but they are not edible.

SOME DANGERS OF MISGUIDED CHEMISTRY

Even when people accept the hard-won concept of food as the source of the raw materials of life, a mythology can attach itself to the chemicals. Let us consider how much of the population deals with two known, real values in the chemistry of nutrition, vitamin C and iron.

Recently, vitamin C has been given great emphasis in some popular ideas about better health. There is no question that vitamin C is essential in human nutrition. (Its functions are described in

Chapter Twelve.) But there is a question about the popular view of how much vitamin C we need and the health value of extras.

In essence we should keep in mind the nutrition principle, which will be carefully explored, that once the body has all that it needs of a nutrient such as a vitamin, more will accomplish nothing and may cause harm. We should also remember that our newest and best surveys of American nutrition suggest that vitamin C is not often lacking in the American diet.[21]

Yet advertising treats vitamin C as if it were a critical factor in the diets of American children. The average child is quite likely to start his day with some juice or fruit which supplies from 100 to 200 percent of his recommended allowance of vitamin C. And he is likely to get more all through the day. But while children tend thus to become surfeited with vitamin C, other nutrients are often ignored, nutrients which surveys have shown to be lacking to an appallingly common extent.

For example, the Ten State Survey of the Federal Government indicates that more than a third of U.S. children under the age of six are so low in iron consumption that they suffer from various levels of anemia.[22] Yet there is little publicity given this common shortage, or the foods which can meet it. For about a decade, a proposal to add more iron to flour has been stalled, despite the willingness of industry to cooperate.[23]

CAN'T INDUSTRY DO OUR THINKING FOR US?

Much of our nutrition confusion is blamed on industry. But industry is in many ways a passive force—amoral but not really immoral, if you will—trying simply to turn out a decent product and make a profit. Basically, industry responds to what we *think* our needs are. It is incredibly expensive to try and create public demands; it is much cheaper simply to find out what people want to buy and give it to them.

The broad food-industry use of added vitamin C is a recognition of the public's distorted idea of the need for this vitamin. General Foods sells its *Tang* (a flavored sugar mixture with an orange taste) on the basis that it has "twice as much vitamin C as orange juice." It does so because the public believes that vitamin C is badly needed, and the more the better. Meanwhile, the Florida citrus industry ballyhoos its oranges as having "natural vitamin C from the Florida sunshine tree." It does this because so many people mistakenly believe that there is a health difference between "natural" and synthetic vitamin C. While neither sales effort may be in the public interest, both are realistic to the extent that they give the public what the public thinks it needs.

There is no real protection against such myths. A primary finding of one panel at the 1969 White House Conference on Food, Nutrition and Health was that "The American people falsely believe that they are well protected by both government and by the ethics of commerce."[24]

Why can't the food industry protect us from nutrition illusion? Theoretically, it could. But the industrial reality is that, while production methods are controlled by technologists of great sophistication, the businesses are guided by marketers. Their training is in the economics of producing and selling. Their information about nutrition is minimal. Their primary interest lies in what will sell, and this is determined by what the public wants. Their foremost research effort is to determine public wishes and to meet them.

The industry's promotion people often know even less about nutrition. Their aim is to express as dramatically as possible the idea that the product furnishes what the buyer thinks is important. Essentially their sales message is that "What you want is what we have to sell."

To see how ironically this system works, look again at the granolas. The vast majority are made by the same companies which sell conventional cereals, with the usual additives. But while one part of the company heralds its granolas by implying that additives are always unhealthful, that sugar is dangerous, and that "natural" products are somehow superior, other parts of the company spend millions to convince us that additives and preservatives are valuable and harmless, and that ordinary cereals give us better nutritive content. In an individual, such behavior might be called "schizophrenia." In a cereal company, it is simply a matter of "market identification" and "market penetration"—in two markets.

PUBLIC ILLUSIONS AND GOVERNMENT ACTION

In terms of nutrition, politicians follow the example of industry. In an effort to give the public what it wanted, the Federal Trade Commission recently proposed some new rules for food advertisers.[25] Since the public was so concerned with protein, the rules made protein content an important factor in advertising a food as "nutritious." To be called "nutritious," a 100-calorie portion of a food was supposed to have at least 10 percent of the recommended daily protein allowance for an adult male. With such a rule it would be almost impossible for most grain, vegetable, or fruit products to be called nutritious. Yet as we shall see repeatedly, these are the foods which are often missing from U.S. diets, leading to various nutrition problems.

Another example of unthinking government response to the public's misguided ideas of good nutrition appeared when the Food and Drug Administration (FDA) sought to set some limits on excess dosages of vitamins and minerals. Nutritionists agreed with the proposed regulation of these overdoses, which can be dangerous.

Apparently this information did not reach the Senators considering the legislation; but they did know that Americans would not like FDA to control access to massive vitamin doses. When Senator Proxmire of Wisconsin moved to give voice to the popular thinking, and to stop FDA from regulating vitamins, he was joined by 36 other senators of every political stripe, from Hubert Humphrey to James Buckley, from George McGovern to Strom Thurmond, from more liberal politicians such as Cranston, Mansfield and Adlai Stevenson III, to conservatives such as Eastland, McClellan and Goldwater.[26, 27]

WHICH FOODS SHOULD WE EAT?

In this book the reader will not find a catalog of good foods and bad. For realistically there is no food which is either essential to health or inimical to it. A lunch of hot dogs at a ball game, a dinner of cocktails and canapes, or skipping lunch entirely—none of these things need be outside the pale of good nutrition. Human life is astonishingly flexible. It can flourish on foods from the Arctic to the Equator, from the desert to the jungle, from the school cafeteria to the pizza parlor. It is the whole *balance* of the diet which matters, and that balance can admit of wide variety in foods.

The nutritionist defines a food as, *any substance which is taken into the body to provide the necessary raw materials for the chemistry, structure, or function of life.* By this definition a chocolate bar is as much a food as is a slice of roast beef. And the consuming of either can be consistent wth good nutrition—if only one knows the needs of the body, the composition of foods, and the appropriate role of foods in supporting life, within the context of the total diet.

As a whimsical example—not to be taken as good dietary advice—consider sources of iron, often low in the diets of children. Some three and a half ounces of roast beef will supply a child, or an adult male, with about a third of his recommended daily allowance of iron. But a three and a half ounce bar of bittersweet chocolate would supply *half* of that allowance. Two-thirds of a pound of marsh-mallows, or a pound of jelly beans would do as well. On the other hand, a three and a half ounce bar of milk chocolate would not supply much iron. (But it would offer about a fourth of an adult's daily allowance for calcium.)

Obviously the candy provides quite a few calories along with these desirable nutrients; it is not seriously suggested that we give every child who is short of iron a pound of jelly beans for breakfast. Rather the object is to show that all foods can have useful aspects, and that terms like "junk foods" tend to confuse more than to instruct.

To carry this reasoning even further, let us consider a hypothetical (and unrealistic) problem in world nutrition. Would candy be a good thing to give to a starving child in Bangladesh? Scientifically, it could actually spare such a child from the ravages of protein deficiency. How can this be, when the candy has little or no protein?

Energy, as measured in calories, is the first need of the body. If we run out of fuel, life stops. So the body gives its first nutritional priority to fuel. If the child in Bangladesh gets adequate protein, but does not get sufficient calories, his body will simply burn much of that protein as fuel. In this way a child who gets enough for his needs, but too few calories of energy, can become protein-deficient.

Candy could greatly improve the nutrition of such a child, by performing the function whch is known to nutritionists as *protein-sparing*. Without the candy, or some other food* to supply adequate energy for the continued function of his brain, heart, and other vital organs, the child will suffer from *protein-calorie malnutrition.* The phenomenon is widely known. It is found on the North American Continent, among certain Eskimo children in Canada.[28,29,30] In this

---

*As indicated above, this example helps make the point—but candy would be obviously unrealistic in such a situation; other foods would be better, supplying energy and also other nutrients that would surely be lacking as well.

view, sugar, because it is a compact energy source, is seen by some experts as a possible solution to some problems of world hunger. For sugar yields more energy per acre than any other crop in wide cultivation.[31]

We shall see that it is a premise of scientific nutrition that virtually no cultural circumstance, no limitation of religion or spirit, of taste or preference, should make good nutrition impossible. We shall see that the realities of nutrition are both personal and universal, that they are in some ways always unique, and in some ways always the same.

The central question is, how do we learn what is real?

REFERENCES

1. Tannahill, R. *Food in History,* Stein and Day, New York, 1973, p. 93.
2. Hadas, M. *Imperial Rome,* Time Inc., New York, 1965.
3. Darden, E. *Olympic Athletes View Vitamins and Victories,* J. Home Econ., Feb. 1973, pp. 8—9.
4. Smith, N. *Food for Sport,* Bull Pub. Co., Palo Alto, 1976.
5. Hedman, R., *The available glycogen in man . . . etc.* Acta Physiol. Scand. Vol. 40, 1957, pp. 305—9.
6. *Nutrition for Athletes,* Amer. Assn. for Health, Phys. Ed. and Recreation, Washington, 1971.
7. Bergstrom, J. and Hultman, E. *Nutrition for maximal sports performance,* JAMA, Vol. 221, pp. 999—1006.
8. Food and Nutrition Board, *Recommended Dietary Allowances,* Nat. Acad. Sciences, Washington, 1974, p. 43.
9. Harper, H. H., personal communication.
10. *Protein Supplement Health Hazards and Marketing Deceptions: a staff report to the Federal Trade Commission,* FTC, Washington, 1975.
11. FDA, *A Study of Health Practices and Opinions,* Contract No. 66-193, June, 1972.
12. Calverton, V.F., ed. *The Making of Man,* Modern Library, New York, 1931.
13. Childe, C., *What Happened in History,* Pelican, New York, 1946.
14. Lowenberg, M., et al., *Food and Man,* Wiley, New York, 1974.
15. Weyer, E., *Primitive Peoples Today,* Dolphin, New York.
16. Crawley, E., *The Mystic Rose,* p. 137, Spring Books, London, 1965.
17. Frazer, J.G., *The Golden Bough,* Macmillan, New York, 1971.
18. Temkin, O., *Nutrition from Classical Antiquity to the Baroque,* In Human Nutrition, Historic and Scientific, N.Y. Acad. of Medicine, New York, 1960, pp. 78—97.
19. Deutsch, R. *The Nuts among the Berries,* Ballantine, 1967.
20. *Cereal market to grow,* Advtg. Age, Apr. 22, 1974, p. 2.
21. Ascorbic acid, in *Recommended Dietary Allowances,* Nat. Acad. Sci., Washington, 1974, p. 63.
22. Center for Disease Control, *Ten-State Nutrition Survey in the United States,* V— Dietary, DHEW Pub. No. (HSM) 72-8133, 1972.
23. *Enrichment,* Amer. Bakers Assn. Report, Vol. 6, No. 2, Mar. 1972.
24. White House Conference on Food, Nutrition and Health, final report, U.S. G.P.O., Washington, 1970.
25. Food Advertising, 16 CFR Part 437, Federal Trade Comm., Federal Register, Vol. 39, No. 218—Nov. 11, 1974.
26. Congressional Record (re: S.548) Feb. 3, 1975.
27. *FDA efforts to Regulate Vitamins as Drugs Hit by Proxmire, Schweiker,* Nat. Health Federation Bulletin, Apr., 1975 pp. 16—28.
28. Sabry, Z.I., ed., *Nutrition Canada,* Information Canada, Ottawa, 1973.
29. Pearson, W.N., *Biochemical appraisal of nutritional status in man,* Amer. J. Clin. Nutr. 11:426, 1962.
30. Viteri, F.E. and Arroyave, G., *Protein-Calorie Malnutrition,* in Modern Nutrition in Health and Disease, Lea & Febiger, Phila., 1973, pp. 604—624.
31. Stare, F., *Sugar in the diet of man,* World Rev. of Nutrition and Dietetics, vol. 22, Karger, Basel, 1975, pp. 239—247.

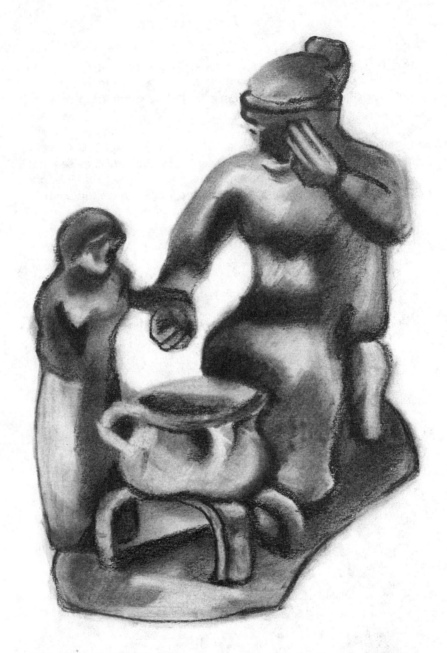

The ultimate reality of nutrition rests with the chemistry of the food we eat and its effects on the processes of life. *The Cooking Lesson. Beotian terra cotta figure, sixth century, B.C.*

chapter 2

THE TESTS OF REALITY

A few years ago, Dr. Henry G. Bieler announced that he had discovered the true cause of the common cold, measles, and polio— and that he could cure them.[1]

Of course, medicine has long been confident that all of these illnesses were caused by specific viruses. But Dr. Bieler explained that medicine had been fooled. True, the viruses actually were in the bodies of the sick, but they were merely feeding on "stagnating waste products," which were the real cause of the trouble.

"Years of laboratory observation and experimentation have taught me," he reveals, "that germs do not cause disease . . . Improper foods cause disease; proper foods cure disease."

Bieler gives examples: the common cold is more common in winter because people overeat during the holidays and are less active, thus building up body wastes. Polio can come from a number of foods, he says, but especially ". . . from the putrefaction of ice cream in the bowels. Polio strikes most viciously at children who eat large quantities of ice cream. One indication of this is that the majority of cases occur during the peak of the summer ice-cream season.''

These ideas may seem patently absurd in the light of current knowledge. Yet until his recent death, Bieler was physician to many of the Hollywood famous. His book, *Food Is Your Best Medicine,* was bought by over 100,000 Americans in the hardcover edition, and by many more in paperback. Evidently his ideas about food chemistry and its effect on health have seemed reasonable to a lot of people.

We can easily test the medical realities of Bieler's ideas, by referring to the enormous body of scientific evidence on contagious disease. [2,3] But what if, as commonly happens, food causes and cures are proposed for illnesses for which the causes and cures are not understood? For instance, Bieler identifies certain foods as the causes or cures of cancer. How can we test his nutritional claims or those of others who promise or threaten much in the name of nutrition?

Food Composition as a Testing Device

Perhaps the most worn volumes on most nutritionists' bookshelves are the handbooks of food composition. For our first interest in foods, scientifically, is as sources of nutrients. Composition tables tell us which nutrients are present in foods and to what extent. And a quick look at the composition of a food is often enough to determine the sense or nonsense of a nutritional claim. For the nutrient content of a food is a basic reality.

If we look closely at Bieler's statements about nutrients, and weigh them against our knowledge of food composition, we quickly find that his chemistry is sadly lacking. He lays heavy emphasis on vegetables (certainly excellent nutrient sources, but within well-defined limits), and calls upon the classics for support: ''When Hippocrates formulates the maxim, 'Thy food shall be thy remedy,' he certainly must have had in mind the medicinal qualities of vegetables.''

Bieler is especially interested in the zucchini squash as ''a cure-all.'' Why zucchini? Because, he says, sodium is so important in treating the toxicities which he thinks cause disease, and ''the zucchini is an especially sodium-rich vegetable, as are other members of the squash-cucumber-melon family.''

At this point we have a specific statement to which we may apply a test, by turning to one of the U.S. Department of Agriculture (USDA) food-composition books, such as Handbook Number 456.[4] This book, along with the earlier USDA Handbook Number 8,[5] is in worldwide use by nutritionists. For it represents great amounts of data, averaged from large numbers of chemical analyses of foods. Only the analyses which follow standard, approved methods are incorporated. (Portions of Handbook Number 456, referring to some common foods, are included in Appendix A of this book.)

Looking up zucchini squash in Handbook 456, we find that a cup of it (raw) contains one milligram of sodium, and that a cup of cooked squash contains 2 milligrams. The sodium values for other squashes are similar. A cup of cucumber contains 6 milligrams, and a cup of muskmelon has 19 milligrams.

Is this a great deal of sodium? Looking through the tables, we find that it is precious little compared to a cup of green peas at 458 milligrams, or a cup of beef stew with over 1,000 milligrams. Plainly, the amount of sodium in Bieler's "sodium-rich" vegetables is minis-cule. His chemical information is wrong in the most obvious way— without even considering the additional fact that all evidence indi-cates that most American diets actually contain too much sodium.

Do these realities disprove Bieler's theories of disease? To some extent they do. More clearly, they suggest that his information about nutrients is grossly in error. But in any event it shows that the rationale for his food "cures" is spurious. Reliable scientists make mistakes, of course, but not such basic ones; and they are protected by *peer review,* that is, letting colleagues review and criticize their work before publishing it.

Let us use food-composition to test some other ideas. For example, recall the survey question FDA asked, about the supposed inferiority of foods grown with chemical fertilizers (an idea which 57 percent of those surveyed thought was true). The idea has been popularized by such writers as Adelle Davis, who said that we can't get enough vitamin A from ordinary foods, because it is destroyed by chemical fertilizers. But if we check the food-composition tables for vitamin A values, we find that they are still there. These values are not hypothetical; they are derived from analyses of ordinary market vegetables.

Some natural-food enthusiasts insist that we must get our vitamins from *fresh* foods, and that canned and frozen products are always inferior.[6,7] But if we look at a widely-consumed vegetable, such as string beans, we find that half a cup cooked from fresh sources provide some 540 units of vitamin A, that canned beans offer some 470 units, and that the same quantity of cooked frozen beans provides 580 units. The differences are relatively small—5,000 units of vitamin A is the recommended daily amount for most adults.

An understanding of food composition is a basic reference point in nutrition, an important guide to reality. For example, in the last chapter of this book, the claims for "organically-grown" foods will be considered. Many of these claims center around the idea that these specially grown foods have more nutrients, especially more minerals. But in truth, chemical analyses of these and of ordinary market foods show no such differences.

What Are the Nutrients in Foods?

In testing for nutritional reality, one must know more than just the amounts of nutrients in foods, however. One also needs to have some idea of the roles these nutrients play. As we have seen, most Americans seem to believe that vitamins are sources of energy. But the fact is that the only energy sources in foods are the *macronutrients.*

Nutritional science learned about these nutrients first. And the fact that *macro* means *large* suggests what the three have in common: The body uses them in large amounts; they are the only important sources of energy; and they are the primary sources of the body's main chemical building materials.

The macronutrients are *carbohydrate, fat,* and *protein.* A fourth chemical group, *alcohols,* could conceivably be called a macronutrient because it constitutes a major source of fuel. When alcohol is used in quantity, it must certainly be taken into nutritional account, for it replaces other foods. But because of its limitations, nutritionists tend to consider alcohol separately from other nutrients.

A second large group of nutrients was identified only in this century. These are the *micronutrients,* so called because we use them in very small, sometimes extremely tiny amounts. The micronutrients are the vitamins and minerals. The first vitamin was not identified until 1911; and we are still learning a great deal about the body's use of minerals, and there is continuing speculation about the need for some of them.

Water is a rather special nutrient, constituting the largest component of our foods. While water does not furnish energy, it plays more than a mechanical role in the diet, taking a critical part in body chemistry. We take in more water than most of us realize; for example, fruits and vegetables are usually at least 80 to 90 percent water; bread is about a third water.

The final food factor is *fiber*. Its role and character are explored in more detail in Chapter Seven, but basically, it is carbohydrate, in a form which is largely indigestible in humans. So it tends to pass through the digestive tract, in the process playing an important part in normal digestion. Whether or not fiber should actually be called a nutrient is now being debated. For its chief role seems to be mechanical (although some small parts of fiber can be digested), and the argument is made that it does not participate significantly in life's chemistry.

In all, there are some 50 known nutrients. The exact number is in doubt because the nutritional roles and requirements for some substances, especially the minerals which are known as *trace* elements, are not yet fully understood, and it is suspected that as we learn more, it will be shown that some additional trace elements are essential in human nutrition.

How Much of the Nutrients Do We Need?

Earlier, in looking at Dr. Bieler's zucchini squash and its sodium, we learned how much sodium the squash contained, but we could not tell very much about its significance without knowing something about the size of our needs for this mineral. Let us look at another example—the taking of supplements of vitamin E.

In recent years, vitamin E capsules have become big sellers in drugstores and health-food stores, as protection from smog, heart attacks, and sexual problems. Typically, enthusiasts recommend that 500 units of the vitamin be taken after each meal.

How much E should we really consume? To find out what scientific evidence has shown can be beneficially used, we can refer to tables prepared by the *Food and Nutrition Board*. The Board is assembled under the auspices of the National Academy of Science's National Research Council. It is composed of large numbers of our most respected nutrition scientists, and its membership changes periodically, both to share the burden of the work and to infuse a variety of responsible opinions.

The Board's Committee on Dietary Allowances is composed of subcommittees for each nutrient, or in some cases, for groups of nutrients. The scientists on each subcommittee constantly reassess what is known of the nutrients, scouring the newest research reports. They also study the quantities of nutrients in our food supply, their effects on the body, and all relevant information about the public's health and eating habits.

About every five years (last in 1974), the Committee on Dietary Allowances publishes an updated report called *Recommended Dietary Allowances*. This report sets out guideline recommendations for different population groups, according to age, sex, height, and weight. Thus a Recommended Dietary Allowance (RDA) for 17 different groups of people is estimated—for every nutrient about which there is information enough to make a judgment. The simplified table which summarizes these recommendations may be found in Appendix E.

The RDAs are widely misunderstood to be minimums for survival. In fact, they include generous safety margins. RDAs, under different names, are also set in other countries, such as Canada and Great Britain, and by United Nations agencies, and these are lower than the American RDAs for several nutrients.

If we look at the adult recommendation for vitamin E in the RDA table, we see that it is 15 international units daily. Thus, the 1500-units-a-day supplement (500 after each meal) supplies over three months' RDA for this vitamin.*

Is it likely that the RDA Committee is grossly in error about the amounts of vitamin E needed for optimum health? One "common sense" way of approaching such questions (which might be called a "biological" approach) is to consider that mankind evolved on the food it could readily obtain, and that one should not expect to find large natural barriers blocking access to foods needed for health. Let us see what one would have to eat to get 1,500 I.U. of vitamin E each day.

Looking at tables of food composition, we find that the oils from seeds are among the richest sources of E. Safflower and cottonseed

---

*Later we shall see that there are other reasons why vitamin E supplements are not recommended except in some few special circumstances.

oils have about the highest content among the common oils—some 39 mg. of vitamin E (each milligram roughly equal to a unit) in 100 grams of oil. Since 100 grams is about 3.5 ounces, we can see that to get 1,500 units a day would require some eight or nine pounds of oil, something over a gallon a day.

Among solid foods, nuts are a good source, almonds among the best. To get this amount of vitamin E would require 18 pounds of almonds a day. And wheat germ, much vaunted as a vitamin E source, would provide the 1,500 units if one ate 27 pounds a day. To get an idea of how much food this is, we see in the food-composition tables that a tablespoon of wheat germ weighs six grams and provides 23 calories. Mathematics show us that 27 pounds of wheat germ would be a little over 2,000 tablespoons a day, or over 46,000 calories. Is it realistic to believe that man cannot enjoy good health without either supplements or 27 pounds of wheat germ?

One may wonder at the fact that these enormous doses of vitamin E are advocated and sold by stores which hold themselves out to be "natural food" shops. There is nothing natural about advocation of such superhuman quantities.

Are the RDAs Set High Enough for Good Health?

As the RDA Committee explains: *"RDA should not be confused with requirements.* Differences in the nutrient requirements of individuals that derive from differences in their genetic makeup are ordinarily unknown. Therefore, as there is no way of predicting whose needs are high and whose are low, RDA . . . are estimated to exceed the requirements of most individuals and thereby ensure that the needs of nearly all are met."[8] (The exception to this rule is in RDA estimates of calories, or energy. Here, obviously, it would not be a good idea to set a generous excess, since overweight is a widespread problem.)

In practical terms, the Committee makes recommendations which should provide an *excess* of any given nutrient for at least 95 percent of people. Even this is very conservatively estimated, as we can see from the RDA for vitamin C. In the 1968 report, RDA for vitamin C for the average adult male was 60 milligrams a day. In 1974, based on newer information, the Committee lowered this recommendation to 45 milligrams a day.

What is the safety margin for this RDA? The minimal need for a vitamin is considered to be that level which will prevent physical signs of deficiency. Experimental evidence indicates that 10 mg. a day of vitamin C will alleviate symptoms of scurvy, the deficiency disease related to this vitamin. Canadian and British recommendations for vitamin C are 30 mg. a day, aimed at maintaining an ample "body pool" of the vitamin. Our American RDA of 45 mg. thus offers the safety margin allowed by British and Canadian scientists, plus an extra 50 percent for even greater safety.

The Meaning of "Vitamin Deficiency."

There are two basic ways to discuss "deficiencies" of vitamins and other nutrients. And to be able to understand reports on nutritional status, it is important to know the difference between the two. A true *nutritional deficiency* is a state in which a physical disorder (deficiency symptoms) appears for lack of a particular nutrient. For when the body does not have the amounts of the nutrient needed for carrying out normal functions, something goes physically wrong. The person becomes sick for lack of an essential chemical. For example, if we are truly deficient in iron intake, our blood cannot carry adequate oxygen to the cells; we become pale and weak, we wake in the morning feeling tired, and so on.

On the other hand, *dietary deficiencies* are failures to get *the recommended amount* of a nutrient from one's food. Such a failure is not necessarily great enough to cause illness; the body may still be getting enough of the nutrient to function normally. For example, suppose we do not get the vitamin C RDA of 45 mg. a day, but only 40 mg. This does not mean that we will be ill. For chances are that so small a departure from the RDA falls within the safety margins which have been allowed. Remember, if we were following British or Canadian recommendations, at 40 mg. a day we would still have a third more vitamin C than was recommended. So we have simply fallen below a mathematical line.

To suggest the problems of dealing too rigidly with the RDA, as if they were absolute minimums for physical health, consider a Londoner who consumes an average of 30 mg. a day of vitamin C. He would be rated in a British study as having no problem with this vitamin. But by the criteria of the U.S. Department of Agriculture such a person would be rated as having a "poor" intake of vitamin C. Why?

Because USDA considers a diet to be "poor" in a nutrient if it falls to one-third less than the American RDA.

So it is that nutrition surveys which merely apply mathematical standards to people's reports of what they eat may be less meaningful than examinations which look for physical signs of deficiency. And when we look at studies of the quality of nutrition, we must keep these factors in mind, to be able to assess the seriousness of the findings.

Testing a Diet for Safety

We have now learned some basic methods for evaluating the quality of nutrition, and how to use two of nutrition science's most basic tools. With this information, we can begin to test the quality of any diet plan, and to predict pitfalls which may be involved. To see how this works, let us take an unusual diet from recent history, analyze it, and make some judgments about it.

Late in the 1960s, the teachings of Sakurazawa Nyoiti, better known to his Western devotees as George Ohsawa, began to attract much attention, particularly on some American campuses. As one journal reported, "Wherever young people congregate, from Boston to Berkeley and on to the Hawaiian Islands, macrobiotic communes have sprung up."[9]

What was the *macrobiotic* dietary concept? Ohsawa described it as follows: "Disease is not necessary. Adherence to a macrobiotic regimen would not only ward off all human ailments, but could arrest, and even cure these ailments, no matter how seriously advanced the condition . . . I could prescribe specifically for such ailments as heart disease, cancer, diabetes, venereal disease, kidney trouble, and even ailments in the area of psychiatry—schizophrenia, paranoia—with assurances of cure within an astoundingly short time." Ohsawa promised that his diet would "eliminate fatigue, renew sexual potency, cure insomnia, increase memory . . ." He said that his diet would protect women from unwanted body hair, and that, "A macrobiotic person cannot be killed by an atomic bomb."

Of course, such claims seem absurd in retrospect. But they were convincing to many people, and they accepted Ohsawa's first premise, which was that, "Natural unpolished brown rice is the perfect food . . ."

Why is brown rice so good? Ohsawa answered by first explaining his concept of health and disease, saying that, ". . . all disease is caused by an imbalance of yin/yang in the body." We have met this idea before, among the ancient Chinese. But Ohsawa offered a scientific explanation for it, saying that the yin is represented by the *potassium* content of food and the yang by the *sodium.*

The most extreme yin foods, according to the system, include eggplant, figs, potatoes, oranges, and sugar. Among the most yang foods are meat, fish, pumpkins, carrots, apples, and strawberries.

We can check these assertions with our food-composition tables (Appendix A). For example, looking at fish, carrots, and apples—which Oshawa said should be much higher in sodium than in potassium—we find that the reverse is true. Fish tend to average about 4 times as much potassium as sodium (which ought to make them yin, not yang), carrots have more than 6 times as much potassium as sodium, and apples have 110 times more potassium than sodium.

Brown rice is supposed to be the only perfect support of life because ". . . it has the perfect natural balance of yin/yang." Ohsawa set this "perfection" as five times as much yin (potassium) as yang (sodium). The facts of chemical analysis? Raw brown rice has about 26 times as much potassium as sodium. If it is cooked in salted water, however, sodium is added, the ratio is reversed, and the rice has about four times as much sodium as potassium.

From such examination we learn that the scientific basis Ohsawa claimed for his system is in doubt. In fact, if we look up sugar, which Ohsawa erroneously condemned as a violent yin food, sure to destroy all masculinity and cause disastrous health problems, we find that table sugar has no potassium or sodium at all. So wanting was Ohsawa as a nutritionist, and so outrageous were his claims, that it may seem odd to pursue the subject further. But the extremes of his diet have a simplicity which provides us with clear examples of how to use some basic principles of nutrition.

Using our food composition and RDA tables, let us appraise brown rice as a sole dietary. At a glance, we can see that while brown rice is a good food and contains several nutrients, at least two important nutrients are wholly missing—vitamins A and C. So we know that in time, eating nothing but brown rice, two real nutritional deficiencies will develop.

The complete absence of a nutrient from a diet is serious business. For example, vitamin B-12 is found almost exclusively in animal-source foods. So we can be sure that it too is missing from the macrobiotic plan, as it is from all severe vegetarian regimes. (Vegetarians who eat eggs or other dairy products are protected from deficiencies of this vitamin.)

Other food essentials, though they are found in brown rice, are limited in quantity. For example, 100 grams of rice would be about ¾ cup. This would provide some 119 calories of energy. The RDA tables indicate than an average young woman should consume about 2100 calories a day. So some 18 servings of rice, or better than 13 cups a day would be needed to supply her with enough energy. Since the same serving of 100 grams also furnishes about two and one-half grams of protein, and since our young woman's protein RDA is 46 grams, we can calculate that it would take about 18 servings a day to supply this amount.

One hundred grams of rice has about half a milligram of iron, compared to a woman's 18-milligram RDA for the mineral. So it would take some 36 servings of brown rice to satisfy her iron needs. If we check other nutrients, we find that the content of riboflavin (.02 mg.), thiamin (.09 mg.), niacin (1.4 mg.), and calcium (12 mg.) are also so low as to require tremendous amounts to satisfy our young woman's needs. We may conclude that true malnutrition is likely to develop if she tries to survive on brown rice alone.

A Human Test of Nutrition Reality

We can match our scientific prediction against a real case history, to see what sort of human story the numbers tell. Early in 1965, Beth Ann Simon entered the macrobiotic world. As she did so, she began a running account of what happened, in the form of a diaristic letter to George Ohsawa. Here are some excerpts from the letter, together with some explanatory notes on the nutritional implications:

"Dear Dr. Ohsawa:
I am 24 years old (born May 22, 1941). Since February . . . I have been observing your macrobiotic directions . . . diet No. 7, with rare yang vegetables *nituke.* Drinking as little as possible."

Diet No. 7 is brown rice by itself. Since the extra vegetables used are not specified exactly, we cannot know just how much extra nutritive value Beth Ann Simon might have received from them.

Would these vegetables have made up some of the nutrient lacks of brown rice, such as the missing vitamins A and C?

Food preparation is always a factor in nutrition, so let us look at *Zen Macrobiotic Cooking,* by Michel Abehsera, to assess this factor. He writes of *vegetables nituke:* "Vegetables are a secondary food, intended to be served in small amounts, mainly as a seasoning or garnish . . . Two tablespoons of vegetables cooked in the Japanese fashion can be the jewel of the meal . . . Properly prepared, there is more flavor in a small sliver of carrot than in a whole mess of frozen, thawed, stewed, brewed and tatooed vegetables."

If we consult food tables, we find that two tablespoons of a vegetable is not much in nutritive terms. Most vegetable serving sizes are from one-half cup to a cup. Two tablespoons make one-eighth of a cup. If we consult the food tables, we see that this quantity of "nituke" will supply little of the missing nutrients, at best.

Moreover, in explaining methods of food selection and preparation, Abehsera advised macrobiotic eaters ". . . to pass by the gorgeously manicured, chemically treated vegetables . . . (and) direct all your impulse shopping to the tired, forlorn vegetables on the way to the refuse bin."

Vegetables tend to lose nutritive value when kept for an extended period after picking. This is particularly true of vitamin C, which tends to be lost to the air rather easily. As for cooking, macrobiotic style calls for *nituke* vegetables to be sliced into "matchstick" pieces, then tossed in hot oil and steamed. The thin slicing exposes greater surface to the air (especially harmful to vitamin C), and during cooking, to the cooking liquid. Vitamins (including vitamin C) which are soluble in water are lost much more quickly from such tiny pieces.

So although Beth Simon was getting some vegetable supplementation, the amounts were small, and little of the missing vitamin C was replaced. Her letter continues:

"Today I am flat on my back in bed. I have been so for three weeks . . . Shortly my knees began to hurt. Walking became painful . . . I began to get weak. I have lost 35 pounds . . . to 90 . . .

"Slowly my legs became painful, stiff, swollen, black and blue. [The black and blue probably represents hemorrhages under the skin, likely a sign of scurvy.] Walking became very painful. Finally I fasted completely for five days. I became very weak but my legs got considerably better . . . My legs are now stiff, black and blue and painful. My back is also painful . . . I am sure that I will get stronger and be free from pain. I would greatly appreciate any comment or advice that you can offer me. I feel I am just beginning my studies and I see Macrobiotics to be the way to happiness, freedom and justice. I thank you very much for making this wonderful way available to us."

One week later, Beth Ann Simon wrote a postscript:

"Now and for the past week I have had an almost constant fever of 100F. to 104F. I have lost another 15 pounds. My legs are almost completely better. I am weak as weakness. Soon I will be well!"

The final result of Beth Ann Simon's macrobiotic experiment is reported in *California's Health:*[10] "Late in 1965, in New York City, 24-year-old Beth Ann Simon died after nine months on macrobiotic regimens 7 and 6. She had a full-blown case of scurvy and had lost 50 pounds. The high-numbered (macrobiotic) diets used for long periods have caused scurvy and advanced malnutrition in a number of other cases."

Beth Ann Simon's case provides bitter confirmation of what we deduced about the macrobiotic diets from our tables. We had noted the total absence of vitamin C from the rice, and noted also that macrobiotic cooking methods and food choices would make it unlikely that supplements would supply much C. Her scurvy was the result.

In 1971 the AMA's Council on Foods and Nutrition issued a warning that the macrobiotic diet was "one of the most dangerous dietary regimens, posing not only serious hazards to the health of the individual, but even to life itself . . . Cases of scurvy, anemia (commonly due to iron deficiency), hypoproteinemia (inadequate protein), hypocalcemia (deficiency of calcium), emaciation due to starvation are likely, and other forms of malnutrition, in addition to loss of kidney function due to restricted fluid intake, have been reported, some of which have resulted in death."[11] (The parenthetical comments have been added.)

SOME SUBTLETIES OF REALITY TESTING

Basically then, we see that asking two questions: What is in the food? Does it supply what the body needs?—can go a long way in helping us test for reality. But we shall find that often we need other information to make valid nutritional judgments.

Some Other Realities of Foods and Their Effects

Often we need more than the information shown in the basic tables. As an example, we could see that brown rice was not a good source of protein. But even if the grain had been richer in protein, or very large quantities had been consumed, there would still have been a problem. For adequate protein *quantity* does not necessarily mean that the protein is adequate for health. Proteins vary greatly in their nutritive *quality*. (We will consider this in Chapter Eight.)

To assess a diet plan, we may need such information—about how fats differ from one another, or carbohydrates, or which forms of the iron that is added to some foods are more efficiently used by the body than others. And we need specific health information about the effects of foods.

For example, we know that sugar has effects on tooth decay. But these effects are misunderstood by many, especially the fact that total sugar consumption may be less important than the form in which the sugar is found or the time when it is eaten. The sugar in soda pop, we will learn, may have little or no effect on decay, while that in caramels which are eaten between meals may be disastrous. The sugar in milk may cause no dental problems for a baby when consumed at meals, yet cause serious difficulties when the baby becomes accustomed to falling asleep with the bottle in his mouth.[12]

Social and Environmental Realities

Characteristics of the society and the environment can have an important bearing on nutrition. A woman may get a diet which is generally adequate but close to the margin of need in certain nutrients. If she becomes pregnant, some of her nutrient needs will increase 30 to 50 percent.

In some nations transportation can be a critical factor in nutrition. Coastal people in Central America may get plenty of high-quality protein from fish, whereas people a hundred miles inland may have to rely chiefly on vegetable sources of protein. A drought may result in protein deficiency, unknown a relatively short distance away.

The natural environment can exert many nutritional influences. Cold climates, for example, may create greater calorie demands for sustaining body temperature. Warm climates with adequate rainfall, as in the South Pacific, tend to make a variety of fruits and vegetables available; an Eskimo or Laplander is not likely to see much in the way of green, leafy vegetables all winter. But in Iceland, a vast reserve of geothermal steam (plus the money to harness it) makes year-round produce available, grown in giant greenhouses. Ironically, many well-to-do American midwesterners live on a soil which is very poor in iodine; so unless they are wise enough to use iodized salt, they are threatened with *goiter* (an enlargement of the thyroid gland), while poor coastal Africans who live by the sea have plenty of iodine in their soil, and no goiter.

Cultural and Psychological Realities

While many scientists give little weight to factors which have no measurable physical existence, nutritionists must be keenly aware of ideas and feelings about food. As we have seen, taboos and mystical beliefs about food can have very real impact. There is a fundamental axiom that food does not become nutrition until it passes the lips.

We do not need to go to primitive tribes for examples. People have refused unfamiliar foods which would have saved them from malnutrition, and they may be so convinced that they will have real physical reactions if they do eat them. Digestive complaints and allergy-like reactions are very commonly triggered by emotion. For example, for decades doctors told ulcer patients not to eat seasoned foods, on the theory that they would cause acidity and pain. And many a patient who broke these rules did indeed experience real symptoms. But now medicine largely holds the view that few foods (mainly coffee and alcohol) actually cause such problems. Told this, many ulcer patients now eat the formerly forbidden foods with impunity.

A number of African people view certain worms and termites as delicious. Physically, these are perfectly good foods and meet some of our nutritive requirements very nicely. But many of us would become genuinely nauseated if we tried to eat them, and our repugnant feelings could induce some real digestive problems. Does this mean that worms and termites cause indigestion?

To choose foods well, we must certainly know something of physical realities—the chemistry of foods, the chemistry of the body, and the interactions of the two. But we must always keep in mind that there are infinite possible shadings of individual differences in culture, environment, our feelings, and the like.

Because all these factors are part of our total personal reality, we will try to integrate them as we examine some of the basic science of food and life. For our essential aim is to help each individual answer the simple question, *What shall I eat?*

REFERENCES
1. Bieler, H.G., *Food Is Your Best Medicine,* Vintage Books (Random House), New York, 1973.
2. Kneeland, Y., *Viral Diseases,* in *Cecil-Loeb Textbook of Medicine,* Saunders, Phila., 1963.
3. Benenson, A.S. ed., *Control of Communicable Diseases in Man,* American Pub. Hlth. Assn., Washington, 1973.
4. Adams, C.F., *Nutritive Value of American Foods in Common Units,* Agriculture Handbook No. 456, USDA, 1975.
5. Watt, B. and Merrill, A., *Composition of Foods,* Agriculture Handbook No. 8, USDA, Washington, 1963.
6. Wade, C., *Instant Health the Nature Way,* Award, New York, 1968.
7. Nittler, A.H. A New Breed of Doctor, Pyramid, New York, 1974.
8. Food and Nutrition Board, *Recommended Dietary Allowances,* Natl. Acad. Sciences, Washington, 1974, p. 3.
9. Nyoiti, S. (Ohsawa), *You Are All Sanpaku,* Award Books, New York.
10. Williams, E., *Macrobiotics,* California's Health, December, 1971.
11. Council on Foods and Nutrition, *Zen macrobiotic Diets,* JAMA, Vol. 218, No. 3, 1971.
12. Finn, S. and Glass, R., *Sugar and dental decay,* World Review of Nutrition and Dietetics, vol. 22, Karger, Basel, 1975.

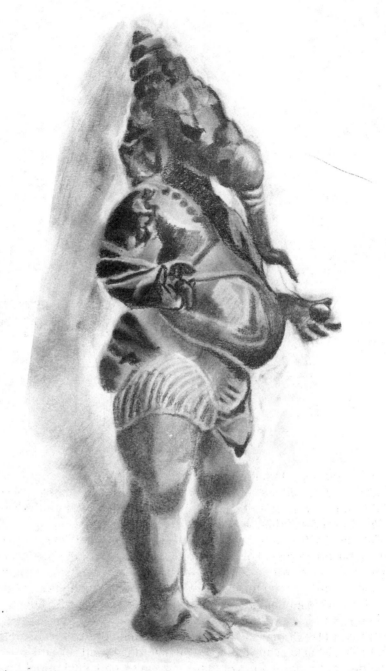

In many cultures, fatness has not been ugly, but a sign of richness and contentment, of prosperity. *Ganesha, the elephant-headed divinity of Hinduism, whose fat belly symbolized good fortune. Indian bronze, possibly 13th century.*

chapter 3

FOOD POWER AND THE FAT OF THE LAND

Americans are tremendously concerned about their individual fatness. According to a recent *Newsweek* report, that concern is so broad that, in a few short years, it has spawned "a soaring $10-billion-a-year diet industry."[1]

Alas, most of the plans and nostrums which that giant industry sells are not based on reality. For example, when the U. S. Senate Select Committee on Nutrition and Human Needs surveyed the weight-reducing plans offered through the land, it found that no fewer than 51 of them were actually variations of the long-discredited grapefruit-and-egg diet.[2]

Clearly, these unrealistic ideas about weight control must lead to failure. But what is even worse, the huckstering which sells them has pervaded our culture with all manner of false concepts about how and why we gain or lose body fat.

The simple truth is that the control of our fatness is chiefly dependent upon understanding how food provides us with energy, and how the body uses that energy potential. For to begin, the fact that we can become fatter is not, as many people tend to see it, a curse upon the race, or a highly visible punishment for gluttony; it is instead an essential mechanism for human survival.

THE BODILY ENERGY CRISIS

Like any other machine, the body must have energy to do work. But the body's energy requirements are complicated by one basic reality: Unlike automobiles or vacuum cleaners, the body is alive.

When we want to go somewhere, we put fuel into a car and start it. When we want to clean up crumbs, we take the vacuum out of the closet, plug it into a power source, and switch it on. When they have finished their work, we merely turn them off, reasonably secure that we can start them up once more when we need them.

But once the human machine has been turned off for more than a few minutes, it is finished. To stop it is to destroy it. It is turned on at the moment of conception, and from that moment it must run continuously until the moment of death. Since this constant running means a constant demand for energy, the machine must have an uninterrupted supply of fuel. If we run out of fuel, we die.

The fuel demand may increase or decrease, but it never decreases below a fundamental "idling" rate. On the obvious level, energy is needed for some rather large muscle systems which are steadily at work. The heart must keep beating. The lungs must keep pumping air in and waste gases out. The intestines need rhythmic waves of motion to keep digestion proceeding day in and day out.

Less obviously, considerable fuel is needed to maintain the function of the body's electrical and communications systems. The brain, contrary to popular belief, functions at much the same level whether we are awake or sleeping. In the process, it alone uses more than 20 percent of all the fuel we need at rest. And from the brain, messages go to every limb and organ, and other messages return, taking still more fuel. If this were not so, when we slept, we would not turn over when an arm is cramped; we would not wake when our ears detect the clock-radio alarm; we would not wake to protect ourselves when we smell smoke; or pull the covers up when a cold wind begins to blow from an open window.

Still more subtly, we must realize that the body is really a cooperative colony of trillions of cells, each of which has an existence and an energy need all its own. It takes fuel for these cells to produce the more than 100,000 chemicals they make, or to let them generate the heat necessary to keep the body at the almost constant temperature it requires.

All of this involuntary and unstoppable energy used to support life at its basic level is known as the *basal metabolism.* The pace at which it goes on is the *basal metabolic rate,* or "BMR." This rate can be measured, and the measurements can provide medical information about the function of the body. (An example would be the evidence of the performance of the thyroid gland, the hormone secretions of which help to govern the metabolic rate.)

Added to these basal energy demands are the requirements of our voluntary activities, just as necessary for our survival. We could not find food or care for ourselves without them.

So our total energy needs are basically a combination of the demands of basal metabolism and of voluntary action. Together they constitute an unremitting energy drain. And no matter how much we restrict our activity, the energy requirement is still quite large. For,unless we do very heavy physical work or are extremely athletic,chances are that basal metabolism accounts for most of the fuel we consume.

If we had to get the fuel immediately for each use, we would be in constant danger. A missed meal or coffee break could mean death. In our affluent and food-conscious society, we rarely are aware of true hunger, or of the fact that, if existence is not to be very precarious, the body must have some sort of fuel storage system. To see how our energy reserve systems work, and at the same time to glimpse the basics of weight control, it helps to look to another era.

The Amazing Neanderthal Diet

For our prehistoric ancestors, food was a sometime thing. It depended on the luck of the hunt and the success of the forage. It depended on the seasons. In summer and fall the land was lush with ripening berries and nuts, flocks of birds were everywhere, and the game grew fat on abundant forage. But in winter the trees and shrubs were bare, the flocks had migrated, and the ground was frozen too hard to be dug for roots. As eating became sporadic, what fueled the body machine through the hard days?

The answer lay primarily in the body's *subcutaneous* (beneath-the-skin) fat. To the naked eye this fat appears to be a yellowish, inert mass. But under the microscope, we see that it is far more complex. It is made up of a crowd of cells, similar to the rest of the cells of the body. The bulk of each of these organisms, which are called *adipose storage cells,* consists of a kind of collapsible, thin-walled tank, which grows larger as it fills with fat and smaller as it is emptied.

The body takes any excess fuel, beyond that needed to meet current energy demands, and converts it to fat, which is then stored in the adipose cells. Fat is used for this reserve because, as we will see, it is the most compact food fuel, with two and a quarter times as much energy value as the same weight of either protein or carbohydrate. As we said, fats provide some nine calories per gram, compared to about four calories per gram for protein and carbohydrate.

So when the hungry days came for the Neanderthal man, his body could simply draw upon the adipose storage cells for fuel. Essentially, the signal for such energy release was, and of course still is, a shortage of ingested fuel—inadequate for immediate needs. It might be triggered by too many hours without eating, or a high fever in illness, or by a lavish expenditure of energy in pursuing game or in being pursued by an enemy (if it were a lengthy pursuit). It is easy to see the urgent practicality of such a fuel reserve system; one would not want to have to make a stop for lunch (fuel) while being chased by a saber-toothed tiger.

The blanket of plump adipose cells under the skin served in other ways, too, and still does. It was an excellent insulator against heat and cold, particularly important when one remembers that the body functions well only within narrow limits of internal temperature (usually 98—99°F.). And the fat is also a good buffer against injury, a shock absorber against blows, a shield to keep a cut from reaching internal organs. This helps to explain why, when we fatten, a fair amount of fat forms around these organs, not only to keep fuel reserves where they may be needed most, but for extra physical protection. One reason why much fat accumulates at the belly may be that organs in this area have no bone shield, unlike the brain inside the skull or the lungs within the rib cage.

The alternating cycles of good and poor eating, of leisure and violent activity probably set up a nice energy balance for the

Neanderthal. Adipose cells filled and emptied, filled and emptied,* and in the end there was probably little Neanderthal obesity. Most studies of primitive people today find little excessive fatness.

But the food supplies of our civilization have affected our delicate fat-storage balance—with supermarkets and refrigerated trucks, with *Whoppers* and *Big Macs* and *Jumbo Jacks* always at hand, and with boxes of corn flakes and *Hamburger Helper* safe in the cupboard. Like our Neanderthal uncles and aunts, we always store each smallest excess of fuel—but the hungry times never come.

Ironically, to empty some of this unwanted storage from our adipose cells, the Neanderthal plan is still the only one that really works. We must either reproduce the prehistoric days of hunger—gnawing celery sticks and trying to think of something other than the telephone number of *Pizza Man*—or recreate the desperate escape from the dinosaur, spending energy just for the sake of spending it, on the jogging track, or swinging our modern clubs and rackets in the mock combat of recreational games.

Even when we are slim, however, our energy reserves are large. Our bodies range from the 5 percent fat of the thin man to the 20 percent fat of the moderately obese, from the 10 percent of the thin woman to the 30 percent of the moderately obese one.

To give some idea of how much stored energy this fat represents, consider the "typical" young American woman, at five feet five inches and 128 pounds. A little over 25 of those pounds are in fat. And this much fat has enough energy potential to meet all the woman's needs for about 45 days, if she gets no food at all.**

This example suggests one reason why it is difficult to make rapid headway against excess fat. For it takes a significant energy shortage, over a substantial period of time, to draw down large excess reserves. Some of the 25 pounds of fat in our example would be "normal," and necessary for activity and general health. But suppose a case of a young woman with 25 pounds of *extra* fat, beyond her normal reserves; it would take at least a month and a half of

---

*The description of fat storage in adipose cells is quite simplified, and will do for purposes of illustration. Actually, "stored" fat does not lie dormant, but participates in continual interaction with body chemicals and processes.

**True starvation is most unwise as a self-treatment for obesity. While a day or two without food is not likely to do much harm to normal people, real progress against fatness would take considerable time and could be dangerous. Starvation has been used successfully among very obese people, but usually in hospitals, with careful medical observation and attention.

complete fasting to dispose of the surplus. And remember that our 153-pound woman (the original 128-pound woman with 25 pounds of excess fat added) is really only at the margin of the usual medical definition of true obesity, which is about 20 percent over ideal weight.

Measuring the Energy of Food and Fatness

Understanding how much energy must be used to make real headway against even moderate fatness—and therefore how much hunger or extra activity is required—we can begin to see why so many people are willing to believe the enticing promises of reducing-plan promoters.

The most common promises are exact contraversions of reality: That fat will be lost quickly, without either hunger or extraordinary physical effort.

Here are some ads which are typical of those recently appearing in such newspapers as *The Los Angeles Times* and the *National Enquirer,* in direct mail promotions, and in magazines such as *Family Circle* and *Family Weekly:*

"FORT LAUDERDALE, FLORIDA (Special Report)—From this Gold Coast City comes word of the GRAPEFRUIT-PLUS Diet and Reducing Plan . . . Practically any *normal,* overweight reader may lose up to 10 pounds in only 10 days . . . You're *never* starved. You eat your fill from a huge selection of pure, healthful foods."

An ad for *Dr. Atkins' Diet Revolution* reads: "You can now command your body to Melt Away Fat." The trick is to eat protein and avoid carbohydrate. The ad says one should lose six to eight pounds in the first week and promises that there will be "not a single hunger pang to suffer through!"

An ad for the *U.S. Olympic Ski Team Diet*—with which the U.S. Olympic Ski Team has disclaimed any connection—says the plan was created to get women skiers back into shape for competition. It says that the buyer can eat special foods, which regardless of activity will provide a 20-pound weight loss in 14 days.

A fourth ad says: "EAT 'FAT-DESTROYER FOODS' TILL YOU GROAN AND STILL LOSE WEIGHT." It soothes any fears of sacrifice with the promise that, "You'll never be hungry or need 'will power' . . . You can even enjoy frequent snacks." It tells us that a businessman named Ronald used the plan to lose 12 pounds in a week.

How can we test the reality of these rosy visions? We can try them out in terms of the basic formula for determining weight accumulation or reduction: Energy intake (food)—Energy expenditure = Fat Gain or Loss

Doesn't the kind of food matter? The body seeks only to meet its energy needs. In this respect it is similar to a battery. It does not matter to the battery whether the electrical energy used to charge it came from the burning of oil, coal, or even wood. And, in turn, the ability of the battery to provide energy for work is simply a question of how many energy units—in the case of a battery, watts—it can take in and hold.

In terms of body energy, the unit of measure is the *calorie*. And this word takes us into a little bit of confusion. First, contrary to popular shorthand usage, food does not "contain calories." It has energy potential, *measured* in calories. The word *calorie* itself, as used in nutrition, is shorthand. Originally, it came from the worlds of chemistry and physics, as a measure of heat—the amount of heat needed to raise the temperature of one gram of water by one degree centigrade.

Heat is a good way to measure food energy, but whereas the calorie as a unit of measurement measures rather small amounts of heat, the heat potential in food is relatively high. The energy in a single peanut can add one degree to two *gallons* of water. An ounce of hamburger could do the same to 20 gallons. A good dinner could provide us with a brief hot shower.

In other words, the calorie is too small a measure to be convenient in nutrition. So nutritionists use the *large calorie,* or *kilocalorie* as a measure, equalling 1,000 of the *"small"* calories of physics.*

Gradually, nutritionists shortened the term back to calorie, but still meant *kilocalorie.* Some, with scientific precision, still use the old names, or use *Calorie, kcal.,* or *Cal* (note the capital Cs) in nutrition notation.

You may encounter this variety of expression, and so should know

---

*The problem has been further confused lately in the shift to metric measures. For one of the few common measures in nutrition which is *not* metric is the calorie. The metric measure for food energy is the *joule.* A calorie equals 4.184 joules. Since a peanut would have over 33,000 joules, again the larger term *kilojoule* (abbreviated as *kjoule* or *kj*) is used.

what it means, but in reality the public, the press, the government, the law, commerce, and food labels all now tend to use the term *calorie,* meaning *kilocalorie.* So will this book.

How do we find out how much energy a food will give to the body? We simply see how much heat is produced when we burn a sample. This can be a little deceiving, for it may seem to suggest that the body "burns" its fuel much as we burn a log on the hearth. This is not true. But when we actually burn a food sample, we find out the amount of its energy potential.

That energy potential is essentially the same no matter how we put it to work. Burning food as we do a log would be an inefficient way to derive its energy—causing it to combine rapidly with oxygen at a high temperature. If the body operated this way, the fuel would be used up very fast, and without much regard for how much energy we really needed at that moment. It would also be quite uncomfortable for our innards.

The difference in the two processes is not so much in the dissimilarities between the log and our food, either. After all, the log is the stem of a plant. We do eat stems—such as asparagus or rhubarb—and use their energy. Both, we shall see, consist largely of carbohydrate and water, though a serving of asparagus makes a much more appealing dish, and one more physiologically useful than, say, a serving of pine chips.

The body does use its fuel through a kind of chemical "burning," and it does combine with oxygen in the process. But fuel burning in the body is an intricate matter, a kind of extremely slow burning which goes through many steps and is exquisitely controlled.

The point, however, is that the energy is elicited from a fuel—for example, whether a given amount of gasoline is sipped by a Toyota, gulped by a Cadillac, or exploded in a Molotov Cocktail—the total energy potential is the same. And the body utilizes the potential energy of its special fuel, through its own "burning" process.

So to learn how many calories of energy a specific amount of food will yield, a dried sample of it is burned in an instrument called a *bomb calorimeter.* The sample is placed in an insulated metal container, together with a measured amount of oxygen. This container, or *bomb,* is sealed, and the sample is ignited electrically and burned. The bomb is jacketed by a water chamber, containing a measured amount of water. The heat of the burning raises the water temperature, and the amount of the water temperature increase can be converted to calories.

Using the same scale of heat measurement, we can also measure how much energy the body spends to do work. This method is known as *direct calorimetry.* It is somewhat costly and cumbersome, because it entails closing a person in a similar but larger chamber with oxygen. Again, the resulting heat is reflected in the temperature of a precise amount of water, and the amount of the temperature increase reveals the number of calories of energy expended. Obviously, this method is not very practical if we want to know how much energy the body expends in a mile run, driving a car, or playing a piano. So for such measurements, another technique is used, known as *indirect calorimetry.*

In this method the subject wears a device called a *respirometer.* This measures the amount of oxygen he takes in. And it also measures the amount of carbon dioxide—carbon derived from food eaten by the subject, which has been combined with oxygen—which he breathes out. From such information scientists can determine how much energy has been used. For example, in a typical case each liter of oxygen used indicates that 4.825 calories of energy have been burned.

By such means nutrition science has developed two bodies of basic data. One consists of tables of the caloric values of foods (see Appendix A), the other of tables of the caloric cost of the voluntary activity involved in living, from washing dishes to riding a bicycle (see Appendix F). These two bodies of information are keys to testing the reality of ideas about human energy—and hence, about weight control.

A Confusing Definition of Energy

While the scientist sees energy as power for doing work, the term is also used in another way. For example, a *Family Circle* article[3] on "How to Recharge Your Energy" offers ten tips "for a quick energy recharge."* One of them is to eat sunflower seeds between meals. And later in the article, it is suggested that supplements of vitamin E might be an answer. Similarly, in a book called *"Introduction to Health Foods,"* it is explained that, "When you eat enough protein, you should have more *energy.*"[4]

---

*As we shall see later, some foods can be utilized more quickly for energy—but not those referred to in the article. In any event, the author of the article was confusing the term "energy", using it more in the sense of "vigor."

The point of examples like these is that certain foods and food combinations are popularly believed to be special sources of energy. Yet, as we have seen, the only real relationship of food to energy is that of fuel to work, with energy value measured in calories. The food which supplies greater caloric value supplies more energy.

Part of the confusion here is between the meanings of the terms *energy* and *vigor*. Vigor is, of course, a very real thing, a reflection of one's physical and emotional status, and might be described as a feeling of readiness to do work. The psychological aspects of this feeling can be crucial. Our Hottentot warrior who has just had a lion sandwich, or our tailback who has just had a pound of blood-rare steak, may both feel physically ready to triumph, and for much the same reason. A young man in the best of physical and nutritional states may, on the other hand, not feel he has the strength to "suit up," because his woman has broken a date.

Feelings of vigor may certainly have a nutritional reality. A person who is consuming plenty of calories and who has ample energy reserves of fuel may, through malnutrition, suffer from a condition such as anemia which makes the use of the energy impossible. Conversely, once one has eaten adequately, additional amounts of nutrients will not furnish additional "energy."

Advertising often adds to the confusion. An example is a recent California dairy ad on television which promotes cottage cheese as "low in calories, high in energy." Plainly calories and energy are implied to be quite different—energy is supposed to be good, calories bad.

Because of such ads, and such confusion, the recent Federal proposal to control misleading advertising of food (see Chapter One) provided:

"An advertisement shall not represent that a food or nutrient contains . . . or is a source of "energy" or "food energy" . . . unless it clearly and conspicuously discloses . . . that "energy" or "food energy" is supplied by calories . . ."

Good health may make a person more *energetic* (in the sense of *vigorous*). And nutrition certainly has an impact on good health. But true human energy comes only from fuel, and the energy value of fuel for humans is measured only in calories.

It should now be clear why the statement was made earlier that taking vitamin supplements does not provide energy. For while in the most technical sense vitamins might be said to have some small fuel value, their tiny quantity alone would prevent them from making a meaningful contribution to energy needs.

Because the body's use of fuel is so basic to nutrition, and because all concepts of weight control are so absolutely dependent on how we use and store fuel, it is worthwhile to look still deeper at how food carries and gives us energy potential, and how the body puts that potential to work.

ATP—The Secret of Our Energy

We have noted that the body uses fuel in a slower, more complex way than does a machine—that it does not really *burn* fuel. This problem frustrated scientists for generations. For on the surface, food and machine fuels seem to follow the same natural laws. As we saw, to determine the energy value of either, we can burn them and see how much heat they yield.

Nearly all fuels give up energy from the same basic source— whether they furnish power for a jet takeoff or a 100-meter dash. The energy of ordinary fuels lies in electrical bonds which hold the atoms of any substance together. These bonds are shown in chemical notation as the little links between atoms. *

Most of our machines can use only one kind of fuel, which has been refined for them by man (as gasoline) or nature (as coal). The first difference in the body's use of fuel is that it has its own ingenious refinery system, for in part digestion can be thought of as a fuel-refining process. The body can deal with an incredible variety of foods, breaking them down step by step and sometimes modifying them, until the relatively simple substances which can be used for fuel can pass through the walls of the intestines and enter the bloodstream.

Now the fuel molecules are carried to the cells. Each cell has its own refining ability. In a process called the *Krebs cycle,* which may consist of twenty and more steps, the bonds between the atoms of the fuel are broken. And in the breaking apart and repositioning of the atoms, energy is released bit by bit from the bonds.

How is this energy put to work? The details are very complex. But

---

*The breaking of the electrical bond between two atoms can be a little like cutting an electrical wire which has current running through it. The only fuels which do not yield their energy from the breaking apart or joining together of atoms are nuclear fuels, which provide energy from the bonds between the *parts* of atoms.

fundamentally, the energy is derived from one mysterious chemical, *adenosine triphosphate,* or *ATP.*

As the second word of the name suggests, this chemical has three atoms of the metal phosphorus. And the special way in which these three phosphorus atoms are bonded to the molecule is the essence of the power of this substance. For in the end, our ability to use our fuel for living depends upon ATP.

To get an idea of how ordinary chemical bonds differ from those special ones which hold phosphorus to ATP, draw this picture in your mind: Imagine a helium-filled balloon. It is held to earth by a rope, which is tensed by the pull of the balloon. If we cut the rope, the balloon surges upward in a release of energy. The rope in this case is like an ordinary bond between atoms.

Now picture that the balloon is tethered instead by a cable of twisted rubber. The upward pull of the balloon stretches the rubber, and much more tension is created. If we cut the rubber, the balloon leaps upward as before, but there is the further released energy from the snap of the stretched rubber. The rubber represents the power of a *high-energy bond.* If we think of the phosphorus atom as our balloon, the energy from food fuel is used to draw the balloon down and fasten it to the elastic tether. In this way, the energy from food has been stored as the high-energy bond in the ATP. It waits, ready for instant use.

Let us suppose that this ATP molecule is one of many thousands in a muscle cell, and that the cell is in a finger. We want to scratch an ear. A signal goes from the brain to the nerves, and is flashed to the muscle cells in the hand. At once the high-energy bond in our ATP molecule is released. The phosphorus atom is released. As thousands of cells are similarly energized, with many thousands of energy bonds breaking, the finger bends.

Then immediately stored fuel is used to restore the phosphorus atom to each ATP molecule. Like a gun which has been cocked, the molecules are ready to "fire" again, "burning" energy.

THE COST OF USING ENERGY

Getting energy from fuel is always somewhat wasteful. Even in the burning of gas in a furnace, more than 20 percent of the potential energy of the fuel is wasted.

Partly because the body must refine its own fuel, breaking it down from complex food substances, and partly because of the controlled ways in which the fuel is then delivered to the cells and used by them, the human energy system is even less efficient. Dr. Krebs, for whom the energy cycle is named, estimates that, at most, some 40 percent of the energy potential from fats and carbohydrates can be used for doing such work as scratching an ear or making a heart beat. The energy potential of protein is used even less efficiently, at a level of about 34 percent.[5]

What happens to the rest of the energy? It follows many paths. Much of it is dissipated as heat, for example, which is one of the reasons we may feel warmer after eating.

Some of the generated energy is put to subtle, but important, uses by the body. It takes energy to refine our fuel. It takes energy to assemble the chemicals and structures of the human machine—to build enzymes and hormones from the chemical raw materials, or to construct a cell wall. And all of the chemical reactions involved release heat. Some of this heat is not wasted. As pointed out earlier it is the source of energy for keeping our bodies at the even internal temperature necessary for basic life processes.

Some of the more wasteful heat losses of energy, which follow eating food, are grouped together under the name *specific dynamic action,* or *SDA.* Lately, some scientists have begun to refer to these losses in terms of the *thermogenic effects of feeding* (*thermogenic* meaning "heat-yielding").

Because in these processes proteins are used less efficiently, some people believe that high-protein eating is a way to make the body store less of the potential energy (fat). And this is the source of many ideas about "high-protein reducing."[6] Unfortunately, the energy losses of SDA are fairly small. Also, protein is really a rather small part of the diet (and, as we shall see later, is almost always accompanied by fat). On the average, in a mixed diet—and it is nearly impossible to eat ordinary foods without getting a mixture of nutrients—there is an average SDA loss of about 10 percent, which changes little no matter how we modify our eating habits.

TRIAL BY CALORIE

All these refinements of human energy use are mainly of interest to the laboratory scientist. In most energy formulas and charts which we may encounter—the standard calorie and energy expenditure tables—they have already been taken into account.

They do help us to see, however, that there is no energy magic in any food. Whether a glass of milk is drunk straight from the cow, pasteurized, or allowed to become a home for a lot of bacteria (as in yogurt), it is the same source of fuel for the body's refining system. Its energy value will either be used up, if needed by life processes and activity, or it will be stored as fat, if there is already enough energy available for the body's needs at that time.

The *laws of the conservation of energy* tell us that energy is never really lost. It has to go somewhere, be used somehow, and add up to a neat balance at the end. If ideas about weight control cannot account for an energy balance, they cannot be real. Let us look at some of the simple tests of reality with which our energy knowledge can protect us.

A key number in weight control is 3,500. This is about the number of calories of energy in a pound of body fat. Thus, it takes 3,500 *extra* calories consumed to make a pound of stored fat. It takes 3,500 *extra* calories of energy burned to use up a pound of stored fat.

Converting these calorie numbers to food terms, we have to eat, as extras, some four loaves of bread or some twelve pounds of baked potatoes to gain a pound of fat. Therefore, fat gain and loss cannot be very great within a short period of time. Gaudy claims of reducing plans must be suspect, as is the common idea that a person has gained or lost a few pounds of stored fat over a weekend. Most likely any sudden change of weight will be due to a shift in fluid retention.

If we return to our sample ads for weight-reduction schemes, we can begin to see, in everyday terms, how testing with the laws of human energy can separate reality from illusion. In the Atkins and grapefruit diet ads, it was suggested that we can lose about a pound a day. If this were true, and if what we lose were fat, not water, then analyzing these diets should show us that they would result in a deficit of some 3,500 calories daily.

It is simple common sense that, unless we step up our energy output with more exercise, before we can create a food deficit of 3,500 daily calories, we must be eating at least this much food to begin with. We can test this in two ways: We can add the caloric expenditures of our BMR and voluntary activity, or we can consult the RDA tables (Appendix E), and see that our caloric needs just don't add up to 3,500 calories per day. The typical calorie need for the reference American woman is only 2,000 a day; the need for the reference male is only 2,700 calories.

So even if these reference people ate nothing at all, they could not lose a pound a day. The only people who could hope to accomplish such a weight loss without greater exercise would have to be much heavier than average—people who use at least 3,500 calories in the course of their ordinary daily routine. We saw that there is a relationship between "average" daily caloric expenditure and weight: We can compute the amount by referring to the RDA numbers, comparing the recommended calories for our reference man and woman with their weight in pounds, and we see that they need (for a woman) 15.5 calories per pound of body weight, and (for a man) 17.5 calories per pound. (These numbers are only averages. They do not take into account differences in activity, differences in efficiency of fuel use, and so on. But they work fairly well for most adults.)

The RDA reference woman weighs 128 pounds. Let us consider a woman who has 25 pounds of excess fat, who weighs 153. Can a diet make her lose a pound a day? Multiplying her weight by our guide number of 15.5, we see that she probably uses only about 2,370 calories daily. So even fasting, she cannot lose a pound in 24 hours. To do this, she would have to be about 100 pounds overweight and weigh some 226 pounds. This of course is if she takes in *no* food.

But remember that all of these ads tell us that we will not feel hungry, that we can eat satisfying diets. These foods must have some caloric value. So one would have to subtract the energy value of the food from the 3,500-calorie deficit the woman must maintain to lose her pound a day.

Protein and the Weight-Loss Illusions

If the popular reducing diets make claims which do not conform to the laws of energy, we may well ask, why are so many people satisfied with them? In 11 months, Dr. Atkins' book[7] sold over a million copies; and then broke records in paperback. And it was not alone, in principle; for its high protein-low carbohydrate plan was nothing more or less than a host of predecessors, such as Stillman's *The Doctor's Quick Weight Loss Diet*[8] and Taller's *Calories Don't Count.*[9]

Since we know that proteins and carbohydrates offer the same caloric values, that calories are the only key to fatness, and that the rapid-weight-loss claims tend not to add up calorically, what makes these diets seem to work?

We will see more precise explanations when we discuss how the body uses the macronutrients. But for the moment, we need only note that carbohydrates are the body's primary fuel. On a low carbohydrate diet, the body must substitute a rather small amount of protein and a rather large amount of fat. This shift forces the body to use less efficient chemical processes to derive energy, and results in certain waste products which stimulate the kidneys. The kidneys respond by increasing their output of fluids to carry off the wastes.

In this way, the body loses some of its normal large content of water. With some water gone—perhaps five to eight pounds in the first week—the midsection is a little less plump, and the body is most definitely lighter. But the lost water has nothing to do with body fat. Though the scales go down, and the dieter is pleased, he is scarcely less fat. He is merely drier.

True, the water loss cannot continue at such a rate for long. But on the other hand, most of us do not stay on a diet very long. Naturally, as the dieter returns to normal eating, the kidneys resume their normal function, and the lost water and pounds are rapidly restored.

There is another reason why people may in the short term lose weight on such diets. If one stays on such a diet for any period of time, even though the rapid water loss stops, the high-fat, monotonous food plan tends to diminish appetite, with nausea for some people. Eating may diminish because the dieters can't stand the food. And the lower caloric intake does begin to use up some stored fat, at a fairly predictable and unspectacular rate. But for reasons which will become clear, the diet plan is considered to be so medically unsafe that the American Medical Association issued a warning to doctors about it.[11]

LOOKING FOR MORE WORK

The alert reader will be asking by now whether the necessary calorie deficit for rapid weight loss could come from greater activity. The question is automatically answered with respect to those diets which promise that "no exercise is necessary." But in other cases the question is a sound one, especially since some reducing plans de-emphasize dieting and suggest that special exercise is the best way to fat loss. Believing in these exercises, Americans pump many millions of dollars into books, gadgets and costly courses in gyms and salons. Let us examine some facts of this effort.

Almost any of us can quickly imagine how we can increase our output of energy. We can run around the block, walk to work, take up hiking, biking or swimming. But the prospect is a gloomy one for many. So they are receptive to claims of painless shortcuts.

As an example for easy energy expenditure, over 1,500,000 Americans are said to have bought a device developed by a Californian named Joe Weider, who is described as a "builder of beautiful bodies since 1936." A full-page ad for the "Joe Weider Original Scientifically Tested 5 minute Body Shaper Plan" tells us that one 218-pound man lost 13 pounds in 14 days this way.[12] It also shows us six women who lost an average of about eight pounds each during the same period.

The crux of the program seems to be a gadget of ropes and pulleys. We fasten this to a door and put each foot and hand into a rope loop, while we lie on our backs on the floor. Since feet and hands are linked together by the ropes, when the right hand and left leg go up, the left hand and right arm go down. We keep on alternating, one pair up, the other down, and so on. It is a little like walking and swinging one's arms at the same time—but while lying down comfortably. We are to do this for two five-minute periods each day.

Before we consider the energy cost of this exercise, first let us look at the reducing diet which comes with it. The ad says, "Eat anything you want (Just 20 percent less)." And we see a photo of a woman who is said to have gone from 145 pounds to 136 in 14 days. We can estimate that, at the start, she would have needed some 2250 calories daily to keep her weight constant (*145 pounds times 15.5 calories*). If she gave up 20 percent of her food, as advertised, she would have a calorie deficit of about 450 calories a day. With such a deficit she should lose a pound in about eight days. So to lose the claimed 9 pounds should take some 72 days.

But elsewhere the ad gives us a conflicting message. It says the dieters were allowed only "850 to 1,000 calories a day"—quite a Spartan diet, and a reduction of more than half our sample woman's food intake. This mini-diet would give her a daily deficit as high as 1,400 calories. So she could lose a pound of fat in some 2-½ days (*3,500 calories divided by 1,400*). In the 14 days allowed, the woman might thus, although very hungry, lose 5.6 pounds. Since the ad claimed she lost 9 pounds, exercise with the "body shaper" must have burned off some 3.4 pounds of fat in 14 days.

How effective is this exercise? If we put a respirometer on the lady for her daily ten minutes of action, we could learn the true energy cost by indirect calorimetry. Since we cannot, we must make some estimates instead. Let us consider some basic facts of energy expenditure through exercise.

WHAT DOES ACTIVITY COST?

We have seen that the production of heat is one way to measure energy output. Another is to measure the distance a weight is moved. The greater the weight moved and/or the greater the distance it is moved, the more energy is spent. For example, a 128-pound woman who climbs a 10-foot ladder spends 1,280 *foot-pounds* of energy (128 × 10) which can be converted to calories. A 154-pound man climbing the same ladder spends more energy, 10 times 154 pounds, or 1,540 foot-pounds.

In caloric terms, by respirometry, one researcher finds that a 134-pound man uses 261 calories to walk three miles. But a 218-pound man uses 408 calories for the same walk, because he is moving more weight.[13]

Many factors can increase the weight-distance effect. For example, walking uphill means pulling more against gravity. So if a 140-pound man uses some three calories every minute while walking on the level, his energy cost increases to well over five calories a minute going up a 10 percent grade, and to some eight calories a minute on a 20 percent grade. Heavy clothing can restrict movement and add work. Air temperature may alter the energy cost. And if we walk on snow or sand, slippage may make us waste energy with each step.

Does the intensity of activity count? Yes. As an example, in the case of the two men of different weights who walked 3 miles, suppose the smaller man walks twice as fast. Essentially, he does the same work in half the time, traveling the 3 miles at about the same total cost.

If one person rides a bicycle at a little over 5 miles an hour, he uses some 4.5 calories a minute. If another person of the same weight rides at a little over 9 miles an hour, he uses some 7 calories a minute. If both ride for an hour, the faster man does spend more energy—mainly because he has moved his weight a greater distance in that time, but not entirely.

An increase in the rate of energy expenditure can increase the total caloric burn. For it can increase body heat and require more rapid breathing and heartbeat. Faster action tends to mean less efficient fuel use, as we see with the extra gas burned by a car driven at very high speed. On the other hand, vigorous activity is not likely to last long.

However, the fatigue of vigorous or difficult activity can be illusory; it makes us feel as if we have spent a great deal of energy. But basically, if we lift a barbell equal to our own weight, we are spending only about as much energy as if we moved our bodies one step. The weight lift costs a little more, because we are moving the weight in a more awkward way and more directly against gravity, and we may be sweating and breathing hard. But remember that we take some 2,000 steps in a twenty-minute walk. 2,000 weight lifts would be heroic.

There is an obvious moral: exercise does not have to be painful, and indeed it had better not be if it's to be regular and long-lasting.

Let us look again at the Body Shaper exercise, recalling that for the woman in the ad, it appeared that her 10 minutes a day with it must have been responsible for 3.4 pounds of fat in 14 days, if the ad were to be believed. Remember, in the exercise we are only moving our arms and legs. Let us estimate that these limbs represent perhaps half of total body weight. In the case of our 145-pound woman, she may be moving roughly 75 pounds in each exercise motion. The weight is moved perhaps three feet. (Actually, a physicist would protest that she is not really doing so much work, because of the use of the pulley, the opposing balance of the limbs, and the effect of gravity to ease the work of each downward motion. But for the sake of an example let us ignore these factors.)

To equal the energy she would spend in walking a mile (which we can estimate from the energy expenditure tables on p. 397) she would have to move her body weight 5,280 feet. If each movement is three feet, this means 1,760 movements (1760 yards per mile, 3 feet per yard). However, our subject is moving no more than half her weight. So she must make twice as many movements, or 3,520. If her exercise is to total only 10 minutes daily, she will have to make 352 of these moves every minute.

But say she did it—how much energy would be burned in this way? About 70 to 80 calories. So we can calculate that this violent 10 minutes a day would theoretically produce the loss of a pound of fat in about 44 days. (*3,500 calories divided by 80.*) In the advertised 14 days, she would lose less than a third of a pound through exercise.

From such calculations, we can see that calisthenics do not tend to be big calorie burners. They can tighten muscles, so that we stand straighter, pull in muscles, and have smaller measurements. And they can provide health benefits other than fat loss. But their impact on obesity tends to be small.

Most commercial exercise programs overestimate the energy cost of activity. But worse, many a gym or salon makes promises for the effects of machines. If the machine does the work, *it* burns the energy, not you. The reserves of your electric company may be depleted, but yours are not likely to be much affected.

Exercise can be an important factor in weight control. But there are no magic exercises, just as there are no magic foods.

THE PERSONAL DIFFERENCES

The fact that the laws and the mathematics of energy are essentially always the same does not, however, mean that we will all have the same experience as we take in fuel or put it to work. When we apply these laws and mathematics to our lives, we quickly learn that there are many personal factors involved in weight control, that each of us is at least a little different. And we also learn that these small differences can ultimately have large effects.

Let us see what these differences are. For in them we will find some key principles of nutrition, some insights into why each of us is as we are in terms of fatness—and just what we, as individuals, can really do to change or stay the same.

REFERENCES
1. *Dietmania,* Newsweek, Sept. 10, 1973, p. 74.
2. Schanche, D., *Diet books that poison your mind,* Today's Health, April, 1974.
3. McGrath, L., *How to recharge your energy,* Family Circle, Nov., 1972, p. 60.
4. Miller, M. *Introduction to Health Foods,* Nash, Los Angeles, 1971.
5. Krebs, H., in *Mammalian Protein Metabolism,* Munro, H. and Allison, J. eds., Academic Press, New York, 1964.
6. Bradfield, R. and Jourdan, M., *Relative importance of specific dynamic action in weight-reduction diets,* Lancet, Sept. 22, 1973, p. 640.
7. Atkins, R., *Dr. Atkins' Diet Revolution,* McKay, New York, 1972.
8. Stillman, I. and Baker, S., *The Doctor's Quick Weight Loss Diet,* Prentice-Hall, Englewood Cliffs, N.J., 1967.
9. Taller, H., *Calories Don't Count,* Simon and Schuster, NY, 1961.
10. Kosover, T., *How the Beautiful People Stay Slim,* Ladies Home Journal, Nov. 1975.

11. Council on Foods and Nutrition, *A critique of low-carbohydrate ketogenic weight reduction regimens,* JAMA, Vol. 224, No. 10, June 4, 1973.
12. *Slim Down Safely,* advertisement, Los Angeles *Times,* Nov. 22, 1975.
13. Pollack, H., *Obesity,* Food and Nutrition News, May, 1964.
General References
14. Kleiber, M., *The Fire of Life,* Wiley, New York, 1961.
15. Durnin, J. and Passmore, R., *Energy, Work and Leisure,* Heinemann, London, 1967.
16. Ball, E., *Energy Metabolism,* Addison Wesley, Boston, 1973.
17. Harper, H., *Review of Physiological Chemistry,* Lange, Los Altos, Cal., 1971.
18. Food and Agriculture Organization of the U.N., *Nutrition and Working Efficiency,* Basic Study No. 5, Rome, 1962.
19. Mayer, J., *Overweight,* Prentice-Hall, Englewood Cliffs, New Jersey, 1968.

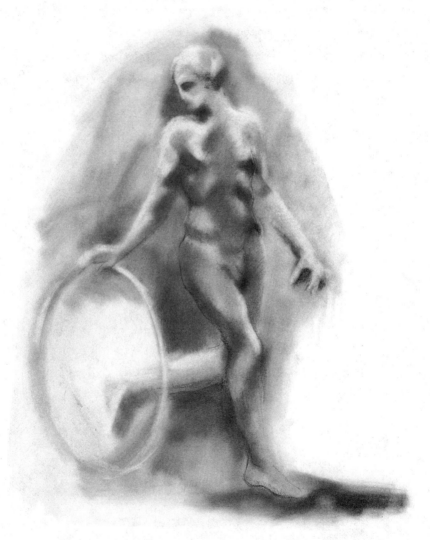

The energy of life follows specific laws, not magic. *The Hoop Roller, Greek stone relief, from the Golden Age, about 400 B.C.*

chapter 4

PUTTING THE LAWS OF ENERGY TO WORK

One of the most widely believed nutrition ideas is that "Americans eat much too much." As one consumer group, the Center for Science in the Public Interest, puts it: "Most Americans are eating themselves to illness—and death. For example . . . some 40 percent of all Americans are overweight."[1]

While the actual prevalence of fatness in the U.S. is unknown, it has been agreed for a generation that obesity is one of our most important public health problems.[2,3,4] And while there has long been a great expenditure of effort and money in trying to deal with this basic health threat, so far there has been relatively little success in preventing or curing the plague.

The public seems to have as many ideas about how to cure obesity as it does about the common cold. But it appears to share one basic concept of the cause—gluttony. Comments anthropologist Margaret Mead: "As the obese so often describe themselves (echoing the beliefs and attitudes of those around them), they are people who can't resist indulging their gluttonous greed."[5]

This idea is worth testing. For it looks as if most of us are already eating somewhat less than we would like, and disdaining a number of foods in the belief—often mistaken—that they "make fat." This, of course, is especially true for those who are already a little fatter than they would like to be. Thus it can seem that, even in their restraint, they are self-indulgent; so that, to maintain their weight, let alone to reduce it, they must resign themselves to a bleak existence of gustatory self-denial, a life of eating without joy.

Such a depressing point of view can discourage people from even attempting to deal with what is a very real problem. For just facing a need for weight control can evoke deep feelings of shame and guilt, in addition to the prospect of unending self-sacrifice.

There is a global implication to this perspective as well, which can add to the guilty burden of sensitive people. For our purported orgies of indulgence at the table are said by many to be at the expense of the world's starving. As the Center for Science in the Public Interest expresses the concept: "American eating habits, promoted by industry advertising, contribute . . . indirectly to the heart-rending plight of millions in famine-stricken nations."[1]

How real is the idea that gluttony is the central cause of our obesity? When the nutrition scientist applies the facts of energy to the question, he finds that gluttony must actually be quite rare. He also finds that very small differences in our intake and use of energy can make great differences in fat storage. From this analysis we can learn much about how to manage our fatness.

AN ANALYSIS OF GLUTTONY

"Gluttony" is a vague word. Let us imagine a very limited sort of glutton, one who, in addition to the food energy he needed each day, ate an extra two ounces of choice porterhouse steak. Very roughly, this could amount to about 250 calories.

Using our energy data, we divide these calories into the 3,500 which approximate a pound of fat and find that every 14 days, this man would gain a pound. In a year he would gain 26 pounds.

If we start him on this pattern at age 20, when he weighs 180 pounds, by the time he is 40 he will have gained some 520 pounds and will weigh 700 pounds. You have only to think of how many people you know who weigh 700 pounds, and you will see how many people are gluttonous to the extent of two extra ounces of steak a day.

What about one extra ounce of steak a day? Still a bit high. At 40 our subject will weigh 440 pounds.

The typical overweight American is perhaps 10-20 percent over ideal weight. Thus, in reality, our 180-pound young man might weigh between 200 and 220 pounds at 40—and think of himself as fat. If we put our equations into reverse, we can find how much extra daily food he would have eaten on the average. He would have gained one or two pounds a year during 20 years. That averages out to an excess of less than 10 to 20 calories a day. For a smaller person, say a 128-pound woman who gets a little pudgy, the excess would be even less.

To measure the caloric value of the dietary to an accuracy of perhaps 5 to 20 calories a day is virtually impossible in ordinary life. It is no small problem even in the laboratory.

Of course, in practical terms our food intake tends to vary from day to day. Chances are that any excesses are sporadic, that we sometimes overeat and sometimes (less often) undereat.

We should be reminded, too, that all our neat tables of caloric values are averages. The same food will vary in caloric value according to the variety grown, the soil, the climate, fertilization, the amount of sun, and many other factors. One of the reasons why wines differ so in different vintage years is that changes in climate change the sugar content of the grapes.

Consider a recent study of the potato. Experiments showed the water content of the potato to vary from 63 percent to 87 percent.[6] This means that the solids, which supply the energy, can vary some 300 percent, and with them the calories in the potato. Moreover, careful as we may be, how accurately can most of us guess the exact serving size of a mound of mashed potatoes? How many of us can guess the weight of a steak within an ounce? And remember what a difference an ounce of steak can make.

Character and discipline are not the only determinants of just how much we eat in relation to what we need; there are individual differences in how our bodies use food and energy. After all, even two cars of the same make and model can use energy at different rates. And not only are we a good deal more subtle and complex than automobiles, but each of us is a different make and model, generally from a different manufacturer.

Not all of the differences are yet fully understood. But there is far more knowledge than most people suspect about how fat we are, how we got that way, how lean we should be, and what we can do to change ourselves. For while few of us are gluttons, many of us are losing some of our potential for health to our own fat-storage cells.

THE GENETIC PUZZLE

In recent years we have learned that fatness has a strong hereditary component. To measure the importance of this effect, consider your odds of becoming fat. If neither of your parents is obese, your risk of obesity may be less than 10 percent. If you have one obese parent, the risk of fatness rises to some 40 percent. And if both your parents are obese, your chance of becoming so is some 80 percent.[7,8]

At one time, this genetic factor was largely attributed to the bad eating habits of obese parents, which supposedly determined the food choices of their children. To an extent, this factor probably has some reality. A child who is taught to savor fatty foods may favor them in adulthood. Meat, for example, simply may not taste right without gravy. Potatoes may not seem good without lots of butter.

But whatever our food tastes, selection may not be too important, in light of the enormous weight-gain effects of routine caloric overconsumption. Today the eating habits taught by parents are thought to have more impact in terms of the *ways* in which food is used, rather than the kinds of food selected.[8,9,10,11]

For example, the habit of eating everything on one's plate—like it or not, want it or not—is seen as more destructive of energy balance than what's on the plate. Then there is the effect of accustoming a child to use food as a way of dealing with stresses. (As in, "There, there, I know you feel bad. Have a little ice cream—or a piece of Mother's cake or homemade soup—and you'll feel better.")

Learned personality patterns can also lead to the use of foods for dealing with stress. The fostering of a strong sense of dependence, with symbolic nurturing seen as a way to deal with one's frustration or depression, is believed to teach a person to "mother" himself in upsetting times. Such a person may engage in episodes of overeating as stress increases.

But aside from such factors, inventive studies have shown some clear genetic bases for obesity. For example, records of identical twins brought up separately, in different environments with different adult models, have shown a remarkable tendency toward similar fatness or thinness.[12]

What causes this similarity?

A Capacity for Fat

The work of such researchers as Drs. Jules Hirsch and Jerome Knittle has established that there are some differences in our bodily facilities for storing fat.[13,14,15] Some of us tend to have more *adipocytes* (fat-storage cells) than do others. Much of the multiplication of these cells appears to take place during the first two years of life. And the tendency seems to be exaggerated by overfeeding during infancy.[16] For example, obese children often equal adults in the number of adipocytes by adolescence or before. Knittle has observed a six-year-old with as many cells as an adult.

At age 10 to 11, there appears to be another critical period for the multiplication of the storage cells. But if a person becomes obese after about the age of 20, the number of cells does not increase; individual cells merely enlarge.[16]

This is one of the reasons why obesity experts believe that fatness which appears early is hardest to deal with. For even if weight is lost, the cells do not decrease in number; they merely become emptied of some of their reserves—smaller, but always ready to enlarge again.*

Differences of Body Type

Another genetic factor is our inherited body type or somatotype. For the shape, and perhaps to some extent the composition of our bodies can be as predetermined as the color of our hair, the family nose, or the family chin.[17] Body shapes are generally assigned to one of three categories, although most of us are a blend of all three, with a preponderance toward one or two of them.

The *ectomorph* is slight of frame, reed-like when seen in profile. He has long, thin hands and feet, narrow, tapering fingers, and a

---

*From these concepts, two classes of obesity are now seen by some—*hypercellular* (obesity with unusual numbers of adipose cells) and *hypertrophic* (with normal cell numbers, but individual cells enlarged in size).

tendency to develop wiry or stringy muscle. He has a low fat-storage capacity. The fashion model who wears a 9AAA shoe is likely to be ectomorphic.

The *endomorph* appears almost as an opposite—softly rounded in style, often with narrow and sloping shoulders, and a torso which bulks toward the abdomen and hips, suggesting a sort of pear shape. The hands and feet are likely to be pudgy and short and, like the fingers, rather flame-shaped. Muscle tends to be soft and not well defined, and there is usually much fat-storage capacity.

Mesomorphs are sometimes described as between the other two groups, but this is not really accurate. They are the football types— broad shoulders, deep chests, with heavy bones and sturdy legs. Their hands are likely to be squarish, with blunt-shaped fingers, and they have bunched, well-formed muscle. Their fat-storage is greater than the ectomorph, but less and more evenly distributed over the body than that of the endomorph.

While pure body types are rare, there is a tendency to speak of people according to predominant type or types, as "endomorphic" or as "a meso-endomorph," for example. Probably it would be more proper to use a term which suggests the preponderance, as "meso-morp*hoid.*"

It is probably obvious that there is a relationship between inherited body style and numbers of fat-storage cells. But there is another important link between body style and the way energy is used.

Of Shape, Substance and Energy

As we have seen, for most of us energy need is mainly governed by our basal metabolic rate (BMR), the exceptions being extremely active people. This rate varies widely, depending on many factors. But one key is the shape and composition of the body.

For example, the rate of basal metabolism, or idling energy need, is between 10 and 20 percent higher for men than for women. One reason for this is that men have more muscle and less fat than women do, again about 10 to 20 percent. Some of this lean may be due to muscle development, but some is definitely a sexual characteristic.

Leaner people of either sex have a higher basal rate. Suppose we have two men who weigh about 150 pounds. One is thin, and the other is not really fat, but plump. At rest the thin man burns about 1.26 calories per minute, and the plump man 1.16 calories.

The difference, a tenth of a calorie per minute, does not sound like much. But if both men eat the same amount of food, the plump man treats that tenth-of-a-calorie difference as an excess and stores it. That is six calories per hour, or 144 extra calories a day, which theoretically could add a pound every 24 days.

Thus an inheritance of muscularity can mean an ability to accommodate greater caloric intake without fattening. But heredity goes further. For the shape of the body helps to determine the total body surface. A long, thin person will have much more body surface than will a short, plump person of the same weight. (A comparison can be seen in packaging. A pint of soda pop may come in a tall thin bottle, a pint of cream in a squat little carton.) Since the greater the body surface, the greater the heat loss, greater skin surface contributes toward higher basal metabolism. It may also influence how many calories of energy are lost during activity.

We can see a vicious circle emerging. The hereditarily thin and lean have more muscle and body surface, and burn more calories at idling speed. A huskier, stockier person, or one who has gained extra fat, spends *less* energy when similarly inactive. In this way nature tends to exaggerate the problems of the heavy and perpetuate them. There can be reality in the plaint of the stocky man married to the slight woman who says, "She eats what she wants and doesn't gain; I eat less and get fat." More often, because of the hereditary greater fatness of women, the complaint is the reverse, with females burning less energy for each pound of body weight.[18]

THE EFFICIENCY OF THE BODY MACHINE

A number of other factors affect the way we use fuel. For example, the older we get, the less energy we need. How much of this is due to changes in body chemistry, and how much is due to activity changes, no one can say certainly. But both elements seem to be involved.

The weather has an effect. If the body is exposed to either high or low temperatures, it must spend energy to compensate for them, for the body must stay at a fairly even temperature to survive. One has only to remember how bad one feels with an extra couple of degrees of temperature. The body becomes seriously threatened when its internal temperature is changed by more than a few degrees.

In cold environments, the body must spend more energy to generate heat, often by shivering—a way to use vigorous muscle activity to generate warmth. If the weather is hot, the cooling processes take energy, in pumping more blood to the skin surface, so that heat can be spilled out. Even sweating takes energy.

And there are endless subtleties. Tests were made of people wearing seven layers of clothing. Their energy needs increased, in part because of the drag exerted upon movement by their clothes.[19]

A United Nations agency concluded: "The energy requirements of individuals depend upon four variables interrelated in a complex way: (a) physical activity, (b) body size and composition, (c) age, and (d) climate and other ecological factors."[20]

Yet even the consideration of these broad variables does not seem to be enough. As Dr. Hegsted of Harvard recently pointed out: "There is . . . no obligation to assume that different individuals, or even the same individual at different times and under different considerations will utilize energy in the food consumed with equal efficiency."[21]

Hegsted is referring, of course, to special differences in the efficiency with which we use fuel, and he suggests ways in which such complex factors as the workings of ATP might differ. In general, while it has been common in nutrition to speak of the energy balance as a rather tidy and precise matter, advanced thinking now challenges such tidiness and precision.

As Hegsted sums it up: "There are abundant data which indicate that the energy needs of individuals, or the efficiency with which individuals utilize energy, vary greatly and cannot be predicted on the basis of current knowledge."[21]

On the other hand, what this really means is that we cannot predict energy use, storage, and the like as accurately as we might wish. It does not mean that we cannot predict and plan energy use in approximate ways which have great practical value.

CALCULATING YOUR BASAL RATE

There are many methods for finding an approximate basal metabolic rate (BMR), some of which are quite complex. All begin with one's body size and apply this to tables which show averages.*

But however carefully these averages are determined, they encompass a rather broad range. For example, in making its calcula-

*Most such tables are adapted from the data of Durnin and Passmore, or more recently, from U.N. data.

tions, the Food and Nutrition Board uses a BMR for the reference 154-pound man of from 1.0 to 1.2 calories per minute, and for a reference 128-pound woman of from 0.9 to 1.1 calories per minute.[18] These ranges cover variations of 20 percent and more. And we have seen what a difference in fuel use and storage can result from even smaller differences.

If you have not had a basal metabolism test, you might get a fairly good idea of your BMR from a simple rule of thumb:

For women: Add a zero to your weight in pounds. Add to the result your weight in pounds.

For men:

Add a zero to your weight in pounds.

Add to the result twice your weight in pounds.

Let us see how close our rule of thumb gets us to other ways of calculating. By our rule, a 128-pound woman would add a zero, making 1,280 calories, and then add her weight (128) to this, for a total of 1408 calories a day.

Applying a widely-used table (adapted from Durnin and Passmore), we see that a 128-pound woman would come under data for a weight of 60 kilograms (132 pounds), if she was of average fatness. The table shows a BMR of 0.98 calories per minute. Multiplying by 1440 (the number of minutes in a day), we get a total daily basal need of 1411 calories, only three calories different from the result of our shortcut method.

To test again, we might refer to a table from the Food and Nutrition Board.[18] It shows the BMR for a woman of 129 pounds (plus or minus 10 pounds) as 1530 calories a day. This shows the variability of such calculations. But it also reflects a refinement, a difference of about 10 percent between waking and sleeping BMRs. The Board recommends using 90 percent of the table number as the sleeping BMR. Ninety percent of the 1530 calories shown would be 1377 calories, only 34 calories less than our shortcut result.

If all of this seems a little confusing, try looking at the subtleties of more precise calculations. Yet no matter how careful the method, we are still approximating.

Correcting for Age

BMRs change with age. Whether this reflects an increase of fatness, a decline in muscle, a change in the function of two sets of glands which influence BMR (the thyroid and adrenals), or other factors or combinations of factors, no one really knows.

To correct your BMR for age, simply reduce it by two percent for each decade of adulthood. That is, a person of 30 would have a BMR which was 98 percent of his need at 20, at 40 a need which was about 96 percent, and so on.

Basal rates in children are a special matter, especially those of infants, and the energy calculating methods shown here will not work for the youngsters. Among other things, their body shapes are different, and the factor of growth enters in. The small, growing body uses an impressive part of its fuel as building material. This is one reason why a child can take in so many more calories for his weight than an adult can. An infant, for example, will use some three times as many calories per pound as will typical parents.[15]

WHAT ACTIVITY COSTS

We have already had some glimpses of the number of calories burned by activity. And we have only to glance at tables which show the caloric costs of different activities to see how hard it can be to add up how much energy any individual spends in the course of a day. Moreover, we have to contend with the fact that the cost is different for each of us, and that the conditions and exact nature of the activity can change from day to day.

For example, suppose you play an hour of tennis a day. If we use Passmore and Durnin figures, we see that the energy spent is some 7 calories per minute, or 420 calories for the hour. Or is it? First, these numbers include basal metabolism and the energy costs of digesting and otherwise putting to work the food we eat. So we cannot really add this to our basal rate; we must deduct an hour's BMR.

Next, tennis is not always tennis. Suppose you are much better than your opponent. You serve and he chases the ball. You return his shots while standing at the net, and he runs a lot. But next day you are outclassed. Now it is your turn to run. You hit harder, stretch further and perhaps stop more to wipe away perspiration and pant. The third day you play doubles, and one of the partners is a lawyer, who frequently stops to discuss violations of the rules and asks the score after each point.*

---

*An unpublished motion study by Braden et al. found an average of six minutes of actual activity in one set of tennis.

You can begin to see how tricky it is to calculate the energy cost of activity. How long do you wait for a chance to play the next hole in golf? How far do you walk between holes, and how steep is the course? If you played baseball for three hours, how much time was the other team at bat? If you played the outfield and your pitcher racked up 15 strikeouts, you spent fewer calories by far than did an infielder on the other team whose pitcher gave up hits every inning. And we must remember that differences in weight, climate, and other factors could make the same activity cost more to one person than to another.

So practical-minded nutritionists usually lump activities together in groups to make a general estimate of energy need, because accurate refinement is so individual a matter, and so difficult to compute. Here is how the Food and Nutrition Board groups activities and puts them together to give an idea of a day's energy expenditure:[18]

Very light. Seated and standing activities, painting trades, auto and truck driving, laboratory work, typing, playing musical instruments, sewing, ironing.

Light. Walking on level, 2.5—3 mph, tailoring, pressing, garage work, electrical trades, cannery workers, washing clothes, shopping with light load, golf, sailing, table tennis, volleyball.

Moderate. Walking 3.5—4 mph, plastering, weeding and hoeing, loading and stacking bales, scrubbing floors, shopping with heavy load, cycling, skiing, tennis, dancing.

Heavy. Walking with load uphill, tree felling, work with pick and shovel, basketball, swimming, climbing, football.

Look back at these lists and reflect a bit, and you can see what wide variation is possible within each activity. Dancing could mean a whirling polka, or a slow sliding to a ballad on a crowded little dance floor. Swimming could mean a lazy social crawl in a pool, or a struggle through the break of a big California surf.

These variations are shown in the use of a range of energy loads for each category. These are averaged and used to calculate average caloric expenditures, for the reference man and woman. The following have been adapted from the Foot and Nutrition Board charts.

It is this pattern by which the Board arrived at its calorie allowances for people in "light occupations," and which forms the basis of the calorie figures used in the RDA tables.

Table 4-1.

Activity	Time (Hours)	MAN (70kg, 154 lbs.)			WOMAN (58 kg, 128 lbs.)	
		Rate (Calories per min.)	Total (Calories)		Rate (Calories per min.)	Total (Calories)
Sleeping, Reclining	8	1.0–1.2	540		0.9–1.1	440
Very Light	12	up to 2.5	1300		up to 2.0	900
Light	3	2.5–4.9	600		2.0–3.9	450
Moderate	1	5.0–7.4	300		4.0–5.9	240
Heavy	0	7.5–12.0	0		6.0–10.0	0
TOTALS	24		2740			2030

MAKING A PERSONALIZED ENERGY BUDGET

There are many such ways to analyze energy output, and all of them will tend to lead ultimately to general approximations. Nevertheless, it is possible to personalize this information to some extent.

If we go back to our rule-of-thumb calculation of basal need, for example, there is a simple way to make this reflect our individual body shape and our fat-lean composition. It goes like this:

If you are thinner than average, *add* five percent to what you would otherwise calculate to be your total basal need. You need more calories for your weight.

If you would consider yourself pudgier than average, so that you might describe yourself as "plump," then you are probably some five percent higher in fatness.* So *subtract* five percent from your basal calorie need.

If, sadly, you would have to describe yourself as "fat," or about ten percent higher in fatness than the average, then you should *subtract* ten percent from your basal calorie need.

---

*Note that percentage of greater fatness is quite different from percentage above desired weight in pounds.

Next we want to add the calorie demands of our activity, which gets tricky because of the variability of individual activity. But there is one fairly dependable constant (in addition to the constant of our BMR, for which we have provided a shorthand method of computation). It might be called our daily activity minimum.

Compare the situation to that of an automobile. BMR is similar to the car's idling engine. But a second component for measuring the car's energy use is its *cruising speed.* This is the time when the engine is moving the car, but not under heavy demand—not overcoming inertia to get moving from a stop light, not trying to accelerate and pass, and so forth.

In our body's operation, once we are up and about, we also have a kind of cruising speed, which might be what the Food and Nutrition Board calls "very light" activity. Whatever our other activities, we have a low level of action as an undercurrent—driving a car, sitting at a desk, waiting for a bus, standing in an elevator, and so on. One group of nutritionists has estimated that this basic activity rate averages about 30 percent of our BMR for the day.[22]

For our reference 128-pound woman, whose BMR we figured at 1408 calories a day, this basic activity rate would be about 420 calories (1408 × .30). So if she were quite sedentary, and seldom if ever exceeded the "cruising speed" of "light activity," she would need 1408 calories plus 420 calories, or some 1828 calories daily.

Adding Higher Energy Output

For many of us, energy output rarely averages more than "very light" activity. In fact, the Food and Nutrition Board concludes that, "The physical activity of people in the United States is generally considered to be light to sedentary." As the Board's RDA Committee points out, it is the higher levels of activity that create the biggest differences in energy use.[18]

We may recall (Table 4-1) that, in estimating the energy needs of the typical American, the Committee assigned no time at all to "heavy" activity. Indeed, it gave only an hour a day to "moderate" exercise.

So for most of us, any difference from the norm for caloric expenditure through activity is due to what we do during a relatively short period of each day. And from this we can see that one of the most important things we can do to change our personal energy balance is to intensify the activity of that short period, perhaps an hour—which we should remember is commonly an *aggregate* of a few minutes here and there—or to extend the total time during which we speed up the bodily engine.

Since the time period (which may be a product of short periods of climbing stairs, hurrying to an elevator or a bus, quickly carrying groceries to the car, and so on) is so critical to our energy use, and so individual a matter, it would seem that this is where we should be most accurate in computing energy use. So take a close look at Table 4-2, Measuring Surges of Energy.

In this table (adapted from standard references) the following energy costs have been removed—the basal metabolism, the specific dynamic action of foods, and the "cruising speed" of the very light activities of the day. All that is left is the extra added surge of "moderate" or "heavy" activity. Using such a table, it should be fairly easy to get a close approximation of what energy you spend over and above the "idling" and the "cruising" expenditures which characterize most of our days.

To adjust these figures for greater weight than that shown in the reference sample, add 7 percent for each 11 pounds (5 kg.) above reference weight, and subtract 7 percent for each 11 pounds below reference weight. This modification will be only approximate, but again, all of these numbers are only averages.

HOW FAT SHOULD YOU BE?

Usually, the question which heads this section is asked in a different way—as, *How much should you weigh?* But in recent years, nutritionists have come to understand that weight and fatness may be quite different.

True, weight is one indicator of the status of our fat storage. But it can be a deceptive indicator. Consider the illusion wrought by water loss in the high-protein, extremely low-carbohydrate diets. Remember, too, the wide variation in human shapes and body compositions. For bone and muscle weigh more than fat. A stocky, burly person can weigh half again as much as the spare ectomorph of the same height.

Does this mean that the burly person is "overweight"? Does it mean that the spare person is "underweight"? In one perspective, the answers to both questions must be, yes. For if we measure these

Table 4-2. Measuring Surges of Energy.

ACTIVITY	CALORIES SPENT PER MINUTE	
	By a Man (154 lbs. or 70 kg.)	By a Woman (128 lbs. or 58 kg.)
Driving an automobile	.47	.43
Washing dishes by hand	.59	.52
Typing quickly	.59	.52
Ironing clothes	.59	.52
Washing floors	.82	.72
Doing light laundry by hand	.94	.82
Playing musical instruments at moderate rate	1.1	.91
Horseback riding, slow	1.1	.91
Painting, light work	1.2	1.0
Playing piano, fast	1.8	1.5
Walking, normal rate	1.8	1.5
Carpentry, average activities	2.1	1.8
Bicycling, easy rate	2.3	2.0
Canoeing, moderate speed	2.6	2.2
Vacuuming	2.6	2.2
Dancing, to moderate music	2.9	2.4
Skating, moderately	3.5	2.9
Swimming, moderate speed	3.5	2.9
Walking briskly (4 mph)	3.5	2.9
Riding horseback, at a trot	4.5	3.7
Ping pong, brisk game	4.6	3.8
Walking upstairs, moderate rate	5.3	4.4
Walking up 10% incline	5.3	4.4
Tennis, average rate	5.6	4.7
Heavy carpentry	6.0	5.0
Running, moderate speed	7.6	6.3
Bicycling, racing speed	8.3	6.9
Swimming hard (2mph)	8.7	7.2
Dancing very vigorously	9.0	7.6
Running cross country	9.8	8.0

*Adapted from various data, especially, Durnin and Passmore, FAO, and Foundations of Nutrition (Macmillan)

people against the charts of height and weight, one is above and the other below some arbitrary number.

As Dr. Francisco Grande summarized the problem in the recent National Institutes of Health Conference on Obesity: "Relative body weight . . . is not a reliable index of fatness except in the extreme situation." (In other words, someone who is five feet tall and weighs 400 pounds is indeed likely to be fat.) "Excess weight over a given standard . . . does not tell how much of the weight difference is accounted for by the accumulation of excess fat.''[23]

As early as World War II, interest in standards for physical fitness led to some studies of the differences between overweight and overfat. In 1942, Behnke and Colleagues[24] made measurements of a group of football players. The athletes averaged well above U.S. Army height-weight standards. But they proved to have a low content of body fat, so they were "overweight," but not obese.

Yet our reliance on height-weight charts continues to this day. In a number of occupations, nutritionally ignorant managements actually discharge people who do not meet these average numbers. Company policy-makers seem to be unaware of the differences in human bodies. Moreover, they tend to use charts compiled as early as 1913 (the date of the first Metropolitan Life Insurance Company charts), for some of these are still in use, despite the steadily increasing height and huskiness of the U.S. population.

Harvard's Seltzer and Mayer have repeatedly pointed out the unrealism of such charts in relation to obesity.[25,26] In 1970 Seltzer made measurements of 1,761 veterans. Using the average weights compiled by the National Health Study, he looked closely at men who exceeded these weight averages by 25 percent. Measuring the actual body fat of the "overweight" men, he found that only 22 percent of them were actually fat enough to be classed as obese.*

And those people who do conform to the charts are not necessarily lean or of average fatness. Brozek and Keys studied two groups of men, young ones with a mean age of about 22 years, and older men with a mean age of about 44 years. There was scarcely any difference in the mean weights of the two groups, much less than one percent. But when they calculated the actual fat content of their bodies, they found that the younger men had a mean fat content of 9.8 percent. The older group had a mean fat content of 21 percent. In other words, while both groups could, on the basis of weight only, be assumed to be of the same fatness, in reality the older men were more than twice as fat.

Are height-weight tables of any value at all to the individual? Their value is limited. For unless a wide range of allowances are provided for, they do not reflect human variation. And if they do embody such a range, it is a very broad one. For example, National Institutes of

*A summary of these studies on fatness criteria is presented by Grande, see ref. No. 4-23.

Health conferees finally adapted life insurance data to make the chart below, showing both an average and a (substantial) range.

Even allowing for the variations, one can quickly compare some of the averages of *recommended* weight to average *actual* weights of

Table 4-3.

FOGARTY INTERNATIONAL CENTER CONFERENCE ON OBESITY
RECOMMENDED WEIGHT IN RELATION TO HEIGHT.[1]

| Height | | Men | | Women | |
Feet	Inches	Average	Range	Average	Range
4	10	—	—	102	92–119
4	11	—	—	104	94–122
5	0	—	—	107	96–125
5	1	—	—	110	99–128
5	2	123	112–141	113	102–131
5	3	127	115–144	116	105–134
5	4	130	118–148	120	108–138
5	5	133	121–152	123	111–142
5	6	136	124–156	128	114–146
5	7	140	128–161	132	118–150
5	8	145	132–166	136	122–154
5	9	149	136–170	140	126–158
5	10	153	140–174	144	130–163
5	11	158	144–179	148	134–168
6	0	162	148–184	152	138–173
6	1	166	152–189	—	—
6	2	171	156–194	—	—
6	3	176	160–199	—	—
6	4	181	164–204	-	-

[1]*Height without shoes, weight without clothes. Adapted from the Table of Metropolitan Life Insurance Co.*

Americans and see the extent of national fatness. The averages of actual weight shown below (assembled by the National Center for Health Statistics) are among the best data we have on the subject.

How good are these averages? As statistical information, they appear to be very good, for they match up well with other studies in which careful height-weight measurements are made. For example, if we compare the average weights for men and women from late twenties to early fifties with the average weights of men and women

Table 4-4.

Height (inches)	WEIGHT (pounds)						
	18–24 years	25–34 years	35–44 years	45–54 years	55–64 years	65–74 years	75–79 years
Men							
62	137	141	149	148	148	144	133
63	140	145	152	152	151	148	138
64	144	150	156	156	155	151	143
65	147	154	160	160	158	154	148
66	151	159	164	164	162	158	154
67	154	163	168	168	166	161	159
68	158	168	171	173	169	165	164
69	161	172	175	177	173	168	169
70	165	177	179	181	176	171	174
71	168	181	182	185	180	175	179
72	172	186	186	189	184	178	184
73	175	190	190	193	187	182	189
74	179	194	194	197	191	185	194
Women							
57	116	112	131	129	138	132	125
58	118	116	134	132	141	135	129
59	120	120	136	136	144	138	132
60	122	124	138	140	149	142	136
61	125	128	140	143	150	145	139
62	127	132	143	147	152	149	143
63	129	136	145	150	155	152	146
64	131	140	147	154	158	156	150
65	134	144	149	158	161	159	153
66	136	148	152	161	164	163	157
67	138	152	154	165	167	166	160
68	140	156	156	168	170	170	164

Table title: *Smoothed Average Weights[1] for Men and Women (by age and height: United States 1960–62[2]).*

[1] *Estimated values from regression equations of weights for specified age groups.*
[2] *Adapted from National Center for Health Statistics: Weight by Height and Age of Adults, United States, 1960–1962. Vital Health Statistics: PHS. Publication No. 1000—Series 11, No. 14, May 1966.*

who served as subjects in the classic Framingham Study*[27] of heart-disease risk, we can see a remarkable similarity.

---

*A long-term population study of the physical characteristics and personal habits associated with greater or lesser risk of heart disease, conducted in Framingham, Mass.

Table 4-5.

Height (inches)	Weight (pounds)	
	Men	Women
55	—	126
56	—	127
57	—	128
58	—	129
59	—	131
60	136	133
61	140	135
62	144	137
63	148	139
64	152	141
65	156	144
66	160	147
67	164	151
68	168	155
69	172	—
70	176	—
71	180	—
72	184	—
73	188	—
74	192	—

The table title is: *Framingham Study Data.*[1]

[1] *These weights were the average obtained at the initial examination from subjects entering Framingham Study in 1948–50.*

From these and other findings, it appears clear that we are a somewhat overweight people. On the other hand, looking at the averages, we do not seem to be grossly fat. And contrary to some earlier opinions, newer information suggests that being mildly obese—say 10 percent over ideal weight—has no great impact on health. For example. the NIH reports on obesity indicate that fatness alone probably does not markedly predispose to heart disease until one is some 25 percent over ideal weight.

Similarly, while obesity can be related to arthritis, to diabetes, to difficulties in pregnancy and childbirth, and to many other health problems, there is considerable question about whether *mild* obesity is very significant. Mild obesity, which is probably the sort of obesity about which most of us are concerned, appears to be more of a social than a medical problem.

It may well be that this limited fatness—which is seen as a sign of beauty or affluence in some parts of the world, such as in Polynesia— has its primary physical effect in terms of activity. Whether it is mainly the result (of sedentary physical habits) or the cause (of a lazier physical life), no one can say certainly. But there is little medical question that the person who does not use his body does not maintain it in its best and most disease-resistant state.

Mild obesity seems to have greater effect when it appears early in life. From a reluctance to appear publicly in a bathing suit to the greater indolence of the chubby baby, obesity and inactivity are related.[8,28] Indeed the two enter into a vicious circle. For example, using time-lapse photography, Bullen, Reed, and Mayer found that chubby teenagers engaged in the same games as their leaner contemporaries moved much less.[29] Thus, the chubby child is programmed to become the fat adult.

The fact is that the truth about the impact of obesity, and on how great that obesity must be before it has real medical meaning, is not yet known. As Dr. George Christakis points out: "While there is little doubt that an epidemic of obesity exists in contemporary Western and some island civilizations, the question of its public health significance remains to be fully explored. There has, in fact . . . been lively controversy . . . as to whether obesity represents a social embarrassment or a public health problem."[30]

HOW FATNESS IS MEASURED

Because weight and height are not dependable ways to judge moderate fatness, other methods have been developed. While there are some very subtle ways, such as measuring chemical phenomena which occur when there is a good deal of body fat, some simple techniques have proved more generally useful. Of these, none is more widely accepted or better documented than the "pinch test."

Repeated experiments by Seltzer and Mayer have shown that there are areas of the body in which the thickness of fat deposits under the skin rather accurately reflect the total amount of fat stored in the body.[26] A scientific "pinch" in these areas is now considered the easiest way to judge how fat you are.

Most widely used is the area halfway between the elbow and the shoulder on the back of the arm. This is named the *triceps* area, after the muscle which underlies the fat. And it is difficult, but not impossible, to reach without help. Bend your elbow, and ask someone to measure the halfway point between elbow and shoulder. Then drop your arm so that it hangs straight down. Now ask your helper to grasp that midpoint between thumb and forefinger, then draw the skin away from the muscle underneath.

The fat adheres to the skin which is drawn away. Light pressure with the fingers now gives an approximate measure of the thickness of a double layer of fat and skin. For more accurate results, researchers use special calipers, which exert a constant pressure and make an exact measurement.

Because of the differences between the fatness of men and women, and because of the differences in fatness associated with age, there are some wide variations in terms of what measurements constitute obesity. A table for making this estimate, according to age and sex, is shown in Table 4-6.

Seltzer and Mayer, who developed this table, found that while the obesity standard for the 18-year-old man was a pinch of 15 mm. (0.6 inches), for his 18-year-old twin sister obesity would produce a triceps skinfold almost twice as thick, 27 mm. (more than 1.1 inches). With advancing age that difference dwindles, until at 30 obesity is indicated by a pinch of the male triceps which is 23 mm. thick (about 0.9 inches), and 30 mm. (or about 1.25 inches) for the female of the same age.

In using the table, keep in mind that 10 mm. equals about .40 inches.

Although this table is set up for "white males" and "white females," the numbers, though perhaps not perfectly accurate, should be generally useful for humans regardless of race. The table can also be regarded as a good indicator for at least two other types of pinches.

One of these is almost impossible to make by yourself. It is known as the *subscapular,* or, below the shoulder blade. It is taken about an inch below the center of the angling bone which is so prominent on the upper back. Easier to make alone, though somewhat less accurate, is the pinch which is sometimes called the *subcostal,* or, below the ribs. For this test, locate the midpoint of your side, above the waist. Then measure two or three inches toward the front of your body, and take the pinch just below your lowest rib.

Even easier than pinching, however, is a look in the mirror with

Table 4-6.

OBESITY STANDARDS FOR CAUCASIAN AMERICANS.[1]

(Minimum triceps skinfold thickness in millimeters indicating obesity).[2]

	Skinfold measurements	
Age (years)	Males	Females
5	12	14
6	12	15
7	13	16
8	14	17
9	15	18
10	16	20
11	17	21
12	18	22
13	18	23
14	17	23
15	16	24
16	15	25
17	14	26
18	15	27
19	15	27
20	16	28
21	17	28
22	18	28
23	18	28
24	19	28
25	20	29
26	20	29
27	21	29
28	22	29
29	23	29
30–50	23	30

[1]*Adapted from Seltzer, C. C., and Mayer, J. A. simple criterion of obesity, Postgrad Med. 38('): A 101–107.*(24)
[2]*Figures represent the logarithmic means of the frequency distributions plus one standard deviation.*

your clothing removed. Look at yourself from the side, as well as head-on. And look for real fat, not for fashionable thinness. Keep in mind that heredity and muscle development have probably played a key role in determining the size of your shoulders, thighs, chest and buttocks, for example. If you are in doubt about what thickness is due to bone and muscle, and what to fat, use the pinch technique to check suspected fat accumulations. And remember that palpable fat can be lost, but your basic body style can never be changed.

REALITIES OF LOSING FAT

In theory, tipping the balance of energy, so that the body loses some of its fat reserves, could hardly be simpler. You have only to achieve some mix of increased energy expenditure and decreased food intake.

Increasing the output of energy is a fairly obvious matter, although we have seen that, unless one is familiar with the facts of energy cost, one may easily select an activity which is tiring but does not really burn many calories. Once an appropriate activity is chosen—usually one which involves a constant energy expenditure over at least the better part of an hour, and which involves the moving of a lot of weight over a long distance, such as walking or bicycling—the problem is chiefly one of persistence.

But unless controls of food intake are also effective, the effort to spend more energy may not accomplish much. One fact about exercise which is a surprise to many people is that a moderate increase in activity, by one generally leading a sedentary existence, can actually reduce appetite.

Mayer and his colleagues discovered this phenomenon in experiments in which animals were allowed to eat as much as they wanted. When one group of animals was exercised for about an hour a day, they began to eat *less* than animals which got virtually no exercise.[3–19] Unfortunately this phenomenon disappears as the animals get still more exercise. Increased energy expenditure beyond this moderate point seems to signal the body to demand more food. So no matter how we approach the problem of losing fat, in the long run we have to confront and somehow deal with that villain of obesity—appetite.

Appetite is a still rather mysterious phenomenon which is compounded by two major factors, the physical and the emotional. And a key reason why appetite remains such a mystery, defying many experimental efforts at analysis, is that these two factors are subtly and complexly interlocked.

APPETITE AND THE BODY

Until rather recently, appetite was thought to be controlled mainly by the mechanical effects of food and digestion—as we can see from such old phrases as "the full stomach." For example, it was believed that the contractions of an empty stomach were among the main cues for eating. It was noted, for instance, that fats, which leave the stomach more slowly, seem to have greater value for long-term satisfaction. But the theory had to contend with the fact that the stomach is emptied usually in from two to four hours after eating, depending on the composition of the meal, without any clear correlation with the arrival of hunger pangs. And more sophisticated studies have shown the process to be a much more complicated one. Food in the stomach does not necessarily stop the wish to eat, and an empty stomach need not start it.

A key factor is now known to be an area deep in one of the oldest parts of the brain, which has been called the *appestat.* The area, known as the *hypothalamus,* is the seat of some of the most basic reactions for survival; it has to do with the control of body temperature, with certain sexual phenomena, and with the primitive "fight-or-flight" reflexes.

This brain area appears to have two centers, one to turn on appetite and the other to turn it off. Both of these switches seem to work by responding to changing blood levels of *glucose,* the simple sugar which is the main fuel refined by the body from carbohydrate and protein foods.

Some researchers suspect there are some other bodily mechanisms for assessing how much fuel is coming in, so that perhaps the "appestat" mechanism really involves a number of body reactions and controls which are related and have a joint net effect of leading us to eat or to stop eating.

Whatever the exact mechanisms, the *appestat* does not seem very responsive to fatty substances in the blood. So the fact that big reserves of stored fat are available for energy and perhaps being put to work does not necessarily shut off the drive to eat. The "appestat" seems to concern itself mainly with whether or not enough fuel is *coming in* to take care of the energy being spent. So the fat person feels just as hungry as the very spare person when lunchtime passes without food. And for similar reasons, the person who is trying to lose weight may feel unsatisfied if he consumes less fuel than his body is burning.

On the other hand, contrary to popular belief, experimental evidence makes it rather clear that the fatter person does not have an unusually active appetite, find taste extremely stimulating, or have very different patterns of appetite.* One exception to this apparent rule, however, is a difference observed by Mayer among people of different body styles. The thin ectomorph seems to have a sharper cut-off of appetite than does the bulkier endomorph or mesomorph, who appears to be more inclined to accept some additional food after he feels satisfied. ("I couldn't eat another bite—but did you say chocolate?")[3-19]

Moreover, the body's appetite mechanisms may create a kind of vicious circle of eating for the overweight. For the demands of appetite in terms of calories seem often to be related to the energy needs. And as we have seen repeatedly, the more of us there is, the more fuel our bodies need. This problem can be compounded by the greater physical effort and awkwardness involved in fatness. The fatter people become, the less active they are likely to be. Further, the less active they are, the less their bodies will consist of muscle and the more of fat, reducing their BMR.

There is also a chicken-and-egg question here. Are fatter people more fat because they are less active, or are they less active because they are more fat? Infants who tend to obesity have been observed to move less in the cradle. And endomorphs have been observed to move less in the same pursuits than ectomorphs.

And through all these themes there runs a strong emotional influence, which blurs logic all the more.

APPETITE AND THE EMOTIONS

We have seen that few people who are fat are truly gluttonous—rather that they are likely to be the victims of small steady excesses of intake over need, or perhaps occasional episodes of extreme ex-

---

*Though there is evidence that overweight people are more sensitive to external cues which remind them of food and may lead to eating. Schacter, S., and Rodin, J., *Obese Humans and Rats,* Lawrence Erlbaum Associates, Potomac, MD, 1974.

cess. So it is easy to see how even minor emotionally-oriented distortions of the appetite might lead to obesity.

And the wish to eat has a powerful emotional aspect. Feelings of all kinds, from joy to pain, can override the physical signals of a need or lack of need for fuel. Feasting is an ancient way to celebrate. And conversely, in the emotional disturbance known as *anorexia nervosa,* young women may suddenly stop eating at all, until life itself is seriously threatened, with no feelings of hunger.

The psychological effects on appetite are well known to have a strong *placebo** effect for many. Almost any system of dieting, or any kind of pill, will magically wipe away hunger for a number of people, if that is what they are told it will do.

This powerful link between appetite and emotion begins in the first hours of life—as a child has his first taste of both love and food in his mother's arms. Without this maternal nurturing, there is no survival. Love and food are interwoven; the need for both becomes a part of our very will to survive; and food becomes a potent symbol of this whole basic emotional system.[8,31,32]

The giving of food quickly begins to symbolize the giving of love, but also it begins to embody the sense of healing, and the relief of stress and pain. Contrarily, the withholding of food becomes a sign of love denied, of rejection, hostility, and an important kind of punishment. Anthropologists note that almost every culture greets its guests with food or drink. And they see as no accident the fact that the business lunch has become one of the basics of our working life.

As the child develops, a reverse image of these emotions appears. That is, to be loved, one must accept the gift of nurture. How would you feel if you invited someone to dinner, and he sat without eating, saying he just wasn't hungry? In some primitive tribes, the rejection of proferred food or drink is tantamount to a mortal insult.

So, in addition to being a way to soothe and please ourselves, eating also becomes a way to please others. For many parents, the good child is the one who cleans his plate. ("See, he likes Mommy's Hamburger Helper that she made just for her baby boy." Or, "Eat your casserole. Don't you care that Mother spent the whole day over a hot stove just for you?")

---

*A placebo is an innocuous substance such as milk sugar, which is administered to a patient to create the illusion of medication, either for test purposes or to pacify him. The word comes from the Latin, meaning "I please."

This subtle kind of reward-and-punishment game can be used in other ways. ("Are you catching cold? Mother will make you some nice chicken soup.") Or perhaps it is *menudos* or taro paste, depending on the culture. ("You won't eat your spinach? All right, no chocolate pudding for you." "Be good at the dentist and Mother will buy a whole bag of peanut brittle just for you.") A child can thus be taught to view foods as palliatives for the pains and stresses of living.

One of the most widely accepted theories about the emotional development of humans is the *internalization* of our parents and their ideas. In a sense, growing up is partly the business of *becoming* our parents in many ways. We learn symbolically to slap our own hands if we want to reach for something that does not belong to us. We abuse ourselves if we have been wrong and feel guilt—voluntarily offering, perhaps, to pay for the window we break. We learn to soothe our own pains, and we learn to reward ourselves for behavior that we think is good.

If our parents have used food for these purposes, then the internalized parents who live in our minds will also use food. Similarly, our early training tends to dispose us to see any deprivation of food as emotional evidence that we are being denied love, or perhaps even being punished for some sin.

Some psychologists have theorized that such feelings on the part of the reducing dieter help lead to repeated episodes of painful crash dieting. It is as if the feeling that we are expiating some crime of gluttony is more important than an adult, rational wish to look and feel better because we have adjusted our energy balance.

With these physical and emotional effects of appetite in mind, let us see how people seek to control appetite.

TRYING TO MANAGE APPETITE

Drugs (prescription). A true and dependably anorexic (appetite-killing) drug is not yet known.[33] Some success has been achieved with drugs classed as "uppers"—stimulants such as the *amphetamines*. How they work, when they work, is not truly understood. They are effective for some people, usually for a limited period of a few weeks. However, they also commonly produce side effects such as nervousness and sleeplessness.[34,35,36]

Over-the-counter drugs. These are rarely very effective and have led to a number of Federal prosecutions for misleading labels and advertising. The drugs used are usually very mild relatives of the stimulants described above, most often *phenylpropanolamine hydrochloride.* Sometimes, however, these supposed appetite suppressants depend on *benzocaine,* a weak anesthetic which is supposed to work by killing the responsiveness of taste buds in the mouth.

Diuretics. These "water pills" stimulate the kidneys to dump body fluid. Some patients who are given these drugs to encourage the idea that they are successfully losing weight seem to think they are also appetite suppressors. And true to the placebo effects common in appetite control, a number of the patients think the pills make them less hungry, at least for a while. But there are some medical hazards in the indiscriminate use of such drugs. And since adequate hydration is necessary for health and vitality, these can be very counterproductive, especially for the athlete. The AMA's Council on Foods and Nutrition has pronounced their use in weight control to be "irrational."

One justification for the use of diuretics in weight reduction is the common phenomenon for many people, of abnormal fluid retention when they start to lose fat. Although fat reserves are shrinking, the change does not show on the scale, because the body replaces this weight with water. If no pills are taken, however, within two to three weeks the body readjusts and dumps the water.

Other Drugs

Some drugs are given for weight control on a mixed theory of both appetite control and a supposed stimulation of the body to burn more fat. Two examples are heart stimulants (such as *digitalis* and its relatives) and thyroid extracts (on the theory that stimulation of the thyroid will speed up metabolism). While some evidence has been offered that such drugs have an effect on fat storage and use, there is far more evidence that any such effects are not dependable, and that they are achieved at some considerable risk. Medical authorities have firmly opposed the use of such drugs for weight reduction.

Because of the common placebo effect of any medication given to control appetite, a long list of drugs has been given testimonial accolades which have not proved to be medically justified. One is

HCG (human chorionic gonadotropin), a sex hormone which has been the feature of chains of medical weight-reduction "clinics." Medicine knows of no reason why HCG should be helpful for weight reduction. The drug's proponents have pointed out, however, that patients who receive regular injections invariably lost weight—*as long as they persisted on a 500-calorie-a-day diet.* Obviously they will lose weight when they eat so little.

"Appetite-killing" Diets

As we have seen in some of our advertising examples, many reducing diets are offered with the promise that, though they are low in calories, they are fully satisfying. There can be a thread of truth to such claims, but it is generally exaggerated.

For example, we have noted that, because fats tend to stay longer in the stomach, they are thought by some to be more satisfying foods. The phenomenon has some reality. But there is the further reality that fats are more than twice as caloric as proteins or carbohydrates.

Many of the very narrow "crash" diets, such as those which are extremely low in carbohydrates and high in fats, seem to act as limits on calorie intake to some extent simply because they quickly become boring, and no one can stand to stay on them or overeat on them for very long. A surfeit of almost anything seems to be a sure way to arrive at some caloric reduction. A diet of nothing but bread seems to work. And one can postulate that probably a diet of nothing but maple creams would soon become effective, too.

Changes of metabolic function have also been claimed for distorted crash diets, again with a thread of truth. *Ketosis,* a toxic state which derives from forcing the body to obtain its energy mainly from fats (as in the extremely low-carbohydrate diets) does, for example, often produce mild nausea. But altering the body's chemistry in such ways is generally considered to be unsafe for many, especially if the abnormal state is continued for long.[3-11,37]

What makes a good reducing diet? The simplest answer, of course, is a diet with fewer calories of energy than are used by the body. But understanding how much time it takes to have much real impact on stored fat, we can readily see that a good reducing diet must also be adequate nutritionally (except for calories).

We have seen that there is little that the physician—and certainly that the self-treating dieter—can do to speed the process up, despite the breathless stories in hundreds of magazines about magical foods and diets.

A recent popular diet is one augmented with cider vinegar, lecithin, kelp, and vitamin B-6. The explanations for why this diet is supposed to work, as expounded lengthily in *Family Circle,* are complex. For example, explaining the role of lecithin, the author writes: [38]

"It isn't that lecithin *reduces* you (your low-calorie or low-carbohydrate dieting does that). On the contrary, it appears simply to shift your weight around to where you want it. And if, perchance, you are skinny, but have lumpy hips or thighs . . . it seems to streamline them." Reporting on a friend who tried this, the author says: "This particular guinea pig is thrilled and vows that it is the first time in her ever-thin life that she was able to be thighless. Not thinner—just not lumpy."

There is no scientific basis for these claims—lecithin won't "shift your weight around." You will still be lumpy.

The explanations for the use of the vinegar, B-6, and kelp are equally convincing and scientific-sounding. However, there is one strategy of the diet which does seem to help—the fact that one must limit oneself to 1,000 calories a day, " . . . but, precisely that amount and not one calorie more . . ."

Are 500 to 1,000 calories a day enough? We have already seen that in terms of pure survival one can go a long time without eating anything and still have energy reserves to draw upon. And most of us would be likely to stop dieting when we became emaciated.

But energy is not all there is to nutrition. For one thing, without some of the micronutrients, our bodies cannot make use of the energy. Instructions for most crash diets include the warning to see a doctor first—although few people do (and there is usually also the soothing statement that whatever the diet, it is perfectly safe)—and to "take a vitamin pill."

Yet only a minority of needed nutrients are available in vitamin-mineral supplements—and we also need the "structural materials," for the building and repair of tissue—the macronutrients and some micronutrients. Extremely obese people who are treated with complete fasting burn not only fat but muscle tissue as well. In a sense, the body consumes its own meat to get needed protein.

So pills and potions are not the answer to a reducing diet which is nutritionally inadequate. To be adequate, most dietitians agree that a diet usually requires at least 1,200 calories a day of food, and more for people who are larger than average. Even at this level, care is needed to insure sufficient intake of the fairly narrow range of foods which are especially potent sources of micronutrients such as iron. For a comfortable, varied diet which is nutritionally adequate, it is hard to plan daily meals for a long period of time which total much less than 1,800 calories.

In designing weight-reduction diets, two key principles are usually followed. The first is the avoidance of "calorie-dense" foods, that is, foods which have high concentrations of energy. Foods rich in fats and oils, and sugars are typical.

Foods with low caloric concentrations are usually substituted for those with high concentration—for example, chicken can be substituted for beef. Foods with high content of water and fiber, such as fruits and vegetables, are usually favored. Their high bulk, relative to their calories, makes them good reducing foods.

A second principle is that of the *"compact* dietary." Foods are chosen which return a high nutritive value for the energy they contain. This is sometimes expressed as *nutrient density.* The simplest way to understand the principle is to picture calories of energy as money. We want to use a limited "budget" of calories to buy as good nutritive value as we can.

This concept explains why sugar is usually restricted in such diets. For in effect, it "dilutes" foods nutritionally. If we compare two servings of canned peaches, one with heavy sugar syrup, and one

Table 4-7.

Nutrient	150 kcal of peaches in syrup	150 kcal of peaches in own juice, or water
Protein	.77 grams	2.0 grams
Calcium	7.7 mg.	20.0 mg
Iron	0.6 mg	1.7 mg
Vitamin A	837 I.U.	2233 I.U.
Thiamine	.019 mg	.033 mg
Riboflavin	.038 mg	.133 mg
Niacin	1.1 mg	3.0 mg
Vitamin C	5.8 mg	13.3 mg

packed without sugar, we see the portions with the same number of calories will have very different nutritive value. Thus, for reducing purposes, we would choose the more *nutrient-dense* peaches, without syrup.

Psychological Aids to Weight Control

The fact that emotions can provide such great impetus to appetite, or such great restraint, suggests that influencing the emotions is an important factor in weight reduction. The theory is good. But it is no more easily put to work in obesity than is the nutritionist's injunction to "eat less and exercise more."

We have noted that the use of food to deal with emotional stress is inculcated very early, and early psychological imprintings run deep. This helps to explain why traditional psychological therapy in depth, such as *psychoanalysis,* may or may not be successful in motivating a patient to weight control. If a patient's deeply rooted "oral" personality patterns—powerful tendencies to depend on nurturing situations and relationships as ways of dealing with pain or fear—can be dealt with, his reliance on managing stress by eating or drinking can be reduced. Such a patient may find the courage to deprive himself and lose fat.

Sometimes, however, psychiatrists have observed that the state of being fat itself may be the unconscious aim. *Hirsch* and others report that some patients who have lost large amounts of weight become seriously depressed and anxious and continue to think of themselves as fat people. Why would a patient unconsciously *want* to be fat? A classic instance is the person who uses fatness as an excuse for avoiding relationships with the opposite sex.

Attempts to make such basic changes in psychological orientation and function are both costly and time-consuming, however. So there have been many recent efforts to find more practical short-term routes to deal with obesity. These attempts fall into two broad categories.

One category uses the psychological pressures of the group—in classes or club-like meetings of the obese. Of course, they also attempt to teach the principles of diet-construction and of nutrition in a limited way. Such programs vary widely in quality. Some have gone to the trouble and expense of getting the nutrition advice of experts. Others have, unhappily, espoused and taught some of the greatest nonsense. But for all of them, the approval-disapproval power of a group of peers and the sharing of common problems is an important part of the method.

In many cases, however, as soon as the participant is out of the group, he founders. The situation can be much like the child who behaves very differently when his parents are not watching.

The second category tends to be labeled loosely with the popular term "behavior modification." The term itself is, of course, a very broad one. In a sense, anything we teach people about nutrition is intended to change behavior for the better. "Behavior modification" usually refers to a special kind of training, in which desirable behavior is rewarded and undesirable behavior is punished. In practice, the methods vary widely. In some cases, they depend, regrettably, on a kind of cold-blooded *Pavlovian conditioning*— Pavlov being the Russian scientist who found that he could ring a bell when feeding dogs, and eventually, when no food was given, and the bell was rung by itself, the dogs would salivate.

An extreme example is the work of one physician who gives unknowing patients a drug which produces mild nausea. He then shows them photos of films such as a plate of spaghetti with worms in it. The idea is to make foods repulsive. On a more humane level, subjects may be taught to count bites of food, for example, with the aim of each day reducing the number of bites taken. This can be useful in making people aware of their eating, so that it is not a kind of blind, unthinking behavior.

In more sophisticated programs,* certain requisites are set up for eating. For example, the subject may be persuaded to keep records of when, how, and what he eats, for greater awareness of the experience of eating. Then he is instructed not to eat food out of hand, or standing at the kitchen counter. He may make a contract to eat nothing except from a plate, with a tablecloth, a setting of silver, and so forth.

Psychiatrists argue that one problem with all "behavior modification" programs, however, is that eating for many obese people may represent a way of dealing with stress. By closing down that technique of adjustment, without managing the underlying cause, the

---

*As examples of sounder and more scientifically based plans, see those of James Ferguson[39] and of Levitz and Jordan.[40]

therapist may only be forcing the patient to adjust by some other behavior which conceivably can be less desirable than eating.

The fact remains that some weight-loss programs utilizing behavior modification techniques have achieved better results for substantial numbers of people, in terms of long-term success, than have more traditional methods.[41,42]

Special Foods

Any number of commercial food products are available, which reproduce commonly consumed foods at a lower caloric value. The product may be an artificial sweetener, such as saccharin. It may be a cola drink sweetened with saccharin instead of sugar.

Such products may be useful, because they allow the dieter some of the satisfaction of familiar tastes. A person who is used to beginning each day with two cups of sweetened coffee may be uncomfortable when told to drink the coffee black.

But when research has examined the effectiveness of such products in actually reducing calories consumed, results have been poor. For example, the use of artificial sweeteners has *not* been shown, in most experiments, to reduce caloric intake. One reason may be that the body's controls over caloric intake are fairly good. If we shortchange ourselves on calories at one meal, or with one food, we seem to make up for it with another.

Calorically reduced products are often somewhat deceptive. A "low-calorie" beef stew may be one with more water in it. A "diet bread" proved to have fewer calories per slice only because the slices were thinner. Certain "specialty" brands of foods, specially promoted to dieters (and often indistinguishable from food not thus promoted), such as skim milk or cottage cheese, or frozen dinners, or dishes with low calorie counts, may be sold at higher prices. But one skim milk is much like another, and some calorie-lowered convenience foods may simply contain less food at a higher cost.

The person who would lose weight in a nutritionally and medically sound way, and without being cheated economically, must accept the unpleasant truth that he will be eating less than he would like to eat; he must understand the insurmountable facts of energy balance; he must be able to compare nutritive values as well as calorie counts. And above all, in a number of ways, he must understand what is in his food.

In the long run, shortcuts are likely to be only self deceptions.

REFERENCES

1. *Food Day* Brochure, Center for Science in the Public Interest, Washington, 1975.
2. Bray, G. et al. Introduction to *Obesity in Perspective*, National Institutes of Health, DHEW Pub. No. (NIH) 75-708,1975.
3. *Final Report, White House Conference on Food, Nutrition and Health*, U.S.G.P.O., Washington, 1970.
4. *Obesity and Health, a source book, etc.,& U.S. Public Health Service Publication No. 1485*.
5. Mead, M. *Why Do We Overeat?* Redbook, January, 1971, p. 28.
6. *Nutritive Analysis of the Potato*, a preliminary report, The Potato Board, Denver, 1976, unpublished.
7. Mayer, J. *Genetic factors in human obesity*, Annals of the N.Y. Acad. of Sciences, Volume 131, p. 412, Oct. 8, 1965.
8. Mayer, J. *Some aspects of the problem of regulation of food intake and obesity*, New England J. Med., 274, Mar. 17, 24, 31. 1966.
9. Jordan, H. *Psychological Factors Associated with Obesity*, in Obesity in Perspective, NIH, DHEW Pub. No. (NIH) 75-708, 1975.
10. *Stunkard, A. The Pain of Obesity*, Bull, Palo Alto, 1976.
11. Bruch, H. *Eating Disorders*, Basic Books, New York, 1973.
12. Newman, H., et al. *Twins: A Study of Heredity and Environment*, U. of Chicago Press, Chicago, 1937.
13. Hirsch, J. and Knittle, J. *Cellularity of obese and nonobese human adipose tissue*, Fed. Proc. 29:1516-21, 1971.
14. Knittle, J. *Obesity in childhood*, J. Pediatr. 81:1048, 1972.
15. Fomon, S. et al., *Normal Growth, Failure to Thrive and Obesity in Infant Nutrition*, Saunders, Phila., 1974.
16. *Endocrine and Metabolic Adaptations to Obesity*, Summary 7, Vol. I, *Obesity in Perspective*, DHEW Pub. No. (NIH) 75-708, 1975.
17. Seltzer, C. and Mayer, J. *Body build and obesity*, JAMA 189: 677—84, 1964.
18. Food and Nutrition Board *Recommended Dietary Allowances*, Nat. Acad. Sciences, Washington, 1974, pp. 25—36.
19. *Energy Balance*, Summary 5, Vol. I, *Obesity in Perspective*, DHEW, Pub. No. (NIH) 75-708, 1975.
20. FAO, *Energy and Protein Requirements*, FAO Nutrition Meetings Report Series No. 52, Rome, 1973.
21. Hegsted, D. *Energy needs and energy utilization*, Nutrition Reviews, 32: No. 2, Feb. 1974, p. 33.
22. Bogert, L. Briggs, G. and Calloway, D., *Nutrition and Physical Fitness*, Saunders, New York, 1973, p. 39.
23. Grande, F. in *Obesity in Perspective*, Vol. II, in press.
24. Behnke, A. et al, JAMA, 118:495, 1942.
25. Mayer, J. *Obesity: diagnosis*, Postgrad. Med. 25:469, 1959.
26. Seltzer, C. and Mayer, J. *Simple criterion of obesity*, Postgrad. Med., 34:190, 1963.
27. Gordon, T. and Verter, J. *Serum Cholesterol, Systolic Blood Pressure, and the Framingham Relative Weight as Discriminators of Cardiovascular Disease*, DHEW, NIH, 1969.
28. Mayer, J. *Physical activity and anthropometric measurements of obese adolescents*, Fed. Proc. Vol. 25, No. 1, Jan—Feb., 1965.
29. Bullen, B., Reed, R. and Mayer, J. *Physical activity of obese and adolescent girls appraised by motion picture sampling*, Am.J.Clin. Nutrition, 14:211, 1964.
30. Christakis, G. in *Obesity in Perspective*, Vol. II, in press.
31. Freud, S. *A General Introduction to Psychoanalysis*, Boni and Liveright, London, 1924.
32. Deutsch, H. *The Psychology of Women*, Grune & Stratton, NY, 1944.
33. FDA Drug Bulletin, *Anorectics Have Limited Use in Treatment of Obesity*, DHEW, Washington, Dec. 1972.
34. Fazekas, J. *Anorexigenic agents*, New Engl. J. Med. 264:501, 1961.
35. Modell, W. *Status and prospect of drugs for overeating*, JAMA, 173:1131, 1960.
36. *Appetite suppressants in the treatment of obesity*, Nutr. Rev. 20:38, 1962.
37. Rickman, F. et al., *Changes in serum cholesterol during the Stillman Diet*, JAMA 228:54, 1974.
38. *My amazing cider vinegar, lecithin, kelp, B6 diet*, Family Circle, Jan. 1974.
39. Ferguson, J. *Habits, Not Diets, The Real Way to Weight Control*, Bull, Palo Alto, 1976.
40. Levitz, L. and Jordon, H. *Manual for the Analysis of Energy Intake and Expenditure*, in Appendix V, *Obesity in Perspective*, Vol. I, DHEW Pub. No. (NIH) 75-708, 1975.
41. Levitz, L. and Stunkard, A. *A therapeutic coalition for obesity, behavior modification and patient self-help*, Amer.J. Psychiatry, 131:423, 1974.
42. Stunkard, A. *Presidential Address 1974: From explanation to action in psychosomatic medicine: The case of obesity*. Psychosom. Med. Vol. 37, No. 3, pp. 195—236, 1975.

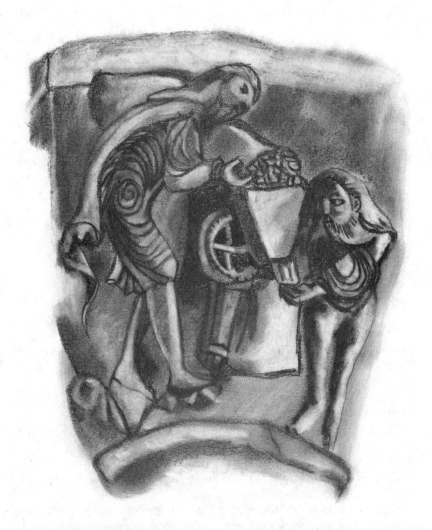

The content of food has long been a mythical symbol for truth. *St. Peter Grinding Out the Grain of the Old Testament to Seek Its Core of Truth. Stone Capital Relief, from a pillar of the Church of La Madeleine, Vézelay, France, 12th century.*

chapter 5

WHAT'S IN A FOOD?

The television butcher, neat and smiling in white, took a jar of peanut butter from his cold room, brought it to the counter and began his commercial pitch—about protein. The peanut butter in this ad, he told us, was "the sirloin of peanut butters."

What did that mean? He explained that, ounce for ounce, his peanut butter had as much protein as hamburger.

The audience reached by such a commercial may be guessed to total in the tens of millions. That audience, believing as most Americans do that meat and high protein are virtually synonymous, was troubled by the high price of meat. It would listen well to the offer of a cheap substitute protein source.

Had the audience been fairly taught about peanut butter and protein? The question may seem related to a narrow and special case. Yet indeed, it reflects one of the most urgent consumer concerns about nutrition: *What is really in the food we buy?*

93

The commercial told the truth—as far as it went. But it omitted some of the information a consumer needed to make a well-informed buying or meal-planning decision.

Let us consult the food-composition tables of USDA Handbook 8. In the first table, all foods are shown in portions of 100 grams, about 3.5 ounces. Peanut butter is listed three ways, according to the amounts of fat, salt, and sweetener added. The protein content of these butters is shown to be between 25.2 and 27.8 grams. Under "hamburger" (ground beef) we find two listings for cooked meat— *regular* at 24.2 grams of protein and *lean* at 27.4 grams. So peanut butter does indeed, ounce for ounce, have as much protein.

But some other questions should be asked. First, as we shall later see in detail, protein can vary greatly in its quality. For what the body needs from protein are the approximately 22 amino acids from which protein is made, and certain ones, which the body cannot itself manufacture, are termed "essential."

When a protein contains all of the amino acids in amounts proportionate to human need, and is easily digested, it is called "high quality." But if one or more of the essential amino acids is present in a quantity less than the needed proportion, the protein is of "lower quality."

In general, the proteins found in animal-source foods are "high quality." What this means in practical terms is that one could grow, survive, and reproduce, if only this protein (and an adequate non-protein diet, of course) were eaten. Conversely, if one tried to exist on vegetable protein from a single source, sooner or later there might be trouble. A child may not develop properly on a single lower-quality protein. (Later we shall see, however, that lower-quality vegetable proteins can be combined or supplemented to make an entirely adequate protein source for a vegetarian child or adult.)

Looking up the protein of peanut butter in a table which shows the content in terms of essential amino acids, and looking at another table which shows amino-acid needs, we find peanut butter wanting.* The essential amino acids *lysine, methionine, and threonine,* and possibly also *tryptophan,* are significantly low.

A second test for this ad is more homely. Three and a half ounces of hamburger is a modest portion. But this amount (almost a quarter of a pound) of peanut butter would be a hefty serving. Imagine this

---

*Among the references for amino-acid content are Orr and Watt,[1] Block and Weiss,[2] Bowes and Church,[3] and FAO Nutritional Study No. 24.[4]

much in a sandwich. In sum, one does not generally eat peanut butter and hamburger in similar quantities; they are not really interchangeable.

A third important test uses an essential principle of practical nutrition. Except in rare cases, or for special purposes, one does not evaluate a food in terms of a single nutrient. For example, the same serving of peanut butter and hamburger may be similar in protein quantity, though not quality. But let us look at the very important question of fat content.

100 grams of cooked lean hamburger (approximately 3½ oz.) is shown in Handbook 8* as having 11.3 grams of fat. That is approximately 100 calories of fat. The total caloric value of 100 grams of hamburger is shown as 219. The *least* fatty peanut butter has 49.4 grams of fat in the same 100-gram amount—*more than four times as much* as the hamburger. This portion thus has *almost 450 calories in fats alone, and 581 calories* total.

Draw your own conclusions. There is no intended implication here that peanut butter is not a good food (it is), or even that it is not a useful protein source. The question is whether, as implied, it is a suitable replacement for beef.

Let us turn to an ad in a popular magazine.[5] It shows an upset woman with a telephone, a shouting child, a crying baby, and what appears to be a miscreant dog. Headline—*"Everyday stress."* And we are told that this is why we should know the facts about orange juice:

"Anyone who's ever had 'one of those days' knows about stress," the State of Florida Department of Citrus informs us. "But did you know that emotional stress can accelerate potassium loss?" (Then we are informed that orange juice is a good source of potassium.)**

So it is. In our food-composition tables, we see that this juice offers some 200 milligrams in a serving of 100 grams (some 2/5 of a cup). Is that a lot of potassium? The Food and Nutrition Board RDA for a healthy adult is 2,500 mg a day. So the serving of orange juice can supply less than one-twelfth of our recommended daily intake.

Checking food tables again, we see that the same size servings of many foods can give us as much potassium, or quite a lot more. Rare

---

*Handbook 8, compiled by the Agricultural Research Service of the U.S. Department of Agriculture, has served nutritionists as the basic reference source for nutritive values. Handbook 456, used for Appendix A, contains comparable information listed in terms of familiar household measures.

**In none of the texts in the author's library is emotional stress noted as an important cause of potassium deficiency.

foods? You judge. Against the 200 mg from a single serving of orange juice, compare 370 mg from bananas, 273 mg from bread, 267 mg from broccoli, 341 mg from carrots, 274 mg from chicken, 350 mg from hamburger or liver, 200 from dill pickles, 850 from french-fried potatoes, and over 500 mg even from popcorn. In brief, one quickly begins to suspect that there is no shortage of potassium in the world of common foods—and that it would be a very rare healthy person who would be potassium-deficient.

When they do occur, potassium deficiencies are largely transient, because they are largely due to transient conditions. For example, the Food and Nutrition Board concludes: "Potassium deficiency . . . usually occurs as a result of inadequate intake coupled with excessive loss due to diarrhea, diabetic acidosis [mainly due to the water loss that occurs when inadequate carbohydrate is available to the body chemistry] or to use of certain diuretic [water-loss] drugs or purgatives."[6]

Readers may draw their own conclusions about whether this ad gives valuable information—and about whether its implications fairly motivate the consumer to drink orange juice so as to deal with emotional stress.

In both of the described ads, only two examples of commonplace advertising methods, true statements are made about the nutrient content. Other types of food messages are used in similar fashion. Let us look at an ad in which the point of persuasion is what is *missing* from a food. The simple statement is found in many ads for bread—"No Preservatives." The absence of preservatives is implied to be a plus for the consumer, and often a higher price is charged.

The complex questions of preservatives and other additives in foods are dealt with in Chapter Thirteen. But keeping in mind the basic truism that each additive and preservative is a separate matter—just as the safety of each individual drug is a separate matter—let us consider this single example.

If there is a preservative in bread, it is generally calcium *propionate* (a salt of *propionic acid*). The preservative qualities of these compounds were discovered long ago. They are the naturally occurring preservers of certain cheeses, such as Swiss cheese. We might bear in mind that cheese is an ancient way of concentrating and preserving milk, in effect making milk longer lasting and more easily portable. How much propionic acid is there in cheese? According to Dr. George York of the University of California at Davis, the amount in a single one-ounce slice of Swiss cheese is enough to preserve two whole *loaves* of bread.[7]

This suggests that it is a little self-defeating to buy bread which is advertised as having "no preservatives," and then make a Swiss cheese sandwich. On the other hand, if we can assume that Swiss cheese is not unsafe as a food, it seems reasonable to conclude that bread which incorporates propionates to slow down spoilage is even safer. Conversely, we know that the mold which will probably grow on bread if nothing is done to prevent spoilage, can certainly be unsafe. How then shall we judge the "no preservative" advertising for bread?

FOOD CONTENT, NUTRITION AND THE LAW

To make intelligent nutrition decisions, clearly we must know the nutrient and other content of foods. But just as clearly, we must accurately know the significance of these contents. The three advertising examples underscore this latter need. For though the statements of content—or absence—are true, they are easily given a misleading meaning.

Let us consider the fact that some sodium is lost in the processing of wheat. Some commercial literature which promotes less-refined grain products makes much of this loss. True, sodium is an essential of body chemistry. But there is a missing piece of information; it is that sodium is plentiful in many foods. Also, the original sodium content of wheat is not very high; and most Americans consume several times more sodium than they need, especially in table salt, *sodium chloride.*

Recent changes in the Federal law have attempted to help meet both the consumer's need to know food content and the need to know the meaning of food content for health. Understanding these laws can show us something of how the nutritive content of foods can help us make practical decisions.

The laws that deal with food content fall into three broad areas. These are:

1. Safety and wholesomeness.
2. Fair value.
3. The truthfulness and meaningfulness of information which is offered for choosing and using a product.

These areas are listed largely in the chronological order in which the government has instituted safeguards and controls. In 1902, Dr. Harvey Wiley, then chief of the Bureau of Chemistry of the U.S. Department of Agriculture, began to issue formal reports on what he considered to be dangerous chemicals used in the manufacture of foods. Aroused by these and other similar writings, Congress passed the Food and Drug Law in 1906 (to become effective on the first day of 1907), creating the Food and Drug Administration (FDA).

In 1912, Congress added the Sherley Amendment, which broadened the powers of the Food and Drug Administration, so that those who made fraudulent statements on package labels could be prosecuted. Some time later, the Federal Trade Commission (FTC) was charged with protecting the public from false or unfair advertising of all kinds. In the interim, the courts upheld the right of the Food and Drug Administration in certain instances to construe labels as advertising.

Despite the considerable body of regulation that grew up around these laws, a report of one panel of the 1969 White House Conference on Food, Nutrition and Health found that:

"These laws are not being obeyed or enforced as they should be. Certain bottlenecks must be removed . . . Food label requirements must be expanded in the light of what the consumer actually wishes and needs to know and couched in language which is meaningful enough so that the consumer may make an intelligent choice . . . all foods should be labeled in such a way as to reassure the most skeptical consumer that he is not being deceived by omissions."[8]

Early in 1973, after intensive study, the FDA promulgated a series of new "Regulations for the Enforcement of the Federal Food, Drug and Cosmetic Act and the Fair Packaging and Labeling Act."[9] These regulations were designed to enlarge the amount of information the public got about foods. But more than this, they were an attempt to put this information in a form which would indicate which facts were really important in making choices.

The regulations are still somewhat limited. But most nutritionists seem to agree that they are a major step forward. And if we understand them, and understand why they are framed as they are, we can learn something about the methods and values by which the scientist chooses food.

NUTRITION LABELING*

Nutrition labeling regulations center about a small box of information which is now found on many food packages, under the heading "NUTRITION INFORMATION." Whether or not this information is supplied on a package is optional, except in two instances:

(1) Where any statement is made about nutritive values, either on the label, or in advertising, or in promotional literature. Even phrases such as "low-calorie," "low-fat," or "a good source of potassium" make nutrition labeling a must.

(2) The addition of any nutrient to a food, as in fortification and enrichment. However, there are exceptions to this rule. Nutrition labeling is not made necessary when, for example, a vitamin is added for purposes which are not nutritional. (This happens more often than many consumers suspect. Vitamins C and E are commonly used as preservatives—ascorbic acid (C) to prevent discoloration of fruits and E (*tocopherols*) to prevent the rancidity of oils.) Another example is when a vitamin is added because a commonly enriched food— such as enriched flour—is used in a product. This is partly because Federal standards have been set for such enrichment, so that it is always the same.

Under these labeling rules, any nutritional claim for a food forces a food producer to put very specific information on his product. As an example, the nutritive wonders of yogurt have been widely touted in advertising and in popular journals. But the fact is that the nutritive values of yogurt and of ordinary milk are generally the same. This will now be clear through the required (so long as nutritional claims are made) labels, and a questioning consumer can learn this by simply comparing cartons.

Serving Size—A Key to Practical Comparison

In comparing foods, the nutritionist traditionally compares equal weights—usually 100 grams—of two products. This allows the assessment of the nutritive properties of the food, in terms of the

---

*Under the auspices of the National Nutrition Consortium, a set of guidelines for understanding and using labeling has been prepared.[10]

density of the nutrients present or in terms of caloric value. But this sort of comparison may often confuse, rather than inform, the consumer.

Looking back at our peanut butter-protein example, we saw that serving sizes are better guides to comparison. The equal weight method of comparison there was based on the implicit assumption that either peanut butter sandwiches are made with a quarter of a pound of peanut butter, or that hamburgers are made with an ounce of meat. Neither is very realistic.

FDA concluded that when consumers wanted to know the nutritive values of foods, they really wanted to understand what sort of nutrition they would get from a typical serving. So FDA ruled that nutritive values on labels had to be shown for a serving which is of "average, usual or reasonable" size.

The determination is left to the packer or manufacturer, but with FDA reserving the right to veto unusual or unreasonable choices. And there are other guidelines which help. A serving size must be such as will be "suitable for consumption as part of a meal." And it must be suitable for an adult male who engages in light physical activity. Servings must be shown in household measures, such as a cup, a teaspoon, a slice, or an ounce. And to clarify the amount, the number of servings in a container must also be shown.

Calories and Macronutrients

A serving's content of calories, protein, carbohydrates and fats must also be shown. Because the nutrient values reflected in even some of our best food-composition tables are sometimes broad averages, with questionable origins, FDA requires that labelers make new analyses—based on a special method of averaging. For fresh produce, for example, composite samples must be made up which include different common varieties grown in different sections of the country. The results are still averages, of course. And recognizing the inevitable inaccuracies, FDA rules call for rounding off numbers. For instance, calories are shown in increments of the nearest 10.

Protein, carbohydrate, and fats, along with all other nutrients, must be analyzed by standard methods specified by the Organization of Analytic Chemists. The three macronutrients are shown to the nearest gram per serving.

The averaging technique is admittedly imprecise. But FDA thinking is that, if a consumer eats much of a product through the year, he is likely to get something like the average nutrient values in the long run. Remember, small variations in nutrient intake from day to day, or from week to week, are not likely to have much effect on a normal person. On the other hand, if the product is eaten only rarely, inaccuracies of the average nutritive values will have little impact on the quality of his nutrition anyway.

Some special listings are possible for fats—in terms of the kind of fat in the product and the cholesterol content. The meanings of these listings and the disclaimers which the Government requires will be discussed later in the book, when we examine fatty substances. Following the fat listings, sodium content may also be listed, shown to the nearest 5 milligrams. More detail about this listing will be covered when we look more closely at this mineral.

U.S. RDA—A New Kind of Standard

One of the most unusual, and controversial, ideas in FDA labeling rules is the concept of U.S. RDA, *United States Recommended Daily Allowance* (as distinguished from the RDA, the Recommended Dietary Allowance established by the Food and Nutrition Board, of the National Academy of Sciences). This new standard is a compromise attempt to deal with one of the most difficult problems in nutrition education—*evaluating* nutrient content.

At first blush, adding nutrition information to food labels looked like a simple matter. We had only to analyze the food and then set out the results on the package, as so many milligrams, micrograms, or international units. Then the consumer would know what was in the food.

Or would he? True, the plan would allow anyone to make certain kinds of comparisons. For example, suppose a shopper was deciding whether to buy canned or frozen corn niblets. Under the system of simply showing the nutrients, the shopper would see that a half-cup serving (about 3½ ounces by weight) of drained corn provided essentially the same number of calories, whether canned or frozen.

Looking at the vitamin and mineral contents, however, the shopper would see some differences. The canned would have .5 mg of iron, the frozen .8 mg.* Vitamin A would be the same, but B vitamins would differ, largely due to the cooking process used in canning: the canned corn would show only .03 mg of thiamin, compared to three times as much (.09 mg) for the frozen; the frozen would have slightly more riboflavin, and it would have 1.5 mg of niacin, compared to the canned corn's .9 mg. Plainly, the frozen corn would seem more nutritious.

But if the shopper is thoughtful, even if not nutritionally sophisticated, he completes his comparative analysis and then scratches his head. How much thiamin, he asks himself, is .09 mg?

From what was said above, of course, it is clear that knowing nutrient content is not especially useful unless one also has some concept of human nutritive needs. Let us apply our knowledge of need (taken from the RDA tables of the Food and Nutrition Board) to the corn question.

Thiamin RDA for a young man is 1.5 mg a day. So we calculate that even the superior .09 mg thiamin content of the frozen corn represents only about six percent of the daily recommendation for this vitamin. The amount in the canned corn, of course, is only two percent.

Looking at the frozen corn's superiority in riboflavin we see that the amount at stake is .06 mg, versus the canned corn's .05. In a relative sense, this superiority may seem meaningful, one being more than 16 percent greater than the other. But in terms of the adult male RDA, neither form of corn contains more than a rather insignificant three to four percent of the recommendation. In other words, these are not good sources for these vitamins; if one relied only on sources of this quality, one would have to get 20 to 30 servings a day.

The meaning of these facts? While corn is a useful source of the nutrients we have compared, it is a minor source, and the relatively small differences in content of these nutrients are not important reasons for buying one over the other. If the canned corn is much cheaper, the shopper might as well take it.

But how were labelers to suggest this information about the *importance* of a food as a nutrient source? It is not reasonable to expect the shopper to carry an RDA table and a calculator for every purchase. To be useful, nutrition labeling must be simple. Early

*Some of the nutrients supplied by canned foods may be in the canning liquid, and may or may not be consumed with the basic product.

surveys showed that fewer than 40 percent of shoppers even expressed an interest in having nutrition information on packages.

Could the label simply show the nutrient content in terms of percentage of human need? A theoretical possibility, this did not at first look feasible. For the RDAs include, for each nutrient, 17 separate recommendations for different population groups. Imagine trying to show the percentage of need for a dozen nutrients for 17 different population groups on a package of salted nuts.

Enter the U.S. RDA (Appendix B), a simplified table of recommended daily allowances that made it possible to express the nutrient content in terms of a standard allowance. Even if it had been possible to interpret the needs in terms of each age-sex group, it would still have been only an approximation, at the very least requiring adaptation to individual height and weight, in order to be sufficiently precise.

So the compromise was made, drawing heavy fire from many a nutritionist for its imprecision: FDA decided on a single basic set of daily recommendations, using the largest nutrient requirements for normal adults. Additional recommendations were set for special groups, and four tables were constructed. The main standard was based largely on the needs of adult males. Another was for infants under 12 months of age. Another was for "junior" foods, for children between the ages of one and four. And the fourth was for women who were pregnant or lactating.

How well does the table work? Let us look at some examples.

The Food and Nutrition Board's RDA recommends that males who are eleven or older consume 5,000 international units of vitamin A daily. This amount has been established in U.S. RDA terms as 100 percent for this vitamin. The idea is that, on this intake, very few people would have less than adequate vitamin A. The amount of vitamin A in either canned or frozen corn is then shown on the label, not in terms of international units, but in terms of the percentage of the full U.S. RDA (5000 i.u.) in a standard one-half cup serving. Since that amount averages out to 350 units, it is seven percent of U.S. RDA.

In the required rounding off of percentages, amounts less than 10 percent of U.S. RDA must be shown in two-percent increments. (So the vitamin A content of canned or frozen corn appears on the label as either six or eight percent.)

Because the U.S. RDAs are averages, they are sometimes inaccurate. Some nutritionists object to the inaccuracy, which can become quite pronounced—for 5-year-olds for instance, who are grouped with adults. In some cases, differences are minor. U.S. RDA for calcium is a little low for teenagers of both sexes and a little high for adults. But in other cases, differences are considerable. For example, women of childbearing age need almost twice as much iron as do adult men, and (because the classification with the higher need is used for the general adult category) the feminine need is used as the U.S. RDA. So the Food and Nutrition Board RDA for a typical man is only 56 percent of the U.S. RDA for iron.

Obviously, the plan is imperfect, but so far no one has a better one. Nutrition educators must simply teach consumers how to interpret the percentages of U.S. RDA for each individual. But even without such teaching, the average consumer can still get *some* idea of whether a food is an important source of a given nutrient.

Another problem is that the U.S. RDAs can become obsolete. Ironically, some of them were obsolete before they became law. For the Food and Nutrition Board reviews its RDAs about every five years. While the food labeling rules were still being finalized, some RDAs were changed. But realizing that label changes are quite costly, and that this cost is ultimately borne by consumers, FDA did not change its U.S. RDAs. As a result, U.S. RDAs are much higher for vitamin C and vitamin E, for example, than are the current RDAs, published in 1974. At this writing, U.S. RDAs are based upon the Food Nutrition Board recommendations published in 1968.

The Special Case of Protein

Because of the particular importance of protein, and especially because of the sharp increase in prices for meats in the past few years, FDA felt that this nutrient should not be shown in grams alone. As was mentioned earlier, protein varies in quality, and most Americans are not aware of the quality differences between proteins. So special methods were needed to show consumers what part of their protein need they were buying in a given product.

The ad for peanut butter which we examined earlier is a good case in point. Here was a claim for a lot of protein in a relatively cheap food. Yet this protein was not of high quality. How could the consumer be alerted to this fact? Again the designers of labeling sought a shortcut. They declared that protein must be listed twice—

once in total grams, and a second time, taking quality into account, in percentage of U.S. RDA.

To indicate that some proteins had more quality than others, *two* U.S. RDAs were set. One was 45 grams—for protein of high quality, from animal sources such as eggs, milk, fish, or meat. The second rating was for lower-quality protein sources, mostly from the vegetable family of foods; this was pegged at 65 grams.

In our detailed discussion of proteins we will see some reasons for this distinction. For the moment, let us simply observe that lower-quality proteins are shown on the label as being a smaller percentage of U.S. RDA. Looking at our earlier example comparing the protein content of peanut butter with that of meat, we see that the protein of peanut butter is given a lesser rating than that of meat. The reason, of course, is that the U.S. RDA for high-quality protein is lower.

The table below* lists some common protein sources, together with the percentages of U.S. RDA which a typical serving would provide, according to protein quality:

Table 5-1.

SOME U.S. RDA PROTEIN VALUES	
Higher quality protein sources	**Percentage of U.S. RDA**
3 oz. of cooked hamburger	50
2 frankfurters	30
3.5 oz. of cured ham	50
3 eggs	30
3 slices of luncheon meat	30
8-oz. glass of milk	20
3.5 oz. of fried shrimp	45
2 1-oz. slices of Swiss cheese	30
2 1-oz. slices of processed American cheese	30
Lower quality protein sources	
1 cup of cooked peas	35
1 cup of lima beans	20
1 cup of potato salad	10
1 cup of noodles or spaghetti	10
1 ounce of chocolate-coated peanuts	8
1 cup of whole-kernel corn	6
1 slice of whole-grain bread	4
1 slice of commercial white bread	4

Adapted from Nutrition Labeling, How it Can Work for You. National Nutrition Consortium, Inc.[10]

The mathematical system is, as we have noted, imperfect. What made the FDA planners feel the system was safe? Partly, it was the fact that Americans are such large consumers of proteins, and of such a high proportion of animal-source proteins. FDA found that between 70 and 75 percent of the protein consumed in the U.S. was of the highest quality. The conservative nutritional rule of thumb is that only 50 percent of protein need be of high quality, and indeed, this percentage incorporates quite a large safety factor.

What is the gauge of the quality of protein? It is the biological value of the principal protein of milk, *casein.* How this yardstick is used will be seen when protein is reviewed (along with some reservations that this method may be more demanding than necessary). In essence, protein with a value equivalent to that of milk is considered to be of high quality.

How Proteins, Vitamins and Minerals Are Listed

The percentages of U.S. RDA are rounded off in three different ways. Up to 10 percent of U.S. RDA, the amounts are rounded off to the nearest two percent. Beyond 10 and up to 50 percent of U.S. RDA, the content of the nutrient in a serving is shown to the nearest increment of five percent. And beyond 50 percent the amounts are shown to the nearest 10 percent.

When nutrition information is required, the values of seven vitamins and minerals, in addition to protein, are compulsory listings. These are vitamins A and C, three of the B vitamins (thiamin, riboflavin and niacin), and the minerals calcium and iron (see Appendix C).

A common misunderstanding has arisen, that these seven vitamins and minerals are somehow of paramount importance. The fact is that any nutrient which is essential to our body chemistry must be seen as equally valuable. A consequential lack of any essential nutrient will produce deficiency symptoms and interfere with the successful function of the body.

Why are these seven micronutrients selected as *musts* for nutrition labeling—along with calories, fat, protein and carbohydrate? In large part, it is because they are the best known, and among those most easily analyzed in foods. Perhaps more important, FDA sees these micronutrients as indicators. That is, when these micronutrients are present, it is believed fair to assume that others are also present. However, analysis has shown that this idea is not always true.

It would be a more valid assumption if more foods were eaten in their natural state. But modern technology confuses the indicator value of these nutrients, because they are commonly (and cheaply) added to foods. An example of how basic nutrient balance can be altered is provided by breakfast cereals such as *Total,* which at this writing is advertising as providing 100 percent of our recommended intake of key vitamins and minerals. The serving size for such cereals is approximately one ounce. It is virtually impossible to provide 100 percent of all our needed micronutrients in an ounce of any grain product, unless one actually converts it into a kind of vitamin pill to be consumed with milk and fruit. And we must remember that vitamin pills have limitations.

To avoid the misunderstanding that adding a handful of vitamins will make an ounce of food into a day's nutrition, FDA has invoked some special regulations. One of these is that, if more than 50 percent of vitamin or mineral U.S. RDA is added to a food, it must be labeled as a "special dietary food."

Some Listings of Vitamins and Minerals Which Are Optional

In addition to the mandatory vitamin and mineral listings on labels, twelve other nutrients *may* be shown, if the packager chooses. (U.S. RDAs for the optional nutrients are set forth in Appendix D.) He may list all of these, or confine his listings to any one or more.

These twelve nutrients are just as essential to health as the seven which *must* be listed. Nine of the twelve were selected for the most obvious of reasons—they are the only other micronutrients for which RDAs have been set. These nine are:

Vitamins	*Minerals*
Vitamin D	Phosphorus
Vitamin E	Iodine
Vitamin B-6	Magnesium
Folacin (folic acid)	Zinc
Vitamin B-12	

The other three micronutrients, *biotin* (a B vitamin), *pantothenic acid* (also in the B complex), and *copper,* are approved for optional listings but have no RDAs. FDA concluded that enough was known about them, and that there was enough public interest in them so that U.S. RDAs could be set and should be. Not all nutritionists agree, however, either about the level of information or about the value of such knowledge to the public.

The U.S. RDA for copper, 2 milligrams, is the amount known to be needed to maintain copper balance in the body. Biotin and pantothenic acid share characteristics which appeared to make it safe to set U.S. RDAs, even though information about the vitamins may not be precise enough to satisfy the requisites of science.

It is worth noting some of the reasons for FDA's confidence; for FDA has often been accused of being careless with the public safety, and this was not an unsafe decision. Like many FDA decisions, it embodies the principle that the practical realities of safety can be satisfied even when the meticulous demands of scientific precision cannot be met.

An Exercise in Practical Nutrition

Of both biotin and pantothenic acid, the Food and Nutrition Board's RDA Committee has decided that there are insufficient data for the establishment of RDAs. This is a reasonable conclusion—for the scientist. But let us see some characteristics of these vitamins which are reported by the same Committee, and which bear upon practical *applied* nutrition:

1. Both vitamins are very widely available in an enormous variety of foods. They are easy to get without dietary effort.
2. Average daily intakes of both vitamins can be calculated, and these would seem generally to cover the known use by the body.
3. Outside of the laboratory, symptoms of deficiency, due to inadequate intake, are unknown. To produce clinical deficiency symptoms of either vitamin, an experimenter must give a subject *antagonists,* substances which block the use of the vitamins by the body.
4. When people take in modest amounts of either vitamin, they excrete quite a lot, *often more than they take in.* How can this be? In the case of biotin, it is known that bacteria living in our intestines actually make the vitamin. The RDA committee finds that three to six times more biotin is excreted in the urine than is

ingested. In the case of pantothenic acid, no such evidence of bodily manufacture has been identified, but it looks as if the situation is much the same; more of the vitamin often comes out than goes in.

The reader must judge for himself. But common sense seems to suggest that there is no danger in setting U.S. RDAs for these two vitamins, despite the non-existence of an RDA. And the RDA Committee itself states that the key reason for its reluctance to establish RDAs is lack of information about *just how much* of the vitamins are produced within the body. In the case of biotin, for example, it may be that we do not really need to consume any of the vitamin at all. This would not be unique. For instance, most species of animals do not need to consume vitamin C because their bodies can manufacture it. (The exceptions are found in Chapter Eleven.)

Why include these micronutrients in labeling at all? One reason is that false health claims have been made for them, and in some cases it has been implied that people may suffer from shortages and need to emphasize the vitamins in their diets. Since such claims are unjustified, giving some idea of how much we really need and how that need is met by various foods, is one way to protect the consumer.

Making the U.S. RDAs More Personal

To make the nutrition information on labels work in planning meals or in assessing the quality of an individual's nutrition, it helps to translate the U.S. RDA percentages into more personal terms. For remember that these percentages represent only the broadest sort of averages. How can they be made more specific?

Suppose 10-year-old Mary is what her mother calls a "poor eater." She seems to pick at her food and has very little taste for meat. Mother worries. For she has heard a lot about protein as the key to good health, and she is afraid that Mary's disdain for meat means that the child's protein intake is very low. She does know that milk, of which Mary drinks some four glasses a day, also has protein of high quality. But what protein contribution does the milk really make to Mary's diet?

Looking at the milk carton, Mother sees that the protein listing is nine grams per serving, and that a serving is an eight-ounce glass.

(This listing is arrived at by rounding off the actual protein content.)

How much protein is that? Mother now looks at the protein listing as a percentage of U.S. RDA. This is shown as 20 percent. (Since the protein is of high quality, the U.S. RDA is 45 grams. The nine grams in a glass of milk is 20 percent of U.S. RDA, when rounded off to the nearest two percent.)

The conclusion? Milk gives Mary some 80 percent (four times 20 percent) of her daily protein allowance. Mother decides to worry only on days when Mary does not drink all of her milk.

In developing simplified methods to help consumers use nutrition labeling, the National Nutrition Consortium developed the charts in Appendices C and D. Their aim is to relate the U.S. RDAs to the RDAs for individual population groups. Keeping in mind that even this information is still based on averages, let us put the chart in Appendix D to work for Mary.

First we find the group into which Mary fits, "Children, 7–10 years of age." Looking across to the protein column, we see the heading "Percentage of U.S. RDA which equals RDA." This percentage for Mary's group is 55 percent.

In other words, Mary does not need 100 percent of the U.S. RDA for protein, but only about half as much. So the milk she drinks makes an even more important protein contribution to Mary's diet than Mother was led to believe. Three glasses give her more than her RDA for protein, even though they supply only 60 percent of U.S. RDA. (And of course this does not take into account the protein contribution of Mary's other food.)

What Do Grade Labels Say About Nutrition?

Many people believe that food labels which show the grade of a product have nutritive significance. In general, this is not true. Mainly, such ratings show esthetic, not nutritive, values.

Many of these grades are given under government control standards, a fact which can sometimes be recognized by the appearance of the grade designation in the shield of the U.S. Department of Agriculture. Usually U.S.D.A. standards for such markings make no mention of nutrition.

For example, U.S.D.A. sets three grades for eggs—"AA" (or "Fresh Fancy"), "A," and "B." "AA" eggs look prettier. If you break one into a hot skillet, it will stay in a smaller space, rather than spreading out. It may also have a nicer flavor. But the nutritive values for an "AA" egg and a "B" egg (though it spreads thinly over the pan) are the same. The same is true for poultry. Even an elderly chicken, which cannot earn such high grade names as "Fryer" or "Broiler," essentially offers the same nutritive value. The case is similar for fruits and vegetables, butter, and fish (which, when graded, are under the supervision of the U.S. Department of the Interior).

Indeed, the only nutritionally important grade label is probably that for beef, lamb, and veal. For these grades are affected by the fat content of the meat. The cut-it-with-a-butter-knife tenderness of "Prime" meat, for example, results in large part from a high fat content. Each succeeding lower grade may be assumed to have less fat—in order of grade after "Prime," we find "Choice," "Good," "Standard," and "Commercial." The latter two grades are not often seen in markets.

Private grade labels of meats can be meaningless. And they generally are not used unless the meat is below the quality levels of "Choice." Legally, the butcher or market may put any kind of label they wish on meat, as long as they do not put it in the U.S.D.A. shield. They can call their meat "Swell" or "Socko" if they choose, but this gives no reliable information as to flavor or fat content.

People who need to restrict fat intake do well to buy cheaper grades of meat. In our food-composition tables, we see that the rib roast of beef, "Good" grade, provides 417 calories in a cooked portion of about three and a half ounces. The same amount of "Choice" offers 481 calories. And "Prime" would go even higher. The difference is in the fat content.

Inspection stamps, as for meat and fish, give assurance of health safety, but again have no meaning for nutrition.

Of course, not all foods have nutrition-information panels on their labels. The manufacturer may decide to avoid labeling. He may know that the food will look nutritionally poor. He may not want the expense of analysis. He may not feel that nutrition is an important reason why consumers buy his product, and so has no nutritional message in promotion or on the package.

Some voluntary labeling has surprised nutritionists. Many potato-chip makers, believing their products have unfairly been labeled as "junk food," put their nutrition story on their packages. So do some makers of candies and snacks.

On the other hand, most meat packers and produce people have, surprisingly, avoided the nutrition-information label, which might tell a good story for them. True, it is hard to put nutrition information on a grape or a pork chop. But provision has been made in FDA rules for alternate methods of labeling, such as the display of label information separately, near the display of a food.

Produce and meat shippers come under some special regulations. For example, the meat industry has for many years been under the supervision of U.S.D.A., not FDA, in such matters. And partly because of the wide variations in nutritive values of fruits and vegetables, some producers have ducked the question; labeling is not required unless a fruit or vegetable is packaged for selling, or unless nutritive claims are made in the displays.

What Ingredient Labels Can Say About Nutrition

Ingredient labels, of course, will not be found on a peach or a ham bone. But they do appear on manufactured food products, and they can provide nutritional clues even when specific nutritive analyses are not given on packages. Let's see how.

What Order of Listing Can Mean

Among the oldest labeling rules are those which require that the ingredients of most foods be listed on the package, in decreasing order of their quantity in the product. From this, the consumer can make a number of deductions, especially about value.

Let us look at *Birds Eye* frozen creamed spinach. Chopped spinach is listed first among the ingredients, so this is the main content of the package. As a point of comparison, ordinary chopped spinach in the same freezer cabinet sold for 20 cents. The creamed spinach cost 47 cents for the same size package, a difference in price of 27 cents, or 135 percent.

What did this difference buy? Looking at the package, we see that the creamed spinach contains no cream. In addition to the spinach, it has a sauce. The main ingredient of the sauce is water. Next come margarine, dry skim milk, and dry whey.

The latter three items are intended to imitate cream. The margarine supplies the fat. It gives the greasy feel to the dry skim milk and dry whey, for the latter two have virtually no fat. Margarine is 80 percent fat. Whey is what is left of milk after the curd is removed to make cheese. The curd contains most of the protein and calcium, two of the most important nutrients in milk. Much of the water is needed to restore the dried whey and skim milk to a liquid state.

Is there any other food substance of much consequence added? Unless one knows the rules of ingredient labeling, one might notice wheat flour among the ingredients, and conclude that extra nutritive value came from this. But we know that ingredients are listed in decreasing order of quantity. We note that the flour in the listing follows the salt *disodium phosphate,* a type of preservative which helps maintain certain qualities of milk products. We would be safe in assuming that there is going to be very little of this salt added; and the amount of wheat flour will be still less.

In nutritional terms, and considering the enormous difference in price, should people on limited budgets buy this "creamed" spinach instead of plain spinach? For example, how much whole milk would the extra 27 cents buy, and what sort of nutritional contribution would it make?

Not far away in the freezer case is sliced turkey, at $1.69 for two pounds, or about 85 cents a pound, considerably more than the price of a small whole turkey per pound. But closer inspection of the label shows the ingredients as, "water, turkey . . . etc." We also note that the package is really billed as "Gravy and sliced turkey." Consider that, if there is less turkey than water, the package being bought must consist of less than *half* turkey meat. Thus the turkey must actually cost at least twice as much as 85 cents a pound. (And when we look at the ingredients listing for the gravy, we see that it has precious little nutritive value.)

In the same freezer case we see *Bel Air* Macaroni and Cheese. This is a prepared frozen product grouped with main dishes, and we might think it a reasonable protein source, perhaps because of the cheese. The ingredients list begins with cooked macaroni, followed by water, followed by cheese. Mathematically, how much cheese can there be?

The name *Kraft Macaroni and Cheese Dinner* clearly states what is only implied in the *Bel Air* product: it is supposed to constitute "dinner." An examination of the labeling confirms a somewhat similar ingredient pattern (which differs mainly because the customer prepares the dish from the included ingredients). A serving of

280 calories offers 10 percent of a day's protein. If dinner provides only 10 percent of needed protein, what meal will provide the remaining 90 percent?

Anyone who wishes to make his or her own gallery of such products has only to walk up and down the market aisles, or perhaps look through his own cupboard. Note especially products which include butter or honey in the names. The butter in "butter bread," for example, may be listed as an ingredient after salt. Special breads of all kinds are apt to provide good material for ingredients readers. Note particularly the listing position of whatever special ingredient gives the bread a fancy name and a fancy price.

What Labels Tell About Processing and Nutrition

If nutritive parts of food are left out or lost in processing, often the resulting difference is clear from a comparative reading of labels. Such a comparison may tell us whether it is worthwhile to buy special products which are promoted as "unprocessed" or "natural" (and often sold at much higher prices).

For example, there can be enormous differences in bread prices. Suppose we compare some typical breads, to see how nutrition labels indicate differences. We might consider just the mandatory listings of the percentages of U.S. RDA (calculated from food-composition tables). (See Table 5-2.)

These breads differ widely in cost and flavor. But in terms of nutrition, there is not a lot to choose from, despite the use of such healthful-sounding ingredients as stone-ground unbleached flour, flaxseed, and so on. Indeed, while there is a great deal of popular talk about the protein values of breads, actually the biggest variable in protein content is the amount of very cheap non-fat dried milk used. (One indicator of this is the higher calcium content of the "high protein" bread; for the dried milk also supplies calcium, of which grains have very little.)

Dried milk is so inexpensive that the entire day's protein for a typical adult could be supplied for less than 35 cents at this writing. But using more than a little spoils the loaf.

Nutritive contributions of some other common ingredients of more expensive breads, such as honey and butter, are so small that they would scarcely alter the nutritive analysis. The ability to read and understand nutrition information on labels can tell us that, nutritively,

Table 5-2.

A SHOPPER LOOKS AT BREADS
(Values shown are percentages of U.S. RDA, rounded to nearest 2 percent)

BREAD (One Slice)	Vit. A	Vit. C	Thia-mine	Ribo-flavin	Niacin	Cal-cium	Iron	Protein
ENRICHED WHITE**	*	*	4	2	2	*	4	4
WHOLE WHEAT	*	*	4	2	2	2	2	4
PEPPERIDGE FARM WHITE	*	*	4	4	3	*	4	4
THOMAS PROTEIN	*	*	6	2	2	8	6	4
ROMAN MEAL (MIXED GRAINS)	*	*	4	2	4	2	4	4
CRACKED WHEAT	*	*	2	*	*	2	2	4
AMERICAN RYE	*	*	2	*	2	2	2	4
PUMPERNICKEL***	*	*	4	2	*	2	4	4

*   Indicates less than 2 percent of U.S. RDA

**1–2% non-fat dried milk added.

***Values pro-rated to equal approximately the weight of standard slices (an average of about 23 grams, some ¾ oz., per slice)

it is not worth spending much extra money for supposedly more healthful breads.

Are there differences between breads which are not shown on this chart? Yes, there are (in some of the "optional" U.S. RDA nutrients). In general, they are of the same magnitude as those we see here, however. In addition, there can be some differences in content of trace elements which may not be listed in nutrition information. And the more refined breads omit some of the fiber found in coarser breads. By and large, however, unless one eats a great deal of bread regularly, or unless one does not eat vegetables, fruits, or other grain products, the coarser breads are not necessary for good nutrition:

Do keep in mind, however, that *enriched* flour is used in the more refined breads shown here. Certain B vitamins and iron have been added to the flour, and these do not have to be shown in the ingredients list. Without such enrichment, and some states do not require it yet, the refined breads are poorer sources of nutrients.

Another example may be seen in the buying of dehydrated potatoes of various types. If we check nutrition information, we see that some dehydrated potatoes are missing something which should be found in potatoes—a good deal of vitamin C. The process commonly used in dehydration destroys the vitamin C. Some manufacturers put this back, spraying it on after dehydration. So we should look for vitamin C content of such products.

What if a potato package does not have nutrition information? Remember that one of the factors which makes nutritional labeling mandatory is the addition of a nutrient to a food. If there is no nutritional labeling, we know that nutrients have not been restored.

Additives can make quite a difference in nutritive content. Baby foods are often criticized as inferior to standard foods. But in many ways they can be superior. For instance, manufacturers often use elaborate techniques to preserve nutrients, such as one which zooms the food to high sterilizing temperatures in seconds, then quickly cools them. Label comparisons can show whether processing results in more or less nutrient value.

A combination of ingredient labeling and nutritional labeling can help us to evaluate some other products. Consider breakfast cereals, some with very high percentages of "essential vitamins and minerals" in a serving, or fruit "drinks," which may contain as little as 10 percent fruit juice, but which may boast of high vitamin content.

Again, remember, if nutrients are added, they must be listed among the ingredients (with the exceptions we have noted), and they make nutritional labeling mandatory. In the fruit "drinks" we can see a distorted nutrition profile, often with a lot of one vitamin, such as C, and little else. Compare these labels with those for real fruit juice and you can see the difference. In fact, from the amount of listed nutrients which are not shown to have been added we can actually calculate about how much fruit juice is in the drink.

In the matter of the "high-vitamin" cereals, some of the ingredients, which may read like a pharmaceutical shopping list, quickly tell us that we are being offered a kind of vitamin pill. But the actual food ingredients, mainly an ounce of grains and sugar, make it clear that despite the vitamin and mineral content, this is only a small amount of food, and that more is needed for breakfast. 100 percent of a few of the day's micronutrients may sound good, but it leaves a lot of needed nutrients unaccounted for—which must be supplied by other food.

Some Details of Law

Spices, flavorings and colorings do not have to be listed by name as ingredients, but can be listed generically, just as "spices," "colors," and so forth. If ingredients are part of a "standardized" food—one for which FDA has set certain maximum or minimum standards for limits on content and/or composition, such as "ice cream" or "ice milk"—they do not have to be listed. This includes certain permissible amounts of stabilizers, smoothers, preservatives, and such. Otherwise, all additives must be listed, and their functions must be described as well. After the additive, the packager must use a common descriptive term such as "to retard spoilage," or "to protect flavor."

When must a food be called an "imitation?" It depends on the nutrient content. If the original food has a measurable amount (2 percent or more of U.S. RDA) of any of the listable nutrients (not including fat and calorie content), the replacement food must have at least an equal amount. If the amounts do not equal or surpass those in the original, the new food must be called "imitation." If the amounts in the original food are equalled, the new product may be called by a special new name—such as, "Hoggo Bits," for imitation bacon bits made from enriched soy meal. Note that the name can suggest the relationship with bacon. "Hoggo Bits" might well have less fat than bacon, and so have fewer calories, but this would not be considered nutritional inferiority.

Labeling laws will be reviewed further, as we deal with specific nutrients and needs. But these general outlines suggest how we can use them to make comparisons. Even if the consumer does not use the new labeling to compare products, the FDA rules still protect him. For they also apply to advertising, especially on the package itself.* For example, promoters can no longer emphasize nutrients which are present only in insignificant amounts. A nutrient cannot be emphasized unless a serving provides at least 10 percent of U.S. RDA. Without such rules, advertisers could point up the protein in lettuce; for lettuce does have protein, although it would take about fifteen pounds to supply the U.S. RDA.

---

*FDA rules apply to advertising when it can be construed as an extension of the label itself and mislead as to content, etc.

While labeling provides new protection for the consumer, and clearer information, it has limited value unless the buyer understands the relative significance of the nutrients in a product. There is little to gain from knowing how much of a nutrient is in a food, unless you understand the role of that nutrient in nutrition and in your own personal diet. So let us look more closely at the nutrients, and at their myths and their realities.

REFERENCES
(See Also, References for Chapter Three)

1. Orr, M. and Watt, B. *Amino Acid Content of Foods,* Home Economics Research Report No. 7, USDA, 1957.
2. Block, R. and Weiss, K. *Amino Acid Handbook,* Thomas, Springfield, Illinois.
3. Bowes, A. and Church, C. *Food Values of Portions Commonly Used,* Lippincott, Phila. rev. 1970.
4. FAO Nutritional Studies: *Amino Acid Content of Foods and Biological Data on Proteins,* No. 24, Rome, 1970.
5. State of Florida Dept. of Citrus, *Everyday Stress,* advertisement, Family Circle, Feb. 1976, p. 170.
6. Food and Nutrition Board, *Recommended Dietary Allowances,* Nat. Acad. Sciences, Washington, 1974, p. 90.
7. York, G. Private communication while eating a sandwich.
8. Deutsch, R. ed. *Report of Subpanel on Deception and Misinformation,* Final Report, White House Conference on Food, Nutrition and Health, 1970.
9. FDA, *Regulations for the Enforcement of the Federal Food, Drug and Cosmetic Act and the Fair Packaging and Labeling Act,* FDA, 21 CFR 1.17 and 21 CFR 125.1.
10. National Nutrition Consortium and Deutsch, R.M., *Nutrition Labeling,* National Nutrition Consortium, Bethesda, 1975.

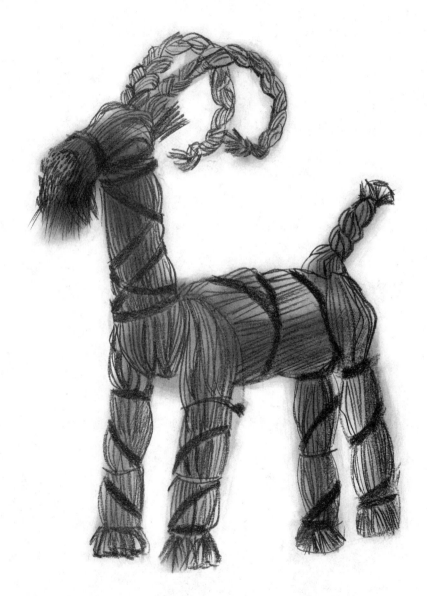

Grain has always had spiritual overtones, for its growth and nutritive quality have meant survival to many cultures. *The Corn Goat, an early Teutonic spirit symbol, fetish of the harvest. Sweden: Such figures of grain straw were carried into Christianity and are much used still at Christmas.*

chapter 6

CARBOHYDRATES AND THE TRAPPING OF THE SUN

One of the popular journals read by patrons of health-food stores is *Let's Live,* which is dedicated to "The Natural Way to Vibrant Health." And a popular feature of the magazine is Linda Clark's column, *Light on Your Problems.* In a recent issue, the *Light* was shed on this question:

"Everywhere I go, and everything I hear or read seems to knock carbohydrates. What's so wrong with them?"—M.L., Kansas City, Mo.

Columnist Clark summarizes her answer with a one-word sentence, "Lots."

Among other things, it is pointed out that eating carbohydrates can result in—"A flabby, rather than a firm body, plus overweight; hypoglycemia (low blood sugar); tooth decay; fatigue; restlessness; depression; insomnia . . ." Ms. Clark—whose breadth of scientific interest is testified to by the titles of her books (such as *Are You*

Radioactive?)—also quotes one Carlous F. Mason's opinions on the effects of carbohydrate eating: "A diet which contains candy, sodas, pastries, gum, pies, cakes, and other carbohydrate foods can lead to nervous breakdown as surely as can drugs, alcohol and the effects of worry."[1]

Much worse about carbohydrates could have been quoted from the popular literature on this subject. For carbohydrates are being widely indicted as being among the serious nutritional threats to life and health.

For example, although *Dr. Atkins' Diet Revolution* is known mainly as a reducing book, it blames carbohydrates for far more than obesity.[3-7] In the capital letters with which the Doctor and his co-author, Ruth West, seem to like to make their most important points, they write: "MANY OF TODAY'S DISEASES HAVE ONE PRE-DISPOSING FACTOR IN COMMON: CARBOHYDRATE INTOL-ERANCE." And they ask: "WHY HASN'T MEDICINE EXPLORED THE DEADLY ROLE OF CARBOHYDRATES?" In lower case, they inquire, "How can so many nutrition 'experts' not be aware of carbohydrate intolerance?" The book concludes: "WE'RE THE VICTIM OF 'CAR-BOHYDRATE POISONING.' The most killing diseases of the twentieth century stem from what I call 'carbohydrate poisoning.' "

Such charges are numerous indeed. There is little doubt that they have had some effect on many people in the making of food choices. And it is hard to ignore these effects when one examines certain changes in food consumption, not only in the U.S., but in the affluent Western world as a whole. For some of these changes appear to coincide with the appearance and popularization of books warning about carbohydrate as a cause of obesity and ill health, and with the publicizing of these ideas in the media.

All of this "anti-carbohydrate" literature began to appear in quantity in 1950 and 1951. Between 1952 and 1972, there was a marked decline of total carbohydrate consumption in Britain. During that time, carbohydrates dropped from 54 percent of the caloric dietary to something less than 48 percent. (This percentage change may not at first seem significant. But on reflection, one can see that it represents a real shift in the balance of the dietary; it is a decrease in carbohydrate intake of over 10 percent.) At the same time—illustrating the fact that, since protein is only a minor part of the dietary, a fall in carbohydrate intake means a rise in fat consumption—Britain's fat intake increased from 34 percent of total calories to 41 percent.[2]

In the U.S., the U.S.D.A. indicates that fat consumption reached a new high during the same period. Our beef consumption per capita rose some 85 percent between 1952 and 1972. And our cheese consumption went up about two-thirds. Meanwhile, in the same period, per capita consumption of wheat declined 17 percent, and that of dried beans, another major carbohydrate source, went down by some 25 percent.[3] These dietary changes have resulted in the consumption of far more fat. And they also suggest that attacks on carbohydrate have been believed and acted upon.

In this light, it seems worthwhile to test the theories of those who decry carbohydrate against some of the realities of human nutrition. It is logical to begin by asking what a carbohydrate really is, where it comes from, and how it plays a role in the chemistry of life.

THE CHEMICAL BIRTH OF FOOD

One of the basic scientific truths about life on our planet is that it is dependent on the sun. That dependence is for more than warmth. It is also for energy.

Essentially, it may be said that all our food energy begins with plants. When man eats the meat of the cow, for example, he gets the energy which the cow stored by eating grasses and other vegetable matter. The same is true of the cow's milk.

Where does the plant get this energy? Its primary source is the sun. The primary process is called *photosynthesis,* which might be literally translated from its Greek roots as "putting together with light."

The light in this case is, of course, the high-energy light of the sun. The things put together are two of the most common chemicals on the face, and in the air, of the earth—carbon dioxide and water. (These two chemicals, interestingly enough, also happen to be the two most important waste products of animal chemistry.) If man could put the two together himself he could create his own energy sources. But it is fairly obvious that he could stand all day in the sun, breathing carbon dioxide from the smoke of a barbecue, and drinking water, and end up with little more than a sunburn and a sore throat.

The plant, however, has the miraculous green chemical, *chlorophyll.* In the presence of chlorophyll, the plant can use the sun's energy to combine carbon dioxide and water. In so doing, it is really combining two basic elements—carbon and hydrogen—each of which is carrying all the oxygen it can hold. For example, when we burn coal, which is carbon, each atom of carbon combines with two atoms of oxygen, when fully burned ($C + O + O = CO_2$). As almost any schoolchild knows, it takes two atoms of hydrogen to hold one of oxygen and thus create water ($H + H + O = H_2O$).

So the plant begins by juggling six atoms—one carbon, two hydrogens and three oxygens. Using solar energy to split apart and reassemble them, it ends up with two products. Two of the oxygen atoms join together to become a molecule of free oxygen gas, just what we need to breathe—and one reason why the air seems so much "fresher" in a forest than on a city street. (There's a lot of oxygen.) What is left over is a mix of one carbon, two hydrogen and a single oxygen atom. In effect, the carbon has been combined with a molecule of water—as $C–H_2O$. It has been *hydrated*.

A hydrated carbon is a carbohydrate.

In actual plant practice, this new hydrated carbon molecule is combined with other similar groupings of carbon, hydrogen, and oxygen into the many forms of the carbohydrate family. One way of grouping these forms is according to the number of carbon atoms in each. Those molecules with six carbons (*hexoses)* are possibly the most familiar to us—as *sugars.*

SUGAR, THE FOOD CHANGELING

To be realistic about carbohydrates, we must first understand what sugar really is. For sugar comes in many chemical arrangements. The simplest of these are among the most basic chemicals of life.

The four six-carbon sugars which have nutritive significance are *glucose, fructose, galactose* and *mannose*. All have the same numbers of the same elements—carbon, hydrogen and oxygen—but differently arranged. The two most widely occurring in nature are glucose (sometimes called *dextrose, corn sugar,* or *grape sugar)* and fructose (sometimes known as *fruit sugar* or *levulose).*

Galactose is not found in a free form in foods, but it is half of an important, more complex sugar called *lactose,* which is one of the primary nutrients in milk. *Mannose* is rarely found in foods, and is more of scientific than practical interest in nutrition.

While we will not make deep forays into organic chemistry here, it may be informative to take a look at the molecules of all four of these sugars—just to see the pattern by which Nature weaves the same few components into very different substances, each with its own special role. In this spirit, let us inspect the sugars closely for a moment. Counting up, we can see how the formula for simple sugars can be noted as C_n $(H_2O)_n$—meaning only what we have said before, that they are combinations of a certain number (n) of carbons and the same number (n) of water molecules. These relatively simple sugars are classed as *monosaccharides*.

These basic sugars are not the smallest carbohydrates. There are some with only three carbon atoms (*trioses*) and some with five (*pentoses*). And by now one may suspect that carbohydrates can be recognized by the suffix, *ose*.

Characteristically, the smaller carbohydrates often appear as indispensable parts of some of the most complex chemicals of life. For example, consider the pentose called *ribose*. It is from this that the B vitamin *riboflavin* takes its name. From ribose also come the names of the key chemicals of genetics, RNA and DNA—*ribonucleic acid* and *deoxyribonucleic acid*.

Ribose, important as it is, does not have to be consumed in foods. The body can make it from other carbohydrates. This suggests a principle. For contrary to what is commonly believed by many, it is not true that carbohydrates serve only the purpose of supplying energy. They also supply some of the important building blocks of life.

When Sugars Get It Together

As plants trap the energy of the sun by making simple carbohydrates, they also use that energy to assemble these basic chemicals into larger molecules. For example, glucose and fructose are extremely common in the plant world. And very commonly they are combined. When one molecule of each joins the other, we get *sucrose*, common table sugar.

It is hard, for instance, to find a sweet-tasting fruit or vegetable which doesn't contain at least a little sucrose. And often there is more sucrose than either glucose or fructose alone. That is certainly the case of the sweet wild grass called *sugar cane*. Its sap runs rich with sucrose. Refining sugar is simply a matter of separating this digestible sucrose from the rest of the grass, which is almost entirely indigestible, as anyone knows who has chewed a stalk. (The same is true, of course, for the abundant sucrose in the sugar beet.)

These double sugars (two simple sugar molecules joined together) are known as *disaccharides,* as distinguished from their component single sugars, the *monosaccharides,* such as glucose and fructose.

Utilizing the Latin names for numbers, there are also triple sugars, *trisaccharides,* and quadruple sugars, *tetrasaccharides.* For example we often find these in soybeans, as well as other types of beans. (All beans are classed as *legumes,* since they, like nuts, are seeds of their plants.) This group of sugars is of limited practical interest to the nutritionist, though there is a practical aspect, due to the fact that the trisaccharides and tetrasaccharides in legumes are not digested by humans. They must be broken apart by appropriate enzymes to be used, and man does not have the enzymes to take apart some of the triple and quadruple sugars. But some of the microbes living in our intestines do have those enzymes. And they do split up some of those sugars, with a waste product of carbon dioxide and water. The carbon dioxide from this bacterial digestion is a cause of some of the intestinal gas that often results from eating beans.

Some scientists refer to all sugars which are more than double as *polysaccharides.* Others use this term only for sugar molecules joined in groups of ten or more; they refer to groups of from three to ten sugars as *oligosaccharides.*

The ability of plants to chain sugars together is great indeed. The chains can be *straight* or *branched,* and they can run to 1,500 or more simple sugars in a single molecule. What are these long-chain sugars? There are two basic groups. The first are the starches, which are complex combinations of sugars formed by plants as a source of energy storage. We taste the results of starch formation in many foods. Older potatoes, for example, are less sweet because more starch has been made from the sugar. The same is true of peas or corn.

Why is starch formed as a vegetable or legume matures? The answer lies in the demands of reproduction, which usually take precedence in the world of biology. The peas, for example, are really seeds for new plants. And until the new pea plants have been able to grow root systems and leaves, so that they can *photosynthesize* their own energy, the infant plants must draw upon the energy reserves of the seed. Starch is a more compact form for such storage. The case is much the same for the potato, which is the source from which the new plant must grow.

Fruits, of course, tend to have less starch. For their seeds are likely to be the parts we do not eat. The function of the flesh of fruits seems more to be attracting animals and insects to dine, so that the seeds will be exposed and distributed over the ground. Thus the edible portion of some fruits will tend to become sweeter with ripening, as starch turns into sugar.

The second group of long chains of sugars made by plants is largely indigestible by man. This is *fiber,* which generally serves as the structural component of plants. For example, the fiber content of celery, rhubarb, and asparagus is high because they are stems. Vegetables such as cabbage and lettuce are also fibrous; they scarcely have stems, and the leaves form the supportive structure of the plant. *Cellulose* is one such fibrous *polysaccharide.* Plentiful in celery, it is also the main constituent of most wood, and is virtually all of cotton. *Hemicelluloses* are other important food fibers; so are *lignins* and *pectins.*

With all the current talk about fiber, it should be pointed out that fiber is not always coarse stuff that gets caught between your teeth. A good example is *pectin,* which tends to make things more viscous than chewy; it is the stuff which makes jam and jellies gelatinize. Pectin fibers are among the common food additives. They hold water, make foods gooey, stabilize, and sometimes emulsify. *Carageenan* is one, which is taken from red seaweed; *algin* is just a long chain of mannoses. Others are *gum arabic, gum ghatti, gum tragacanth* and *locust bean gum.*

Fiber can be slithery. Or it may be quite subtle, so that you are really not aware of it at all. By the time the carrots and turnips and potatoes in your stew have simmered for several hours, you may not suspect that you are eating fiber.

Remember, too, that our definition of these substances as indigestible, is very human-centered. Ruminant animals, like cows and goats, find grasses perfectly digestible and nutritive. One species' fiber is another's meat and potatoes: The shells of lobsters and grasshoppers are made of a long-chain carbohydrate known as *chitin,* which snails (because of an enzyme in their systems) can flourish on. And termites eat well on the cellulose of wood.

Sugar and the Realities of Human Food Use

If the basic facts of how food is digested and put to work by body processes were better known by the public, the most cherished myths about food and health could scarcely survive. This seems especially so in the case of carbohydrates.

Let us suppose that we have just taken a Thanksgiving bite of candied sweet potato. Like virtually all foods, this one is complex. It contains a large number of chemical compounds, some of which play a role in nutrition and some of which do not. But since the chief nutrient substances in the dish are two classes of carbohydrates— starch in the potato, and sugar in both the potato and the candied topping—we can learn some principles by following a bite. For once that bite passes the lips, it enters into what is for most people the very mysterious and rather messy world of human innards.

In the mouth the candied sweet potato immediately comes in contact with two important bodily devices. It quickly encounters small nerve endings, especially in the tongue, known as "taste buds." These transmit only rather rudimentary impressions, which have been variously classified, but which are usually grouped as *sweet, sour, salty, and bitter.*

In practical terms, this rudimentary tasting ability can be regarded either as a kind of early-warning device or as a kind of energy-sensing system. For example, extreme bitterness or sourness might warn (respectively) of high alkalinity or acidity, which might suggest that the food should not be eaten. Extreme saltiness might also be a warning. But high sweetness does not seem to function this way. Some biologists speculate that this is because sweetness is the hallmark of carbohydrate, and that since carbohydrate is the primary energy source, sweetness is almost always perceived as pleasant.

(One might also infer from this speculation that such sensations as the acid fire of *jalapeno* peppers, for example, becomes desirable only by a learning process which contraverts a natural system of defense. This also suggests that taste is not a reliable indicator of safety or desirability in food, but is easily modified by learning. For instance, some peoples savor tastes which most of us would perceive as indicators of rotting. The ease of taste learning is evidenced partly by the many flavors which small children find unpleasant, but which are relished by them later as adults. By the same token, taste research has made it clear that there is no reality to the idea that the body's nutritive needs are reflected in one's taste preferences. Children left to choose foods for themselves do not choose with nutritional wisdom, any more than expectant mothers who develop sudden cravings for hot fudge sundaes.)

Back to the sweet potato. In a very quick reflex, the brain responds to the presence of good flavor and a large lump, by ordering the jaws to chop, grind, and tear the sweet potato apart. At once a second taste factor comes into play: Aromatics are released. (These vapors are usually carried in tiny amounts of oils in foods such as vegetables, or in the large quantities of fat in meats.) The vapors from the food are carried through the mouth and upward into the nasal passages. The most subtle flavor receptors are in the *epithelial lining* at the back of the nose. Here we differentiate between sweet potato and duck in orange sauce, which is why we cannot taste well when we have a stuffy nose. Once again, warning aromas, perhaps conditioned by memory, may give us a chance to reject, say, spoiled meat.

The Saliva and Its Enzymes

If both sets of taste receptors suggest that the sweet potato is indeed an acceptable food, the jaws and teeth continue their work of breaking up the food. This is aided by the presence of liquid, the saliva, from several glands under the jaw.

The moistening action helps to prepare food for its long journey through digestive passageways. But it also does more. In the saliva is an enzyme* called *salivary amylase* or *ptyalin.* It can break apart some starches. That is, it can snap the long chains of sugars, at certain points, into smaller chains. Here we can begin to note some ways to understand nutrition language.

For example, ptyalin is an *amylase.* This word derives from two Greek roots. The suffix *ase* denotes an enzyme, generally one which can decompose a food substance. The first part of the enzyme's name refers to that particular food substance. In *amylase,* the prefix comes from the word *amylon,* simply meaning starch. Once we are familiar with these roots, we can quickly see that *amylase* is an enzyme which decomposes starches.

An amylase does its work by the very basic digestive process known as *hydrolysis.* Let us look at the roots again. *Hydro,* of course, refers to water, as in *hydroelectric* or *dehydrate.* And *lysis* is a root

---

*An enzyme is an organic chemical produced by plants or animals, which promotes chemical reactions in life processes. (See Chapter Eleven.)

which turns up repeatedly in nutrition. It stems from the Greek for *breaking down,* as in the word *analyze.* So *hydrolysis* is nothing more than breaking things down by using water.

This process can be extremely detailed and complex. But in practical terms it is quite simple. Consider the body's problem of pulling apart the long chains of sugars—which we shall see is essential before the body can use the carbohydrates in its life chemistry. Picture the long chain of sugars which makes a starch as though it were a string of beads. But there is no string to hold them together, or any sort of glue. So what can keep the string of beads whole? The answer, of course, is small electrical charges, positive joined to negative.

Let us return to the making of a carbohydrate by the combining of the carbon dioxide molecule (CO_2) and water (H_2O). Recall that in this reaction, two atoms of oxygen were freed. This was one use of the solar energy, the breaking of the oxygen bonds. When the oxygens were broken off—one from each of the combining substances—the remainder of the two substances was left with unsatisfied electrical charges, where the oxygen atoms had been attached, like two tiny magnets. So they snapped together, to form our basic carbohydrate.

Essentially the same sort of process takes place when sugars are joined together to form starches. A bit of each sugar molecule is broken away, leaving the remainder with an unsatisfied bond, with an attractive force. The open bond can be filled by the next sugar molecule in line, which has a similar electrical need. One romantically inclined biochemist has compared the process to the behavior of two lovers who are left alone by a kind of chemical divorce. They tend to fill the gap again.

If the sugars which have joined together are separated again, they will once more be electrically incomplete. Something must be put in the empty places. A molecule of water can serve this purpose. This is one important reason why water is so fundamental to life processes. And it is in this way that an amylase adds water as it helps to break the chains of starch apart, so that shorter chains or individual sugars can stand complete.

In essence, life forms renew themselves and grow by putting simple substances together into the complex forms which give them their structure and which they use to survive. Our foods are just such complex chemicals, developed by other life forms, plant and animal.

To get the simpler chemicals we need, we must first break down the complex food substances into the fundamental parts which our own cells can use. The first step in this process is *digestion.*

From the Mouth to the Stomach

Contrary to earlier belief, the saliva does not do a great deal of chemical digestive work. In the main, except for its physical wetting properties, it makes only a first break in the chains of starch, and does not deal with sugars.

The shorter chains which the amylase makes from the starch are largely the *dextrins.* We see these in some food products, such as those packets of sugar substitute which look like sugar. The *saccharin,* or perhaps the cyclamate, in such products is present in tiny amounts. So it is filled out with dextrins, which have relatively little caloric value, but do add bulk for easier handling.

One old idea about salivary digestion is true. The longer the food stays in the mouth, the better the amylase does its work. For the strong acid in the stomach, only a few seconds' trip away from the mouth, stops the enzyme's action.

As it enters the stomach, our candied sweet potato is a pulp consisting of dextrins, intact starch, and intact sugar. (For the moment, we will ignore the protein, fat, and other chemicals which are found in sweet potatoes and most other foods.)

The stomach is a sort of muscular sack, with three sets of muscles that keep up a churning motion when food is present. Among other things, this churning mixes the pulped food, now called *chyme,* with stomach acid. We might note here that such factors as emotion or alcohol can slow or virtually stop the stomach's churning. This helps to explain why too many cocktails gulped before dinner can leave one feeling as if there is a large inert burden in the stomach. There is. It also suggests why there is a feeling of relief when the stomach returns the meal dramatically, through the route by which it entered.

In more normal circumstances, the stomach can deal very powerfully with food, mainly using its production of *hydrochloric acid* (HCl). This is the same sort of acid one uses to clean mortar from bricks. It is more dilute in the stomach, but still strong enough to break down tissue. Secretions of the stomach lining keep the acid from eating into the stomach itself, and it is usually neutralized as it enters the intestines. But anyone who has had an ulcer in the stomach itself or in the first part of the intestine (the duodenum) can testify to the acid's strength. So will anyone with the "heartburn" we feel when "indigestion" splashes a little up into the esophagus.

The strength of the stomach acid suggests that it is naive to worry much about the much smaller acidity of most foods. That is why few foods are now banned from the diet of the ulcer patient. In such cases emotion is a much more potent factor than *pizza*.

The stomach acid continues the process of breaking down the sugar chains. The process is called *acid hydrolysis,* and the word roots quickly explain the meaning. The acid, rather than an enzyme, snaps apart the chains, and water fills the electrical gap to make stable compounds. For example, *sucrose* can be broken into its two component simple sugars, fructose and glucose. As the chyme leaves the stomach, the respective sugars glucose and fructose are just so many molecules of the same two monosaccharides—regardless of whether the potatoes were candied with raw sugar from the health-food store or with white sugar bought at the supermarket.

The Departure from the Stomach

How long carbohydrates remain in the stomach is governed by many factors. In the case of most foods, the time is likely to be some two hours. Carbohydrates dissolved in liquids move faster. When there is more accompanying fat, the stomach time is longer. Fats commonly remain in the stomach up to four hours.

In this context, it is interesting to note some popular ideas about "quick energy" of the sort held by some coaches. For example, distance skiers and bikers are commonly urged to eat sweets to bolster their energy during an event. The same is true for many hikers and other outdoorsmen. Many of these people reach for a chocolate bar, especially one with raisins and nuts, when they feel energy flagging. If this food does not leave the stomach for hours (especially when fatty foods such as nuts and chocolate are involved) how "quick" is the energy which is supplied?

Once the valves of the stomach have opened to allow spurts of chyme to enter the small intestine, digestion enters its final phase. The *dextrins,* broken from the starches, must be broken further, into shorter chains called *maltoses*. From the *ose* suffix of maltose, we can see that it is considered a sugar. It is also produced commercially, commonly by letting yeast enzymes break down starches in a factory. It is much less sweet than *monosaccharides* or other *disaccharides,* but it has some properties which make it useful in such products as instant foods.

The further breaking down of polysaccharides to maltose and then to single sugars, and also the final digestion of any remaining disaccharides, is carried out by enzymes in the small intestine, especially those from the *pancreas*. Our sweet potato is now quite unrecognizable. Its usable carbohydrate is thoroughly broken apart into the basic sugars, like the blocks of a child's building set. For it is only in very simple forms that nutrients can actually enter into the bloodstream to take part in life processes. Those carbohydrates (fiber) which stomach acid does not affect, and for which we tend to have no appropriate enzymes, travel down the twenty-plus feet of intestine intact, to be eliminated—except, of course, for those which our intestinal bacteria can digest.

How Carbohydrates Enter into Life Processes

In ancient folklore the digestive tract was the innermost center of the human. Once the stomach was seen as the seat of the emotions or of the soul. The reality is quite different.

In truth, the digestive tract can be visualized as "outside" the body. Its mucous membrane lining can be seen as an extension of our outer skin. But it can do things our outer skin cannot do. The cells which line the "inner skin" of the intestine secrete digestive chemicals. And they also admit foodstuffs, including water, into the bloodstream, to reach the vital organs.

This entrance into the bloodstream and the real inner depths of our physical lives is most subtle, a process still not understood in every detail. For our purposes of application, however, the system is abundantly clear.

The inner skin which lines the intestines is far from smooth. It is lined with projections made of *epithelial* (skin-like) cells. Under the magnifying glass these projections, called *villi,* are tightly packed, like dense seaweed along the ocean floor, somewhat tangled, and constantly moving. Each is about one-twenty-fifth of an inch long. And in a similar pattern, each of the villi is covered with *microvilli,* so small that they must be viewed through a microscope.

Because of this complex of irregular projections, the surface area of the intestinal wall is in effect multiplied and then multiplied again, until it is quite enormous. There is a need for this huge total surface, because it is through the cells of the lining that the simple sugar molecules must enter the bloodstream.

Because only the smaller carbohydrate molecules can pass through the microscopic passageways of the cells which make up the villi and the microvilli, it is fair to say that only "refined" carbohydrates may enter the bloodstream. The original source of the carbohydrates matters not at all. Whether we begin with *Fruit Loops,* organically-grown turnips, or our candied sweet potato, what will go into the epithelial cells is mainly glucose and fructose, with perhaps some galactose from the milk poured over the *Fruit Loops,* and a tiny bit of mannose.

These simple sugars then pass through the opposite (inside) walls of the cells, which face upon the bloodstream and the true core of our inner lives. From this moment, the origin of the various sugars matters no more to the organs and cells which will use them than do the origins of oxygen matter to the lungs—whether from sea air, city smog, or a scuba tank. Glucose is glucose. Fructose is fructose. And we shall see that the same is true in the digestive and metabolic processes for all nutrients.

Indeed, the next step is toward even greater simplicity. Like tributaries into streams, and streams into a great river, the little capillaries in the bloodstream which pick up the sugar molecules from the intestinal-wall cells feed into small blood vessels, which in turn pour into the big *portal vein* that flows to the liver. And here is the final simplification. Virtually all the single sugars which are not glucose are converted by the liver into glucose.

If it has ever seemed curious that hospitals often supply energy to certain patients with simple glucose (sometimes called dextrose) as the whole carbohydrate source, the reason should now be clear. Ultimately, glucose is the sole carbohydrate which most body cells use for energy.

This simple sugar, which is released from the liver to flow through all the bloodstream and nourish all of the cells, is what is known as the *blood sugar.* In normal people, the concentration of this sugar in the blood at the standard fasting level tends to be fairly constant—at about 60 to 100 milligrams of sugar in every 100 milliliters of blood.

(To envision this concentration, consider that 100 milligrams is 1/10th of a gram, about 1/280th of an ounce, or about 1/40th of a teaspoon of table sugar. Since a milliliter is 1/1000th of a liter, 100 ml. is a little less than half a cup. 1/40th of a teaspoon in about half a cup is not much sugar in the blood. To get an idea of how much sugar is available in one's entire bloodstream, start with the fact that blood is about 9 percent of body weight. Thus, there is about a liter of blood for each 23 pounds. A person who weighs 140 pounds would have about six liters of blood. So we can calculate that such a person would ordinarily have no more than six grams of glucose available in his bloodstream, or less than a quarter of an ounce.)

Clearly, something else must be happening to most of the glucose which is consumed in foods or converted from other sugars or starches. And indeed there are two chief destinies for the rest of the glucose.

First, the liver converts much of the glucose into a storage form, from which glucose can easily be released into the blood when needed. This storage form is a chain of glucose molecules (a polysaccharide) known as *glycogen.* Typically, about 10 per cent of the weight of the liver is glycogen, around 100 grams, or 3.5 ounces. But glycogen is also stored in other tissues. Heart and muscle tissue hold another 200 to 250 grams, about seven to nine ounces more. The energy value in the body's total carbohydrate may thus be seen as 1200 to 1400 calories. And this suggests how important is this nutrient. Recent research in exercise physiology has developed methods of increasing the capacity of muscles to store glycogen for limited periods, and "glycogen loading" has become a prominent part of preparation for important athletic competition.

Any excess glucose above the blood and glycogen requirements is converted to fat and stored in adipose cells.

WHAT'S THE HARM IN CARBOHYDRATES?

It should be plain from what we have seen that carbohydrates are scarcely poisons, but rather a major part of the food systems of the body. The body produces a large variety and quantity of special chemicals solely to deal with the carbohydrates, and depends upon them for the immediate energy needs of most cells. The only efficient fuel for the brain and other key organs is glucose.

On the other hand, there are people whose bodies cannot deal with all carbohydrates. For example, as we have suggested, each disaccharide must have a kind of matching enzyme which can put it to work. Consider lactose, the special sugar of milk. A disaccharide, lactose is composed of a molecule of glucose and a molecule of galactose, each a single sugar. To use lactose, we must have an enzyme to break these single sugars from one another. Following the system of naming enzymes, this one is called *lactase.*

Lactase deficiency, apparently an inherited problem, is common. In children between 11 months and 11 years, lactase deficiency seems to occur in about 10 percent of Caucasians and some 35 percent of Blacks in the U.S. Moreover, the deficiency tends to grow worse with age. Among Greek Cypriots, Arabs, Ashkenazic Jews, and many other peoples, adults show lactose intolerance to the tune of from 60 to 80 percent. About 70 percent of American adult Blacks share the problem, and the percentage rises to over 90 among Japanese, Thais, Bantus, Formosans and Filipinos. In fact, if one looks at lactase deficiency on a worldwide basis, it really appears that more than half of the adults suffer from it to some degree.

Genetically, any enzyme may be missing or in low supply. But with few exceptions, it is a medical rarity to find deficiencies of carbohydrate enzymes. Nonscientist critics have made much of the fact there are known cases of people who lack *sucrase,* and so have difficulty in putting sucrose (table sugar) to use. But in truth, such people seem to be few and far between. As of 1965, only 63 cases (of those who suffer from what is known as *sucrase-isomaltase deficiency)* had been found worldwide.

Substantial deficiencies of carbohydrate enzymes are not especially subtle. When the double sugar *lactose* cannot be broken down, it cannot be absorbed from the gut, since only the single sugars can enter the cells of the intestinal walls. These and other nonabsorbable carbohydrates tend to draw water into the gut, which then becomes distended. Further along in the intestines, bacteria begin to dine on these unbroken carbohydrates, using their own enzymes. The result is gas (flatus) and lactic acids, which are produced as waste products. And, depending partly on what else the person has eaten, and how much, he is apt to experience cramps and diarrhea, discomforts which are not likely to go unnoticed.

On the other hand, if there are very subtle deficiencies of enzymes, the results are also very subtle. Tiny amounts of undigested carbohydrates do no medical harm and cause no discomfort. We know this because we know that ordinary diets are not perfectly digested, and all of us deal continually with small amounts of undigested carbohydrates. In fact, as we shall see, some undigested carbohydrate is actually important, to provide bulk and to help the intestinal wastes remain moist enough to be moved along. This is the key role of dietary crude fiber, the "roughage" we get from plant foods.

The important fact to remember is that meaningful inabilities to deal with carbohydrates in our food tend to produce signs that something is wrong. Such inabilities do exist. But this does not change the fact that carbohydrates are very fundamental fuels and sources of building materials. So let us look more closely at some of the myths and realities of the effects of carbohydrate on human well-being.

REFERENCES
1. Clark, L. *Light on your problems: What's wrong with carbohydrates?*, Let's Live, Jan., 1974, p. 17.
2. Hollingsworth, D. *Changing Patterns of Food Consumption in Britain*, Nutr. Rev. Vol. 32, No. 12, Dec., 1974.
3. National Food Situation No. 142, USDA, Hyattsville, Md., 1972.

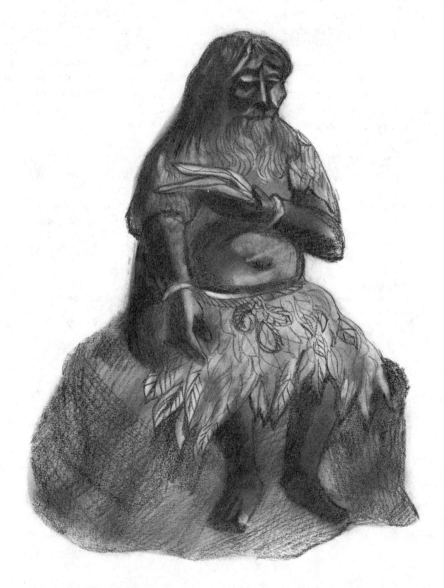

For thousands of years, nutrition has been the cornerstone of medicine, as symbolized by the combined roles of this Chinese god. *Shen Nung, Deity of Agriculture, Medicine and Pharmacy. Early pottery figure. China.*

chapter 7

OF CARBOHYDRATES AND HEALTH

Recently, Drs. E. Cheraskin and W. M. Ringsdorf (authors of *New Hope for Incurable Diseases*) wrote in the trade newspaper *Natural Food News:*[1]

"Refined carbohydrates are . . . reported to play a role in the etiology and progression of these (and other) disorders—diabetes, hypoglycemia, gout, kidney stones, urinary infection, peptic ulcer, cardiovascular disease, dental caries, periodontal disease, overweight, intestinal cancer, diverticulosis, indigestion, hormonal disorders, oral and vaginal infections, osteoporosis, alcoholism and mental illness."

While these charges are not fully explained, a number of them are related to a supposed national health problem of *hypoglycemia,* or low blood sugar. This low level of sugar in the bloodstream is said by Cheraskin, Fredericks,[2] Dr. Atkins,[3–7] Adelle Davis,[3,4] and a host of others to result from a national overconsumption of carbohydrates.

139

The answer to this difficulty is widely purported to be the eating of much less carbohydrate and much more protein. "Refined" carbohydrates are claimed to play an especially important role.

So pervasive is hypoglycemia said to be that Atkins is quoted in *Town and Country:* "The commonest reason for a patient to walk into a doctor's office is that he has hypoglycemia which hasn't been diagnosed."[5] Popular newspaper columnist Dr. Peter Steincrohn concurs, calling hypoglycemia "the most commonly misdiagnosed disease."[6]

Pamphlets and handbills about low blood sugar often emphasize emotional ills and child misbehavior as unsuspected results of low blood sugar. "Do you have one or more of these symptoms?" asks one. "It may be hypoglycemia . . . Allergies—Exhaustion—Fatigue—Alcoholism—Dizziness—Drug Addiction . . . underachievers and/or BEHAVIOR PROBLEMS."[7]

Long lists of symptoms are offered to aid self-diagnosis. *Town and Country*'s list begins:[5] "Exhaustion, irritability, nervousness, depression, vertigo or dizziness, headaches, faintness, cold sweats, cold hands and feet, weak spells, drowsiness, forgetfulness, insomnia, worrying, confusion . . . hostility, belligerence and asocial behavior, indecisiveness, crying spells . . ." etc.

How real are these ideas about sugars in the blood and their medical effects? Because such concerns have been so earnestly believed by so many, the scientific view of blood sugar may be a good place to begin our look at the medical implications of carbohydrate.

THE DOCTOR LOOKS AT BLOOD SUGAR

As we have seen, by the time carbohydrates from food reach the main bloodstream, they have been broken down to simple sugars, either in the form of glucose or chains of glucose put together by the liver, as glycogen.

There are more complex and varied carbohydrate substances in the blood as well. But these have been made by the body's cells, not taken in from food. For example, one finds *glucuronic acid,* a detoxifying agent in the liver, which helps us to deal with toxic chemicals and bacterial byproducts. There is *heparin,* which controls the clotting rate of blood. There are carbohydrate compounds which are key constituents of skin, muscle, cartilage, connective tissue and heart valves. There are carbohydrate compounds essential to the nervous system, to our hormones and heredity.

But because we cannot control the presence of these substances, let us focus our attention on how the body deals with the carbohydrates from the food we do select—on glucose.

The most common glucose-related medical problem is *diabetes,* which often goes unrecognized. The name, from the Greek, means "passing through," a reference to the fact that untreated diabetics urinate often. To this is added the term *mellitus,* deriving from the word for honey, since the urine of the diabetic is sweet with sugar.*

Actually diabetes is of different kinds. About one-fifth of cases are *juvenile onset,* beginning in childhood or adolescence. These are quite different from the far more common *"maturity-onset"* diabetes.

Diabetes can be diagnosed in several ways. The simplest, but least accurate, is by the afore-mentioned presence of sugar in the urine. The most accurate method involves sampling the blood for sugar content—the *glucose tolerance test.*

Most of the time there are about 60 to 100 mg. of glucose in each 100 ml. of blood—medically described as 60-100 *mg/percent.* Just after a meal, the glucose is higher, about 140-150 mg/percent in normal people. Long after a meal, it is lower. If the body cannot handle glucose well, and the concentration of this sugar rises much higher, sugar may spill over into the urine.** Diabetics tend to have much higher sugars. The state in which the blood holds excessive sugar is called *hyperglycemia*— from *hyper* (too much), *glyc* (sugar) and *emia* (in the blood.)

Insulin and the Cause of Diabetes

Back in the 1920s, there was an easy explanation for diabetes. The body lacked *insulin,* and so could not deal with glucose, the primary energy source. The glucose built up in the blood. There were two answers (after Best and Banting isolated insulin): First, cut down carbohydrate intake, so as to minimize the amount of glucose to be dealt with. Second, give insulin to replace what was supposedly missing.

---

*Another illness with a similar name, *diabetes insipidus,* also has the characteristic of copious urination, but is not the result of this same faulty carbohydrate metabolism.
**The level at which this happens is called "the renal threshold."

Unfortunately, not all diabetics did well on this plan. And even though fewer died from the direct effects of diabetes, diabetics did tend to die much sooner than normal, largely from diseases of the blood vessels—and consequently, also of strokes and diseases of the heart. Obviously something else was wrong.

Today the cause of diabetes is described as "unknown." And curiously, this represents a great advance in knowledge. It also changes the methods of treatment.

Insulin is a hormone. That is, it is one of a myriad of messenger proteins which travel through the blood to signal the beginning or ending of biochemical processes. For example, *adrenalin* is also a hormone (note the common ending of the words) and it triggers profound bodily changes which send blood pressure and pulse rate up and generally prepare the body for emergency action, as in anger or terror.

Insulin sets off a number of reactions—such as the release of enzymes—which help regulate the use of carbohydrate. For example, it plays a role in three of the key processes of glucose use: It helps to get free glucose in the blood through the walls of muscle and adipose tissue cells which need this sugar for energy; it facilitates the liver's work of storing glucose molecules by stringing them together into glycogen; and it is intimately involved with the conversion of excess glucose into stored fat.

Insulin is produced in certain cells—the Islands of *Langerhans*—within the pancreas. Recall that this organ is also one source of enzymes which break down carbohydrates in the first portions of the intestines, so that they can be absorbed into the bloodstream. So it is considered a fair bet that insulin may help to release such enzymes from the pancreas. But this is still only a reasoned speculation.

Modern research has shown that some diabetics (maturity-onset particularly) may have plenty of insulin in their blood. And this also leads to some speculation—that the pancreas of some people may be less responsive to signals for releasing needed enzymes—that it *might* take an exceptional amount of insulin to get an impaired pancreas to turn out enough enzymes to manage the glucose in the blood.

Other research has shown that carbohydrates in the diet do not really seem to overwhelm the blood's insulin. Indeed, glucose stimulates the release of insulin. In 1971, the American Diabetes Association issued a statement that, "There no longer appears to be any need to restrict disproportionately the intake of carbohydrates in the diet of most diabetic patients."[8]

There was another reason for this statement. As we have seen, the practical possibilities of protein intake are limited. So carbohydrate and fat must make up the vast bulk of the diet. Repress one and you automatically increase the other. When the traditional diet for diabetics restricted carbohydrate, the fat intake zoomed upward.

Although, as we said, in recent years fewer people have died of the direct effects of diabetes, diabetics have been disproportionately susceptible to heart and blood-vessel diseases. It seemed questionable to push people with such susceptibilities into high-fat diets, since such diets may add to the risk of heart and blood-vessel problems. As the American Diabetes Association report noted: "A liberalized carbohydrate intake . . . will necessarily be associated with a decrease in dietary fat."[8]

Today the management of diabetes aims chiefly at controlling obesity.[9] This, the experts observe, may be the most important part of the dietary treatment. Again, a high-fat diet crams many calories into little food, a poor diet for the obese. And most diabetics in the maturity-onset group tend to be obese.

For these reasons, the modern diet for most diabetics is actually high in carbohydrates—about 45 percent of total calories. In other words, nutrition scientists do not believe that carbohydrate is hard for the human body to handle. They prescribe a diet rather high in carbohydrates *even for diabetics who have a known impaired ability to deal with this basic macronutrient.*

On the other hand, physicians who treat diabetics still limit the intake of simple sugars—such as table sugar, corn syrup, honey, raw sugar, and foods high in such sugars. Why? Chiefly because these foods can go into the blood more rapidly, since they require less digestion. And large amounts of simple carbohydrates, rapidly consumed, cause a surge in blood-glucose levels. This can mean trouble for the diabetic, with his impaired ability to deal with glucose.

Is "Refined Carbohydrate" Dangerous?

The possible hazard of simple sugars for the diabetic is one of the two basic reasons given by popular writers for fearing carbohydrates, especially "refined carbohydrates." In essence, they say that since simple sugars can be harmful for some people—diabetics—they are harmful to all of us.

Can sugar really be toxic? Can carbohydrates in general be toxic? Of course they can, because *all nutrients* can be toxic. Protein, fats, vitamins, minerals, even water can harm us and even kill us—in large enough amounts.

True, these substances are all needed by the body. Therefore, the body has mechanisms for using them, and mechanisms for dealing with excesses beyond need. But eventually, there comes a point of quantity at which the body's mechanisms for use, and for protection against excess, are overwhelmed. What must be clearly understood is that these mechanisms are not equally effective in all people, under all circumstances. So the diabetic, like all humans, must have glucose in his blood, and he must be able to use it. But his limits of tolerance are lower than normal. Knowing this tells us much more about the diabetic than it does about glucose, however.

For one of the primary questions of food safety rests with the conditions of the expected use of a food. In the case of carbohydrates, most nutritionists agree that the typical American intake is well within tolerance. And this intake is far less than that of many nations, some of which consume diets which are 80 percent carbohydrate and more.

Another important factor about carbohydrates is that, if we do not consume *any*—a difficult trick, for there is some carbohydrate in the vast majority of foods, even eggs and meat—the body will *make* carbohydrate. We can make carbohydrate from protein, and we can convert a certain part of fat molecules (glycerol) to carbohydrate. Does this mean we do not really need to eat carbohydrate foods? No, for if the body must rely on the conversion of other nutrients to carbohydrate, problems can arise in the process. The Food and Nutrition Board, while it cannot pin down an RDA for carbohydrate, notes that some must be eaten "to avoid ketosis, excessive breakdown of body protein, loss of cations, especially sodium, and involuntary dehydration."[10]

How much carbohydrate must we have as a minimum? The RDA Committee writes: "50 to 100 grams of digestible carbohydrate a day will offset the undesirable metabolic responses associated with high fat diets and fasting."[10]

This does not mean, however, that such a minimum is desirable. The Committee observes that our consumption of fats is too high, recalls the American Heart Association's recommendation of a diet no higher in fat than 35 percent of calories, and suggests that this would "probably provide a diet conducive to better health in the United States population." A diet this low in fat must be about 50 percent carbohydrate, since protein intake tends to be fairly constant.

Is there any recommendation about the *kind* of carbohydrate? Yes, there is. It is made on the basis that the overconsumption of overly-refined foods reduces our intake of needed vitamins and minerals. And it is for this reason that experts caution against consuming too much of our diet in the form of refined fats or sugars, and too little in the form of fruits, grains, and vegetables.

This injunction can easily be misinterpreted, however. Let us consider one misinterpretation—the idea that relatively isolated sugars and starches are somehow harmful *in themselves,* rather than potentially harmful because they may displace other nutrients. This erroneous deduction leads some popular writers to describe isolated sugars and starches as "poisons." One such writer not only calls sugar "toxic," but says that it is "probably a major factor in the deaths of hundreds of millions of people."[11]

The reality is that a molecule of sucrose remains a molecule of sucrose, no matter what its source. Usually food processing does not change the carbohydrate itself. "Refining" is more properly used to describe what happens to the total food, not the nutrient. So refined carbohydrate *foods* might have had many substances removed, which might or might not have nutritive value. But the sugar or starch is likely to be unchanged. And in any event, before it enters the peripheral circulation of the body, digestion and the metabolic processes of the liver will have brought it all to the "refined" form of simple sugar.

In some cases, the processes either of man or nature do change the form of carbohydrate. Starches may be broken down into shorter glucose chains, to become maltoses, a job the digestion would have to do anyway. Or they may be "modified," as in the case of those from corn or potatoes which are arranged in a slightly different pattern by chemists, so that they serve in baby foods to keep water and solids from separating. Changes can also occur in the way atoms are arranged within a sugar molecule. Certain acids (as in making fruit jams) and enzymes (as when the bee makes honey) can do this. The change does not alter nutritive value meaningfully. It mainly produces new physical characteristics, such as a greater stickiness.

Honey, maple syrup, corn syrup, brown sugar, raw sugar—all are refined foods, separated from much that was in their original sources, either by a tree, a bee or a human refiner. For nutrition purposes, since they are essentially simple sugars, they are no more "toxic" than the same sugars would be in apples or raisins. For example, medicine flatly rejects the popular idea that sugars can alter the heredity of cells so as to cause cancer.

SOME REALITIES OF TEETH, HEARTS AND SUGAR

Not long ago, consumerists petitioned the Food and Drug Administration to ban any breakfast cereal which had more than 10 percent sugar. For, they said, with such cereals "frequent use contributes to tooth decay and other health problems."[12]

Sugar and Tooth Decay

Table sugar is seen by many as the main cause of dental caries. The idea is based on observations that many bacteria in the mouth, like those we met in the intestines, can metabolize carbohydrates nicely. These bacteria excrete an acid waste after dining on our carbohydrates, and this leads to the erosion of dental enamel and cavities. So it is maintained that to eat sugar is to feed mouth bacteria too well.

A good test of this thesis—which has essential scientific correctness in many respects—is a study done at Vipeholm, Sweden.[13] For five years, groups of patients in a mental institution were fed sugars in controlled forms and amounts, and their dental health was closely watched. One group was put on a diet free from table sugar. They continued to develop cavities.

A second group got over ten ounces of table sugar daily, in beverages at meals—over 1,000 daily calories from sugar, or more than twice as much as the high American average. Their decay rate did not differ significantly from the first group's.

A third group got a sticky sweet bread at meals. When served at one daily meal, the bread yielded no increase in caries. Served four times a day, it led to more cavities in males—but not in the females, who brushed their teeth more often.

Four other groups got sugary foods *between meals.* One of these got sugar in beverages for two years, then over two ounces of chocolate instead. Neither the patients nor the 77 employees who also ate the chocolate showed significantly more cavities. But three of these between-meal groups did show more decay. The first got 22 caramels between meals each day. The second got 8 special toffees, which had less sugar than the caramels but were stickier. The third got 24 sticky toffees between meals. Of these groups, the third got most caries and the first, least.

How are these and supporting studies interpreted?—chiefly, to the effect that carbohydrate foods which remain longest in contact with teeth lead to most decay. And the consumption of such foods between meals is more harmful, because total time of exposure to carbohydrates is increased, and there is no accompanying consumption of other foods and liquids to help clean the teeth.

Total sugar content is not so important. If the sugar is in a liquid, for example, it seems to pass the teeth too quickly to do much harm. So soft drinks in ordinary use are not fairly indicted as cavity-causing to any extent. Nor is the source of the sugar especially important. In one of several such studies, Australian children who were denied table sugar but given "natural" sweets such as honey and dried fruits, developed caries at an average rate.[14]

All sugar molecules seem to be good food for the bacteria, hence *cariogenic* (decay-causing). For example, there was more *lactose* (milk sugar) than sucrose in the toffee which caused most damage in the Swedish studies. And it has been shown that babies who are put to sleep with a bottle of milk left in their mouths show a marked increase in early decay.[15] There is evidence that sucrose is especially cariogenic, but the key to decay control appears to be *how* we use *any* sugar.[16]

Since we know that life forms other than man can also break more complex carbohydrates down to simple sugars, we ought not to be surprised that food starches are also good food for many decay-causing bacteria. Indeed, some bacteria can actually convert starches to stickier forms, which cling to teeth.

These facts can help to explain some of the studies done on commercial cereals and decay.[17] In one, 979 schoolchildren were allowed to eat as much unsweetened or presweetened breakfast cereal as they wanted. At the end of the study, there were no significant differences in the incidence of caries between children who chose the different kinds of cereals.[18] Although this study has been criticized for lack of control over the remainder of the diet, it is nevertheless suggestive. And applying some simple practical tests, one can see why sugared cereals eaten at breakfast might not have a lot of impact on dental problems. Let's look at cereals with 10 percent sugar. Remember that it is common for cereals to offer about 100 calories per serving. So we can expect about 10 calories of sugar, a little over half a teaspoon, in a cereal which is 10 percent sugar.

The more one analyzes the matter, the more factors one sees. Let us ask a few more questions about sweet cereals. How concerned should we be about sweeter cereals, say, up to 40 percent sugar, or some 40 calories to a serving? For many youngsters, this is less than 10 percent of their daily sugar. Per capita consumption of sweeteners, including corn syrup, is some 400 to 500 calories a day.

Keep in mind that the content of vitamins and minerals in the cereals is usually greater than that of the other foods in which we consume similar or larger amounts of sugars. We must also remember that often the use of such cereals leads to the consumption of more milk, and possibly fruit. Children and adults alike usually add sugar to "unsweetened" cereals. Moreover "unsweetened" cereals often use malted grains (with starches hydrolyzed to rather simple maltose) to add sweetness without saying "sugar" on the label. Finally, let us not ignore the fact that in many households, without "help-yourself" cereals about, children might have only poorer alternatives, such as sweet rolls or toaster-heated waffles and tarts.

The great question about cereals, realistically, may well be less their sugar content than our national tendency, carefully nurtured by some advertising, to believe that an ounce of grain and sugar can be thought of as a meal. We will look further at our national breakfast problem in Chapter Twelve.

Does Sugar Cause Heart Disease?

While most scientific interest in the effect of diet upon cardiovascular diseases has centered on fatty substances, some popular writers have blamed sugar for this number-one cause of death in the U.S.[19]

Four links are usually drawn between sugar and heart disease. One is that sugar-eating countries have a higher incidence of the disease. But other countries with "remarkably high consumption of sugar,'' such as Venezuela, Cuba, Costa Rica, Colombia and Honduras, have quite low incidence of heart disease.[20] And while Finns and Swedes eat about the same amounts of table sugar, Finns have many more heart attacks.[21]

Another claim is that heart disease increases with sugar consumption. But in the U.S., while sugar consumption has been almost static for 50 years, heart deaths have gone up sharply. In a review of this question, Dr. Ancel Keys found: ''There is no basis in fact for the claim that the trend of coronary heart disease mortality reflects changes in the consumption of sugar.''[21]

Third is the claim that heart patients eat more sugar than others. Dr. John Yudkin, almost the chief exponent of a link between sugar and heart disease, based this claim on 20 patients.[22] On review, these patients proved to consume only about as much sugar as did their English countrymen.[23] And in nine studies, the hypothesis proved false.[24] In two of these it was found that heart patients ate *less* sugar than normals.[25,26] The Medical Research Council of the United Kingdom made its own studies, and concluded that, ''differences were not statistically significant.''[27]

Finally, it has been charged that sugar eating leads to a rise in fatty substances, such as cholesterol, in the blood, increasing the risk of cardiovascular problems. But while such a rise does seem to result from a sharp increase of sugar consumption, it is very temporary, and it occurs in response to a great deal of sugar. Grande, reviewing tests in which subjects got as much as 75 percent of their calories in sugar, noted no ''specific effect elevating the concentration of either cholesterol or triglycerides [another fatty substance which may indicate heart risk] in normal individuals.''[28]

Reviewing all such studies, Zollner and Wolfram reported: ''In our opinion, the total evidence linking sucrose with coronary heart disease is scant.''[29]

There is, however, another side of the coin.

SOME RESERVATIONS ABOUT SUGAR

While we have seen that many of the popular accusations about sugar are not founded in reality, there are also some real questions which have not yet been settled. Why might the body treat sucrose differently than it does other carbohydrates? After all, we know that sucrose is only one molecule of glucose (the body's chief fuel) and one of fructose, the sugar found naturally occurring in fruits and vegetables.

The answer to this question centers about a principle which we have examined before and will stress again, that the body has mechanisms for dealing with any food chemical within a certain range of quantities. But there is an upper limit always, no matter how innocuous the molecule may generally be. We know that the body can handle very large amounts of glucose very nicely. But the thinking of some nutritionists is that there may be much tighter limits for fructose.[30,31]

How Much Fructose is There in Most Foods?

While fructose provides sweetness and energy value to many of our most desirable foods, it is not usually present in very great quantity. The amounts of food one would have to eat (other than sweeteners) to get these high levels of fructose is great. It is certainly well outside the typical U.S. dietary habit. (A pound of peaches would probably contain less than 100 calories of fructose—a pound of grapes only slightly more.)[32]

How the Body Deals with Fructose.

While the general mechanisms for dealing with fructose are known, precise information is lacking. The fructose is absorbed from the small intestine and then goes to the liver. But the question is, then what happens? We know that the fructose can be converted to glucose. But the liver can also use the fructose to make *triglycerides* (the most common form of fat in the body). And some researchers suggest that fructose is more rapidly converted to fat than is glucose.[30,33]

What is the significance of this possibility? Many experts in the nutritional aspect of heart and blood-vessel disease have observed that in a minority of patients (perhaps about 10 percent) there is a tendency to show high levels of common fats in the blood (*hyper-*

triglyceridemia). These experts are convinced that it is not enough to check the blood for *cholesterol* as a warning sign of high risk for heart disease; one must also test the blood for triglycerides.[34]

Whereas—as almost everyone knows, and as we shall see in greater detail in Chapter Ten—it is common to reduce the intake of fats in *most* people with high risk of heart attack, it is not the procedure for all. A small percentage of such patients show a blood pattern which suggests the need for a reduction of carbohydrates, in an effort to lower triglycerides in the blood.

The linkage between this phenomenon and the apparent tendency of fructose to be converted to triglycerides is obscure. In view of this and some other research, some experts see wisdom in limiting sucrose intake.[35,36]

The Realities of a Controversial Decision.

The scientific aspects of the sugar controversy are far more complex than we have suggested here. And the whole subject is further clouded by the enormous amount of unsubstantiated faddist belief about sugar. It is important to distinguish between the genuine scientific concerns and the irrational condemnation of sugar as poisonous, which it is not.

In making a personal decision about sugar, however, we might consider some broad practical realities, which will be presented more fully in Chapter Twelve. For example, we do know that sticky between-meal snacks (which are often quite sugary) tend to lead to dental problems. More importantly, as has been suggested, sugar in quantity can dilute the other nutritive values of the diet; in a sense, it takes up a lot of space, because of its high caloric density. Foods high in sugar *usually* do not contribute a very high concentration of vitamins, minerals, protein, or fiber.

However, there is no evident reason for normal people to be concerned about consuming a *moderate* amount of sugar, especially if it is not eaten in sticky form between meals. But consuming very large amounts of sugar leads to an unbalancing of the diet, as we shall see. The fundamentals seem to indicate some sensible, and not terribly restrictive, limits. Later we shall see what these might be, and how we can comfortably apply them.

Reality and Hypoglycemia.

It is easy to understand the popular belief that, because diabetes is a disorder of sugar metabolism, the consumption of sugar may be a cause. But the American Diabetes Association does not confirm this popular impression. And two authorities, Drs. E. Bierman and R. Nelson—the former having chaired the committee which liberalized carbohydrate intake for diabetics—reviewed the literature and reported: "There is no evidence that excessive consumption of sugar causes diabetes."[9]

Indeed, the evidence points to diabetes as primarily a hereditary problem. A history of parental diabetes increases markedly the risk for a child. And a number of other findings tend to confirm the importance of heredity, such as the fact that infants who weigh more than nine pounds at birth are more likely to develop the disorder at some time in life.

Certain popular authors maintain that our consumption of simple carbohydrates also causes another major health concern—hypoglycemia. Most of these authors maintain, moreover, that the reason for a great increase in hypoglycemia (low blood sugar) is that we eat more carbohydrates, especially in refined forms, than we used to. Their history is bad.

U.S.D.A. finds that our consumption of refined carbohydrate foods has tended to remain constant since 1925, at about 16 to 17 percent of total calories. And they also find that from 1909 to 1972 consumption of complex carbohydrate foods did not grow, but rather declined sharply.[6-3]

There are those, however, who claim that low blood sugar afflicts a major part of our population,[6,7,37,38] and see this disorder as the cause of an endless array of common symptoms. They attribute these symptoms to a supposed phenomenon which looks like the opposite of diabetes—that is, instead of the body being inadequate to deal with glucose, it handles this basic sugar with a kind of overenthusiasm. So instead of the diabetic problem of excess concentration of glucose in the blood, people with low blood sugar are claimed to use up glucose *too fast*—to have an excessive insulin response, or *hyperinsulinism.*

Looking back at the claimed symptoms of hypoglycemia, and then comparing them to certain symptom groups in any textbook of psychiatry, we observe a remarkable parallel.[39] For these are generally the symptoms of *anxiety neurosis,* a personality disorder which embodies an underlying sense of fear. Characteristically, that fear is "free-floating," attached to no cause the patient can discern. There is a need to attribute the fear to something, and there is a high degree of suggestibility.

Physically, the reactions of people with anxiety problems are those associated with bodily reflexes which prepare us for flight or defense. It is not hard to see how these physical reactions, coupled with the headaches and emotional outbursts of the inner conflicts which become involved, can account for much of the symptomatology of "low blood sugar."

Like all *psychogenic* (psychologically caused) physical symptoms, these are quite real. They can be profound, and they can alter body chemistry. For example, prolonged anxiety can actually lower blood sugar levels, though slightly. And, in turn, these lowered blood sugar levels can trigger other physical and emotional symptoms. We all have had some experience with these, for we all experience a true hypoglycemia when we are very hungry. Remember, it is thought that a fall in blood sugar sets off the body's "appestat," a major factor in making us want to eat.

Emotionally, we should keep in mind that, at the core of all anxiety neurosis—or of its acute form, *anxiety reaction,* which can result in actual collapse—is a fear so threatening that we must keep it hidden from our conscious minds. And it can be urgently needed comfort to be able to say, "These feelings are caused by my diet. I don't have to find out what it is that I fear." As Danowski, one physician reviewer of the subject puts it: "We may find it easier to say, 'My blood sugar is low,' rather than, 'I can't cope.'"[40]

Most "low blood sugar" can be confirmed by the *glucose tolerance test,* in which, after an overnight fast, the patient is given a large dose of glucose. The combination of the empty stomach and the liquid form of the glucose serves to rush this pure form of the monosaccharide through the stomach and into rapid absorption from the gut, so that blood-sugar levels shoot up. Hourly blood tests are then made to see if the body has an impaired ability to deal with glucose, especially as in diabetes.

Like all tests, this one is only as good as the way one interprets it. For example, those who worry about hypoglycemia see any fall of blood sugar below 60 mg./percent as diagnostic of "low blood sugar."

Yet Danowski and his colleagues found that between 20 and 30 percent of normal people showed the lows which enthusiasts call abnormal. These *mild hypoglycemia* levels (between 45 and 60 mg./ percent) were found to have no medical significance in the vast majority of cases. In some instances, they might be seen as indicators of a pre-diabetic state; but such a state is usually indicated by sugars between 30 and 45 (*moderate hypoglycemia* on the test). Such *moderate* or *severe* (below 30) low sugars call for further diagnostic work. In themselves, they are not diagnostic of any particular thing, but are merely signs that something is wrong.

What does a true hypoglycemic response mean? It may be a symptom of severe intestinal disease, or disorders of the pancreas or liver, of threatening tumors, or a variety of rare diseases suffered by newborns as well as adults. At the least, it signifies emerging diabetes. *Mild* reactions are usually meaningless, a result of too much emphasis on a finite number system. In any case, medicine does not consider "low blood sugar" to be a real diagnosis but, rather, a symptom, as are a "running nose," "itch," or "pain."

Two factors can contribute to make blood sugar depressed in such a test. One is the fact that people in an anxious state anyway often become more anxious when subjected to any medical procedure. For example, in blood-pressure testing, anxiety commonly sends pressures high. The other factor is the effect of diet: the test is likely to be low when the subject has been on a low-carbohydrate diet for a few days.

Is the theory of Atkins[3-7] and others, that enormous numbers of people suffer from excessive insulin response because of their carbohydrate intake, given medical credence? Dr. Edward Rynearson, studying the question, comments that when *hyperinsulinism* is actually found with a rapid using up of blood sugar, tumors of the pancreas, which produce extra insulin, are usually the cause.[41]

Rynearson questioned each of the past presidents of the American Diabetes Association on how many cases of true "reactive" or "functional" hypoglycemia they had seen. He writes: "These physicians were unanimous; they had seen thousands of patients with diabetes . . . but almost never one with reactive hypoglycemia." And Rachmiel Levine, noted authority on carbohydrate metabolism, writes that treating such a "disease" may be called "acute remunerative therapy."

By 1973, the popular interest in "low blood sugar" had gone so far that the American Diabetes Association, the Endocrine Society, and the AMA felt obliged to issue a formal public statement on the question:[42]

"Hypoglycemia means a low level of blood sugar. When it occurs, it is often attended by symptoms of sweating, shakiness, trembling, anxiety, fast heart action, headache, hunger sensations, brief feelings of weakness, and occasionally, seizures and coma. However, the majority of people with these kinds of symptoms do not have hypoglycemia; a great many patients with anxiety reactions present similar symptoms. Furthermore, there is no good evidence that hypoglycemia causes depression, chronic fatigue, allergies, nervous breakdowns, alcoholism, juvenile delinquency, childhood behavior problems, drug addiction or inadequate sexual performance . . ."

As a general principle of nutrition, it is important to understand that the fact that a symptom can result from a nutritional phenomenon does not necessarily mean that there *is* a nutritional cause. Moreover when a nutritional problem is the cause, one expects to find either an abnormality of diet or an abnormality of body function. Nutritionally-related symptoms do not occur in a vacuum, as we shall see when we consider vitamins and minerals.

In the case of hypoglycemia, we have a multitude of reasons to suspect that the nutritional confirmations claimed by the anti-carbohydrate advocates do not exist. For one thing while hypoglycemia is said to be due to a much greater consumption of carbohydrate foods, the fact is that our total consumption of carbohydrates has been going *down* for years, not up, and consumption of simple sugars seems to have stayed rather consistent. Secondly, if excess consumption of carbohydrates is at the root of this supposed national epidemic of hypoglycemia, then those who consume much more carbohydrates than we do should have more trouble. As Philip White has commented: "It is curious that hypoglycemia does not appear to be a problem in parts of the world where carbohydrate provides up to 80 percent of dietary calories."

Let us apply our reasoning to some of the other health problems attributed to carbohydrate foods.

The Magic of Fiber

Every generation or two for the last 150 years, the meaning of dietary fiber in health has become a popular, and sometimes, a medical issue. We have somewhat vaguely defined fiber as the indigestible carbohydrate in our food. This definition is somewhat incomplete, but usually accepted because scientists have not yet been able to define fiber with much precision.

Fiber is found in the cell walls of plants. While it is mainly a carbohydrate substance, being made of long chains of sugars, it can also incorporate protein and fatty materials, along with other chemical compounds. In any event, it is not a single substance, but rather a family of related substances—cellulose, hemicellulose, lignin, pectin, etc.—as we have seen earlier. Actually, the basic approach to determining just what is fiber in foods has changed little from the work of Einhof, which was done between 1806 and 1809. Ever since that time, fiber has been defined in terms of its function, as the substance in food necessary for the normal passage of undigested food, or the waste products of digestion, through more than 20 feet of intestine, to elimination.

In the late 1800s, nutrition eccentric Dr. John Harvey Kellogg was keenly interested in fiber, or "roughage," as the key to regular elimination from the bowel, which, in turn, he and some of his fellows saw as the key to good health.[1-19] In the 1900s this interest received new popular attention, and fiber began to be known by such graphic descriptions as "nature's broom," suggesting that fiber went through the intestines in large enough particles to tickle the intestinal walls and stimulate movement down the intestines.

Today, while this somewhat curious view of fiber's functions has been modified by scientific discovery, the exact role of fibers in the digestive tract is still something of a puzzle. It seems to be more than just a simple matter of acting as a sort of wedge forcing everything through. For example, a key factor in keeping things moving in the intestines appears to be the ability of some kinds of fiber to hold water (making the stools less hard and compact).

To understand the new popular concern about fiber, we might look at the best-sold book on the subject, *The Save-Your-Life Diet*.[43] It is the work of Dr. David Reuben, known better for his fame in sexual than in digestive matters. Reuben simplifies his claims in *Woman's Day*,[44] in the following manner: "A high-fiber diet may provide protection from: 1. cancer of the colon and rectum; 2. ischemic heart disease (the prime cause of heart attacks); 3. diverticular disease of the colon; 4. appendicitis; 5. phlebitis and resulting blood clots to the lungs; 6. obesity; 7. hemorrhoids and varicose veins."

These claims are based on British research into the diets, bowel habits and general health of African villagers—especially those who are poor and primitive and do not consume the processed foods of civilization. Reuben's science seems to stem mainly from the work of Burkitt and Painter,[45,46] which is not reported quite as Reuben puts it. For Reuben seems to imply that, if only food wastes move through the intestines at a brisk enough pace, harmful food factors of many kinds will neither irritate the intestinal walls nor be absorbed into the bloodstream. He bases many of his conclusions on data suggesting that rural African villagers have shorter intestinal *transit times* than either English schoolboys or sailors.

Unfortunately, Reuben seems to be unaware of research which shows that adding fiber to the diets of people with normal intestinal function does *not* shorten transit time.

At this writing, science has not yet been able to specify what is a desirable amount of fiber. One of the few estimates, made by Cowgill, suggests that about six grams of fiber should be about right— approximately a fourth of what Reuben recommends. But Mendeloff,[47] in perhaps the best current review of the question, sums up: "Since no one can agree on exactly what dietary fiber is or how to measure it, it is impossible to define whether or not fiber deficiency or excess in the diet exists, or can constitute a protective or noxious element in the diet."

Examined in detail, the ideas of the fiber enthusiasts are often erroneous in basic matters. The enthusiasts say that appendicitis is related to the increased consumption of refined foods. But Mendeloff finds data to show that actually appendicitis has "shown a distinct downturn in recent decades." He also finds that colon cancer "has remained constant in the same population, . . . [that] there is no relationship between transit times . . . and the incidence of colonic cancer."

Fiber and the Deceptiveness of Nutrition Research

The attempt to relate a decline in fiber consumption to some of our most serious modern disease problems characterizes the ways in which nutrition research has often been treacherous for any but the most thoughtful of scientists. For food differences among populations are almost always related to a host of other differences, affecting physical and social environments, and it is seldom clear that food differences alone necessarily explain differences of health or of longevity. And differences in the intake of some specific nutrient are often related to broad differences in both eating and living.

Let us look at just one of the health differences between rural African villagers and typical Americans—that of atherosclerosis, the roughening and thickening of blood vessel walls, which leads apparently to so much cardiovascular disease.

Kannel and others have demonstrated that differences in atherosclerotic disease may be related to a great number of life style differences. And there are many obvious differences. Rural Africans do not live as long as Americans do. And cancer and heart disease, along with many other health problems, are primarily disorders of the later years. People who die in middle age or sooner tend to die of other causes. For example, consider most Central American nations, where the age of death tends to be much lower than ours. In these countries, where fiber intake is likely to be high, the leading cause of death is not heart disease or stroke, as it is with us; it is diarrhea, from infections and spoiled foods.

Rural Africans and Americans have different patterns of exercise. Most African villagers do not have cars or television sets, washing machines, or vacuum cleaners. They are much more likely to hunt or gather or grow their food than to buy it in the supermarket. Is this not as meaningful a difference as the disparity in fiber intake? We know from the Framingham studies that physical activity plays an important role in keeping the blood vessels and heart clear of trouble.

Rural Africans also have different patterns of emotional stress, of the type which seems to be related to heart disease, whereas constipation and hemorrhoids seem to be associated with the tensions and frustrations of more civilized living. The rural Africans' high fiber consumption is a result of a different eating pattern. For one thing, their diet is much higher than ours in carbohydrate foods. As we have seen repeatedly, when the consumption of carbohydrates goes up, the consumption of fats goes down. To ascribe a lower level of cardiovascular disease among the rural Africans solely to fiber is to ignore the fact that Americans take in far more fats, especially from animal foods.

We might also, with this same sort of thinking, review Reuben's statement—"Even more surprising is the relation between dietary fiber and obesity." (The *Reader's Digest*[48] has recently given great notoriety to this relationship.) Reuben says: "Most African villagers remain lean and lithe throughout their lives—despite consuming up to 3,000 calories and 600 grams of carbohydrates a day." He says this is because such foods ". . . require more chewing . . . so they produce a feeling of fullness." And he speculates that " . . . roughage may actually impair the ability of the small intestine to absorb calories."

The chewing hypothesis seems gratuitous. For it is well known that when we consume more of our calories from fruits, grains and vegetables, the diet is much bulkier. We must eat a much greater volume of food to get the same number of calories. Indeed, this is the basic precept of the "Weight Watcher's Diet."

Reuben specifies that the Africans get 600 grams (2400 calories) of carbohydrates out of a total diet of 3,000 calories. This leaves only 600 calories of protein and fat. Since a substantial portion must be represented by the protein, fat must represent a lower portion of the African than of the American diet, probably representing no more than about 10 percent of dietary calories, less than a fourth of the typical American consumption.

One cannot say that fiber does not make a difference.[49] But it is naive to claim that it is the only difference.

Reuben, and indeed some of the fiber researchers as well, claim support for the importance of fiber through the fact that African villagers who move to urban areas, and who consume diets much like our own, eventually develop our disorders—those which they see as associated with low-fiber intake. The reasoning is flawed. For the move to the city entails much more than just taking fiber out of the diet—both in what is eaten and in the conditions of living.

Do we need more fiber? No one can say with certainty. It does appear that Americans' consumption of fiber has fallen off in the last century,[40] perhaps by a third, and that much of this decline has occurred since 1900. But this is largely a guess, particularly since we have never defined fiber precisely. At best, we must start by guessing what current consumption is, as a basis for considering any recommendations about fiber. We assume our consumption has dropped, because of the fall in consumption of complex carbohydrates, with which fiber is mainly found.

But there are valid arguments to support an increase in fiber consumption, and most nutritionists recommend that we should eat more fruits, whole grains and vegetables, which will automatically increase our intake of fiber. There is also reason to believe that we consume too much fat, and an increase in carbohydrate eating will inevitably result in our eating less fat. Also, we are short of certain vitamins and minerals which are found in complex carbohydrate foods.

Should we, as Reuben and others urge, simply add bran to our food? This would certainly add fiber. Yet it is never good nutritional design to count on just one food for the purpose of getting just one nutrient. To do so—as, for example, to plan on getting our vitamin A by eating a carrot every day and ignoring all other vegetables—loses the most important safety factor in nutrition, that of variety. You fill up on a few items, and increase the chances that vital nutrients will be missing.

Carbohydrate—The Poor Man's Diet

The high-carbohydrate diet of rural Africans is no rarity in the world. Rather, it is the commonplace of our planet. It is the American-European diet which looks more like the anomaly, in which the bulk of calories come from protein and fat. The world has been mainly carbohydrate-eating for thousands of years, ever since the development of crops made civilization possible and signaled the end of the hunt. According to historians, the change started long ago. An FAO (Food and Agriculture Organization of the United Nations) report puts it: "There are reasonable grounds for supposing that, in the so-called Fertile Crescent of Western Asia, the cultivation of wheat and other wild plants . . . began during the years 8,000 to 6,000 B.C. and perhaps earlier."

Some animal husbandry also developed at about the same time. As the FAO report explains: "The domestication of sheep and goats . . . took place simultaneously." Some of these animals were kept for milk and others for their meat. But much land was required to supply food for each beast, land which could yield the food for many people when planted to grains. The result was not surprising. The animal foods went mainly to the rich, as luxuries.

And the general situation has not changed very much. Except for the hunting peoples of the earth, the poor must live largely on plant foods. Since the world remains mostly poor, the Agency for International Development points out that today some five-sixths of the people on our planet are "mainly dependent on cereal grains—

wheat, rice, corn—for the satisfaction of both their calories and protein needs . . . These cereals cannot do an efficient job of nutrition unless they are fortified.''

Contrary to what many people might expect from reading the writings of Atkins and others who point to carbohydrates as a dietary hazard, this does not mean that five-sixths of the world is in the throes of ''low blood sugar,'' diabetes, crying spells, nervousness, and so forth. It is true that we find most of our real malnutrition among these people. But this is not directly attributable to the fact that the bulk of their food comes from plants. Rather, the main problem is their poverty. For when the world's food supply is short, or when their local crops fail, price drives the poorest from the market. They stand last in line.

Poverty also tends to confine such people to narrow and monotonous diets, with the vast majority of their food coming from just one or two kinds of plants, such as rice. Much of their malnutrition is eloquent testimony to the nutrition principle that variety is the best guarantee of good nutrition and that monotony is the handmaiden of bad nutrition.

Making matters still worse, a poor economy tends to have poor preservation and distribution of food. Transportation is lacking to bring in food. There is no money to support supermarkets or to buy refrigerators. Even when they seem to have adequate overall wealth to survive—in terms of land, crops and even animals—there is little money. Without money, they cannot buy food from other nations, or even from other parts of their own nation. In other words, survival depends upon what happens in their own small microcosm; it is at the whim of the seasons and of local rains and frosts and crop diseases.

Usually, the crucial nutrition issue for such peoples is protein. Generally their basic food is a grain, though legumes may contribute. These foods do supply proteins. And even though such proteins are not of the highest quality, one can survive nicely by wisely combining plant proteins.* But unlike most animal-source foods, plants are not rich providers of protein. The protein is present in a kind of ''dilute'' proportion; the ratio of carbohydrate to protein is high. So one must eat a lot of the food, and will still tend to stay close to the margin of

*The one essential nutrient not found in plant foods is vitamin B-12. Without some animal-source food or supplementation, vegetarians are susceptible to the deficiency symptom known as ''vegetarian back.''

safe protein intake. Thus any cutback in total food quantity may suddenly mean that there is no longer enough protein in the diet.

Exacerbating this problem is protein-calorie malnutrition. A reduced food supply can compromise the body's first need, for energy. Thus some of the protein eaten may be converted to energy use; the combination of reduced calories and a dietary which furnishes only marginal protein even when calories are adequate, can mean a protein shortage. (See Chapter One.)

Of course, protein does not represent the only nutritional difference between predominantly plant and animal-source diets. Each also supplies different amounts of fat and micronutrients. We have seen that predominantly carbohydrate foods contain more than only sugar, starch and fiber.

But protein seems to represent the critical nutrition problem of the world. What is curious to the point of irony for the nutritionist is that we Americans, who are the food-rich of the world, tend to emphasize protein as if we, too, had to take great care to get enough. Let us test this idea.

REFERENCES

General References See References for Chapter Seven.
1. Cheraskin, E. and Ringsdorf, W. *Refined carbohydrates: How much should you eat?* Natural Food News, Feb., 1975.
2. Fredericks, C. *Dr. Carlton Fredericks' Low-Carbohydrate Diet,* Award Books, New York, 1965, pp. 39—40.
3. Davis, A. *Let's Get Well,* New Amer. Library, New York, 1972, pp. 72, 75 and passim.
4. Davis, A. *A Diet for Better Sex,* Pageant, 1971.
5. Wysor, B. *Hypoglycemia: Facts you should know,* Town and Country, June, 1971.
6. *The Hypoglycemia Fad,* Newsweek, Jan. 29, 1973, p. 47.
7. *Low blood sugar: Fact and fiction,* Consumer Reports, July, 1971.
8. American Diabetes Association Committee on Food and Nutrition, *Special Report: Principles of nutrition and dietary recommendations for patients with diabetes mellitus,* Diabetes, 20:632—4, 1971.
9. Bierman, E. and Nelson, R. *Carbohydrates, diabetes and blood lipids,* World Rev. of Nutr. and Diet., 22:280—7, 1975.
10. Food and Nutrition Board, *Recommended Dietary Allowances,* Nat. Acad. Sciences, Washington, 1974.
11. Patrick, J. *Are you on the "stuff"?,* Nat. Health. Fed. Bull., Feb. 1975.
12. Jacobson, M. news conference reported in *The Nation's Health,* APHA, Sep. 1974, p. 1.
13. Gustafsson, B. et al., *The Vipeholm dental caries study,* Acta Odont. Scand. 11:232—363, 1954.
14. Harris, R. *Biology of the children of Hopewood House, Bowral, Australia,* J. Dent. Res. 42:1387—99, 1963.
15. Finn, S. and Glass, R., *Sugar and dental decay,* World Rev. Nutr. and Diet. 22:304—26, 1975.

16. Nizel, A. *Nutrition in Preventive Dentistry,* Saunders, Phila, 1972.
17. Rowe, H. et al. *Effect of ready to eat breakfast cereals on caries experience in adolescent children.* J. Dent. Res., 53:33—36, 1974.
18. Glass, R. and Fleisch, S. *Diet and dental caries,* J. Amer. Dent. Assn., 88:807—13, 1974.
19. Yudkin, J. *Sweet and Dangerous,* Wyden, New York, 1972.
20. Walker, A. *Sugar intake and coronary heart disease,* Atherosclerosis, 14:137—52, 1971.
21. Keys, A. *Sucrose in the diet and coronary heart disease,* Atherosclerosis, 14:193—202, 1971.
22. Yudkin, J. and Roddy, J. *Levels of dietary sucrose in patients with occlusive atherosclerotic disease,* Lancet, ii:6—8, 1964.
23. McGandy, R. Hegsted, D. and Stare, F. *Dietary fats, carbohydrates and atherosclerotic vascular disease,* New Eng. J. Med. 277:186—92, 241—7, 1967.
24. Grande, F. *Sugars in Cardiovascular Disease,* in Sugars in Nutrition, Nutr. Fndtn., Academic Press, New York, 1974.
25. Little, J. et al. *Diet and serum lipids in male survivors of myocardial infarction,* Lancet, 1:923—5, 1965.
26. Begg, T. et al. *Dietary Habits of Patients with Occlusive Arterial Disease,* Atti V Convegno Int. sugli aspetti dietetic dell'infanzia e della senescenza, Vol. 2, pp. -6—75, Rome, 1967.
27. Working Party to the Medical Research Council, *Dietary sugar intake in men with myocardial infarction,* Lancet, 2:1265—71, 1970.
28. Grande, F. *Sugar and cardiovascular diseases,* World Rev. Nutr. and Diet., 22:248—69.
29. Zollner, N. and Wolfram, F. *Sucrose in Human Nutrition,* in The Role of Sugar in Modern Nutrition, Naringsforskning 17 (Suppl. 9):22—25, 1973.
30. *Glucose Versus Fructose,* Lancet 2:1178, l968.
31. Ahrens, R. *Sucrose, hypertension and heart disease,* Amer. J. Clin. Nutrition, 27:403, 1974.
32. Tables in *Sugars in Nutrition,* Nutrition Foundation, Washington, 1974.
33. Naismith, D. *Differences in the metabolism of dietary carbohydrates sutdied in the rat,* Proc. Nutr. Soc., 30:259, 1971.
34. Frederickson, D. *A Physician's Guide to Hyperlipidemia,* Mod. Concepts Cardiovascular Dis., ed. 3, McGraw-Hill, New York, 1972.
35. *Diet and Coronary Disease* (advisory panel report) H.M.S.P., London, 1974.
36. Briggs, G. and Phillips, M. *Sugar, Nutrition and Disease,* addendum to testimony before Cal. Senate Subcommittee on Agriculture, Food and Nutrition, Oct. 8, 1974.
37. Welch, M. *Hypoglycemia,* Ladies' Home Journal, Nov. 1971.
38. Abrahamson, E. and Pezet, A. *Body, Mind and Sugar,* Holt, New York, 1965.
39. Linn, L. *Clinical Manifestations of Psychiatric Disorders,* in Diagnosing Mental Illness, (Freeman and Kaplan, eds.) Atheneum, New York, 1972.
40. Danowski, T. et al. *Hypoglycemia,* World Rev. Nutr. and Diet. 22:288—303, 1975.
41. Rynearson, E. *Americans love hogwash,* Nutr. Rev. July, 1974.
42. Editorial, *Statement on hypoglycemia,* JAMA 223:682, 1973.
43. Reuben, D. *The Save-Your-Life Diet,* Random House, 1975.
44. Reuben, D. *Eating to live longer,* Woman's Day, May, 1975.
45. Burkitt, D. et al. JAMA, 229:1068—74, 1974.
46. Painter, N. and Burkitt, D. *Diverticular disease of the colon,* Brit. Med. J. 2:450—4, 1971.
47. Mendeloff, A. *Dietary fiber,* Nutr. Rev. 33:321, 1975.
48. Reuben, D. excerptions from (36), Reader's Digest, Jan. 1975.
49. *Dietary fiber and colonic function,* Nutr. Rev. 33:70, 1975.

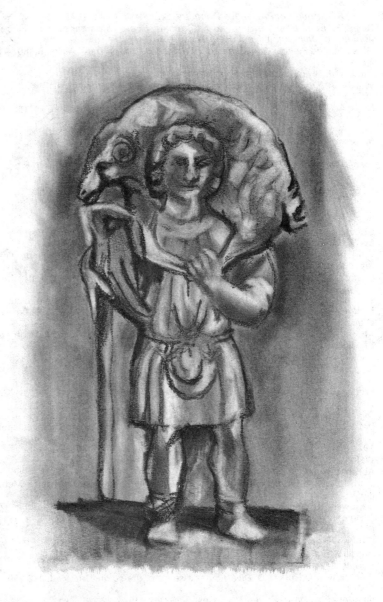

Animal protein has usually been mankind's most preferred food, but costly and hard to
get; earliest agriculture provided domesticated meat animals to the right and noble.
The Shepherd, ancient Coptic sculpture.

chapter 8

PROTEIN AND THE RICH MAN'S DIET

Recently, four groups of teachers—two of professional home economists and one each of health educators and elementary-school teachers—were asked: "If you could add just one nutrient to people's diets, what would it be?"

In all four cases, the overwhelmingly dominant answer was, "Protein."[1]

The answer reflects what seems to be Americans' first nutritional concern. We have seen that protein has become a primary inducement in food advertising, and our attitude appears to be that the more protein we eat, the better. Protein has become the dietary lure to which the consumer consistently rises, like a hungry trout on a quiet morning.

In most people's minds, it appears, the "protein foods" are mainly meats, milk, cheeses and eggs; indeed, it would seem that to many these foods *are* protein. But it is interesting to note that while the very first scientific inklings that there was such a thing as protein are two centuries old at most, the preference for these foods seems to be as old as humankind. The preference, however, has been an expensive one, and its satisfaction has been denied most people by cost.

(There are some obvious exceptions, such as the hunting cultures, which by necessity survive only in unpopulated and relatively un-civilized regions. Some of these cultures remain so largely without choice because, as in the case of the Eskimos, the land cannot be used for crops. Other vegetarian cultures, particularly the Hindu, derive from religious belief. Even among Hindus, however, except for beef, it is only members of the Brahmin caste who abstain wholly, and they are permitted milk and ghee, a clarified butter. It may be meaningful that those religious patterns which ban animals as food tend also to deny the sensual and material bonds to the present real world and aspire to another existence, wholly spiritual and aloof from the physical. Biographers of the late Mahatma Ghandi report that he was deeply troubled by two things—occasional sensations of sexual feeling, and the fact that he was forced by medical necessity to drink goat's milk.)

In food history, Egypt is mainly noted for its grain, and indeed, once ancient Egyptians discovered the tricks of leavened baking, bread was the currency of labor. Workers on the pyramid of Cheops were paid three loaves of bread a day and some beer. Yet animal husbandry was well known. From the time of Egypt's Old Kingdom, there was grain-feeding of cattle—mistakenly believed by many consumerists today to be a new, exploitive idea of beef barons—and the force-feeding of birds to make plump roasts.

But such foods were for the rich. As we have seen, the diets of the Greek and Roman common folk were mainly grains, sometimes flavored with honey or wine. People who could afford to eat what they chose largely disdained such food.

In the Golden Age of Greece, the poet Eubolus writes:

> "I pray you, where in Homer is the chief
> Who e'er eat fish or anything but beef?"

When Alexander the Great swept from Macedonia through all of Greece, an account of one of his dinners recites a start of chicken, duck, goose, ringdove, hare, pigeon, turtledove, partridge and young goat. There follows a great pig, stuffed with thrush, warbler, duck, eggs in pea purée, oysters and scallops. Finally came the main dish of skewered boars.

The cereal foods were not entirely banned from the tables of the Greek wealthy. But the manner of their use symbolized the aristocrat's feeling about such nourishment. The breads were baked and served—to be used as napkins, to wipe the meat and grease from the fingers. (The napkin appeared only when Rome took power.)

The double standard of meat preference may be followed down the centuries. The 1840s in England were known as the "hungry forties." Depression was rife. Wages, for those lucky enough to have jobs, were at a bottom low. In both Ireland and England, the potato—recognized from the 1600s as one of the world's richest yielders of calories per farm acre—was the dietary staple. Supplementary energy value seems to have been supplied mainly by gin or beer. It was in this worst of times that the plant disease struck which decimated the potato fields. The last food resort gone, it was then that so many emigrants began to struggle abroad.

But in this same era—though after the worst of the depression and the hunger had passed—Lord Palmerston, then Prime Minister of England, was chronicled on the subject of his eating habits at home. The start was ". . . two plates of turtle soup; he was then served very amply to a plate of cod and oyster sauce; he then took a pâté; afterwards he was helped to two very greasy looking entrees; he then despatched a plate of roast mutton; there then appeared before him the largest . . . slice of ham that ever figured on the plate of a nobleman, yet it disappeared, just in time to answer the inquiry of his butler, 'Snipe, my Lord, or pheasant?' He instantly replied, 'Pheasant,' thus completing his ninth dish of meat at that meal."[2]

THE NEW RIGHT TO MEAT

One of the inducements which led emigrants to the New World was the availability of land. The land in the Old World was taken by a privileged few. Even the hunting forests were the private preserves of the nobility.

In America there was a chance to get land, either cheaply or free, and this could guarantee that a family would eat. And there was game. A colonist may have endured much, but he could still eat meat. As Tannahill writes: "In the backwoods, until well into the nineteenth century, the visitor still found himself eating plain-cooked possums, raccoons, and other unexpected animals."[3] In many areas, the farms each had a smokehouse, for preserving the game. Especially in the South, the pig flourished on the smallest farms, and the barrel of salted pork was the food staple for many households.

But it was only a matter of time before the cities grew, the forests were pushed back, and the game was killed too freely. In the areas which were colonized first, the poor were driven toward carbohydrate foods—beans in Boston and corn grits in the South, along with molasses and sorghum to fill the belly.

So the westward expansion began as a push toward food security, toward open land for farms and forests to supply meat. Weren't animals raised on the small farms in the first colonies? Yes, but as luxuries. For while grass would feed them in the warm months, the winters required stored animal fodder. It was a luxury to keep corn or grain for a cow and to keep land to grow the animal's food. For many a farmer, animals were investments, one of the few sources of money needed to buy implements and food supplements.

Not until the 1870s did the great western herds begin to have an impact on the national food supply. And even then it took a lot of money to buy meat in eastern cities. For while beef was cheap at the source, it had to travel far. And once it was butchered, it could not be kept fresh for long.

So as late as the Depression of the 1930s, the American poor were used to a high-carbohydrate diet. In those dark years, the poor were hard-pressed to get their carbohydrates, and as much of the middle class joined them on the "bread lines," "A chicken in every pot" became a political fantasy.

Then World War II came, just as the Depression was lifting. There was money now, but there was also meat rationing. So it was not surprising, with the end of the war, that Americans rushed to the butcher shop, hungry for meat, and with the strongly inculcated idea—from the budding nutrition education of the 1930s—that to eat meat was to get protein—and good health.

The postwar economic boom wiped out much poverty. We could also afford a generous welfare program; the poor needed meat, and we could enable them to eat it. Compared to most of the world, even the U.S. poor had become nutritionally rich. (This is not to imply that none were hungry or malnourished in America. It is a relative statement. And it was true then as now, that some of those who were hungry just did not know how to avail themselves of the relief available.)

For the nation as a whole, we have seen that from about 1950 to the early 1970s, consumption of beef and cheese rose dramatically, while demand for beans and grains waned. In that time, chicken and turkey consumption rose 93 percent per capita; but the use of milk, and the eating of fruit, declined by a fourth. By 1973 Americans were each eating some half a pound of meat a day, some two-thirds of it beef. The consumption of vegetables, as a group, stayed about the same. But the identity of the vegetables within the group seems to have changed. School children and adults both seemed to reject the green vegetables. Lettuce, with relatively low nutrient value among the greens, became *the* vegetable on the national menu.

Encouraged by out-of-date nutrition education, and especially by anti-carbohydrate reducing diets and suspicions about sugar and starch, Americans viewed meat as the guarantor of the diet, the assurance of health. What else was eaten seemed to matter little, as long as meat was on the plate.

Then in the early 1970s, food prices rose dramatically, especially the prices of meat. Poorer people felt that they had been deprived of a right—the right to meat—and complained that their health was threatened by the lack of protein.

It was certainly true that the poorest Americans, those on welfare and at the bottom of the income ladder, had been pushed away from the table of steaks and roasts. But setting aside the social and political questions, what are the nutritional realities of this change? As significant as may be the right to share what the culture decrees to be a decent table, what are the protein needs for health?

For, in the face of the social protest, some scientists suggested that a limitation on the availability of meat might actually be an advantage. Why was this said? To understand the answer, we must know something more of the science of proteins, of the foods in which they are found, and of the quantities necessary for health.

EARLY CLUES TO THE PROTEIN MYSTERY

Shortly before Lavoisier made his epochal discoveries about the chemical character of life and food, a French scientist named Macquer made some of the first progress toward a scientific understanding about protein.

Protein is not physically obvious; seldom do we see it in pure form.

Popular belief to the contrary, we do not see it when we look at meat or cheese. This is in contrast to the other macronutrients: We see carbohydrate in quite pure form as table sugar or honey, or even the sap of trees. We are familiar with fats as we prune them from the leaner parts of meat, as we toss a salad with oil, or as we french-fry a potato.

We do see pure protein in the white of an egg. Macquer was struck by some of the now well-known characteristics of egg white. Heat it, and it changes from a viscous liquid to a slippery solid. Agitate it, and it assumes yet another form, as when we whip it to stand in peaks, perhaps for the meringue on a lemon pie. Macquer looked for other life substances with similar characteristics of coagulation. For from Hippocrates' time science had sought a basic nutrient substance. Macquer suspected that this coagulation-prone substance in food might provide an answer; some very essential materials shared the characteristics of the egg—blood, lymph, and seminal fluid for example. Perhaps, he thought, this was the stuff which had been sought for so many centuries. "The gelatinous matter of animals," he wrote finally, "is the true animal substance. It constitutes almost entirely the bodies of animals; it is that which nourishes, repairs and reproduces them."

Macquer was very close to a nutritional truth. Others tried to dig deeper. In 1811, Bertholet found a clue. He found he could treat all these substances so that they gave off ammonia. This was not true of carbohydrates or fats. We now know that the other macronutrients are composed of carbon, hydrogen and oxygen. The ammonia showed that the coagulating substance had something else—*nitrogen,* for ammonia is made of three atoms of hydrogen and one of nitrogen. (Chemically, its notation is NH_3.)

Nitrogen is hardly an uncommon element. It is, in fact, the largest constituent of the air we breath. (There is more than three times as much nitrogen as there is oxygen in air.) But while we can use the oxygen from the air in our body chemistry, we can make little chemical use of the nitrogen we inhale. So our bodily nitrogen must come largely from food.

Until the middle of the 19th century, scientists still thought in terms of a single primary substance of life. For example, one set of widely applauded experiments showed that a gelatine could be elicited from proteinaceous matter. It was thought that this gelatine was *the* basic life chemical. So the stuff was named *protein,* from the Greek meaning elemental or primary. Today science knows that the assumption was erroneous. By 1900, researchers knew that proteins were actually made up of much smaller and more basic molecules—the *amino acids*. And they had identified at least 16 of them, which appeared over and over again in food proteins.

Then, by 1909, Osborne and Mendel had embarked on the monumental work which showed that it was really these amino acids on which life depended—that it was not protein *per se* which was the nutrient, but the amino acids of which it was composed.

WHAT A FEW AMINO ACIDS CAN DO

We now know that there are more than 16 amino acids in food proteins. Nutrition literature now gives the number as "about 22." This seeming imprecision puzzles many. The reluctance to give a firm figure for amino acids is due to some curiosities, some exceptions, and some subtleties of protein chemistry.

Nineteen amino acids are usually listed as being found in foods. But at least five others have been identified in rare cases, sometimes as occurring in only one food. And to make matters a bit more confusing, these rarities have not been shown to be essential to human nutrition. On the other hand, there are amino acids which do play roles in human nutrition which are not known to occur naturally; *citrulline, hydroxylysine* and *cysteine* are examples.

For our purposes of making realistic judgments about foods, we can fairly limit our inquiry to the "about 20" amino acids which recur in food proteins.

The most awesome fact about this handful of chemicals is that they can be juggled into the whole variety of plant and animal life on earth. Consider how they are used in our own bodies. Over a thousand enzymes are made from them, as are enormous varieties of hormones and antibodies. But more than this, they are the principal materials of which our cells are composed—cells of bone and brain, blood vessel, muscle, nerve, skin, intestine, gland, and lung. These cells are estimated to make over 100,000 different compounds from these same few amino acids, not only to produce the chemicals of life processes, but also to repair and reproduce themselves.

Now reflect that we are only one species, and that these amino acids must be used still differently by other life forms—from mosquitos to daffodils, from whales to sparrows, from fur and claw to leaf and bark. How is this possible?

THE CHEMISTRY OF LIFE'S VARIETY

The potential number of variations of which the handful of amino acids are capable, is of course mathematically huge. Keep in mind that our whole language is built from just 26 letters, and that these same few units spell out many tongues.

The rearrangement of these few symbols into such huge systems suggests how a few amino acids may be sequenced to make a whole library of proteins. In fact, since the chains of amino acids are so much longer than our words, which rarely have more than a dozen letters, the possibilities for variation in proteins are enormously greater. For the proteins of life chemistry are usually at least 100 amino acids long, and they commonly range from 500 to 1000 units.

Like our language, the proteins can be affected by the slightest change in sequence. Change the sequence of letters in words and you can change meaning drastically—for example, in going from *baste* to *beats* to *beast.* Thus the same units serve radically different functions when they are differently ordered. And similar differences occur when you substitute one unit for another, as in *six* and *sex.*

Amino acid changes have at least as much impact. Consider *hemoglobin,* which carries oxygen in our blood, to supply all of our cells. It is a chain of well over 500 amino acids. Change just one and you have sickle cell anemia. Such tiny changes can, in many cases, spell the difference between sickness and health, between life and death.

The *sequence* of amino acids in a protein is known as the *primary structure.* But changes of the *geometric arrangement* of that chain can also alter the characteristics of the protein, multiplying possible variations almost to infinity. As a very crude comparison, picture the amino-acid chain of a protein as a thread. If we drop that thread, perhaps with a twirling motion, it never falls in quite the same pattern. It turns and twists and crosses over on itself.

The geometry of protein molecules is far more sophisticated. Remember our analogy of proteins as words, with the amino acids as letters. Suppose that these extremely long words could be written not only in straight lines but, without actually changing the sequence of the letters, in shapes, each of which had a different meaning, like this:

```
R O T
P   E I N
```

Or perhaps, using the name of the amino-acid phenylalanine:

```
          P

     H         E

          N Y L
              A

     N A L
     I
     N E
```

Recalling that these protein words are often 500 letters long, imagine the potential variety of shapes. Also imagine that the meaning of the words can be changed by the formation of links between parts of the word, like this:

```
     P H
     E – A      L A–E
     N Y L      N I N
```

In effect this gives you a whole new set of links, in addition to the links of the primary sequence. (In protein chemistry, the element *sulfur* often helps to form these cross-linkages.)

But the variety does not stop here. So far we have considered the variety of *two-dimensional* geographic arrangement, using only the vertical and horizontal dimensions of this flat page. Imagine that, having written out our immensely long word in this wandering pattern, and having added cross-linkages, we could further change the meaning by folding the paper in pleats. Now still other sets of letters would come out opposite one another and still more linkages could be formed. Indeed, in nature protein "words" are written in three dimensions.

Protein Shapes and Their Meaning in Life

How important are these changes of shape? Sometimes they can be even more important than changes in the amino-acid sequence. For example, there are a couple of amino acid sequence differences between the protein molecule which constitutes human insulin and the insulin of other animals. Yet some animal insulin can work in the human body, because, despite the differences of sequence, the shape and cross-linkages are the same as those of the human insulin molecule.

Shapes may be used to classify proteins. At the simplest level, there are two general classes. One is *fibrous* protein, which, though it may twist, turn and fold, tends to be organized along one axis. Such proteins are likely to be insoluble in water—for good reason. Fibrous proteins make up such structural materials as tendons and hair, and the need for water-insolubility is obvious: If you forgot your hat, rain could put you in the market for a wig.

The other dominant protein shape is generally spherical or ellipsoidal. These proteins are called *globular*. Since they include enzymes, hormones, and such bodily substances as the serum of the blood, it is plain that they must be water soluble.

We have seen that protein molecules can change their characteristics when heated, agitated, or exposed to certain chemicals, as in the case of egg white, or even *Jello*. Such alterations are generally the result of changes in the shape of the molecule, usually the result of cross-linkages being either broken down or created.

Cookery commonly causes such changes, and usually in an advantageous way. For much digestive work is needed to break the big protein molecules down into the constituent amino acids, and cooking often does the first part of this job by breaking some cross-linkages. (This work should not be confused with the very different cooking accomplishment of making more protein available from vegetable sources, by freeing it from the relatively indigestible fibrous compartments in which it is enclosed.)

These changes in protein molecules are known as *denaturing*. The coagulation and color change of the blood and other "juices" on the surface of a broiling steak is an indicator that some of the cross-linkages have broken. If anything, those changes enhance digestibility, and there is little physiological virtue in raw or undercooked meat or eggs.

On the other hand, prolonged intense heat can cause more links to form within the protein molecules, and make them resistive to digestion. For we may not have enzymes for breaking such links. The blackened surface of meat broiled over an open flame is probably less digestible than the rest (although in practical terms, this crust is apt to be very thin, and have little effect on nutritive quality).

Denaturing can inactivate the proteins which are enzymes. And a dim understanding of this has led many well-meaning "health-food" advocates to insist on raw foods, and to worry needlessly about some processing techniques. For example, enzymes in milk are denatured by pasteurizing, so some people insist on "raw" (unpasteurized) milk. The same people demand wheat which has been stone-ground, on the theory that more modern milling methods produce somewhat more heat and inactivate the enzymes of the grain.

But while these critics are correct about the denaturing of enzymes, they fail to understand the processes of digestion and absorption of proteins. For these particular enzymes are treated by the body merely as ordinary food proteins; they are broken down into their constituent amino acids, and have no special use except as tiny contributors to the total amino acid pool.

In general, meat tenderizers are safe, because their effectiveness comes from the action of their digestive enzymes, which help break down meat protein. But clearly, we would not like them to digest *us*. Why do they not? There are several reasons, among them the fact that cooking denatures them, and the fact that digestion breaks them apart.

The shape and chemistry of protein may also be changed by *conjugation*. This merely means the linking of proteins to other chemical substances. When a protein which is broken down completely yields only amino acids, it is a *simple* protein. When it yields amino acids plus other chemicals, it is *conjugated*. The conjugated proteins are classified according to the combining substance. For example, when the latter is a fatty chemical (*lipid*), the conjugated protein is a *lipoprotein*. Protein joined to a carbohydrate structure is a *glycoprotein*.

Conjugations are familiar and often desirable in cooking reactions, as in the case of browning. They can tie up some protein and other food substances to make them unavailable to the body. But contrary to some popular belief, the nutritive effects are usually so small as to be meaningless, as when we toast bread and browning results from the combination of some carbohydrate with some protein. The change is not even enough to alter the caloric value of the bread. However, improper cooking of food in fat can cause conjugations and other effects which can interfere with digestion.

Many conjugated proteins are important to life, and many are nutritionally useful. Hemoglobin is a conjugated protein, and digestion can break it down to yield both amino acids and valuable iron, as when we eat liver.

Digesting and Absorbing Proteins

The processes by which the body breaks the big protein molecules apart, and by which it admits the amino acids to the bloodstream, are elegant and elaborate. But a general understanding of the process can help us to deal with the practicalities of eating.

When we chew up protein-rich foods, little happens other than the mechanical chopping, and a mixing with saliva. Unlike carbohydrates, proteins are relatively unaffected by the chemistry of the saliva. For there are no *proteases* (enzymes which split proteins) in the mouth. And the chemical digestion of protein does not begin until the food reaches the stomach.

In the stomach, the first important digestive factor is the acid produced by cells in the stomach wall. The acid is, however, less important for its direct effect on the protein than it is for putting another substance to work. This is a chemical called *pepsinogen,* produced by certain cells of the stomach lining. The acid breaks it apart, and the result is the important enzyme, *pepsin.* Historically one of the first digestive enzymes recognized, pepsin was named from the Greek word *pepsein,* which means to cook or digest. It causes the first breakdown of protein molecules into smaller amino-acid chains.

In infants, another stomach enzyme also goes to work on protein. Called *rennin,* it modifies casein, the main protein in milk, to form a curd. Why is it useful for milk to curdle in the infant stomach? The baby is on a liquid diet. Liquids move more rapidly through the digestive system, perhaps too fast to be broken down by body chemistry and absorbed fully. The curds, being more solid, slow down. Indeed, anyone who has cared for an infant has seen the effect of rennin in the cheesy substance which babies commonly spit up. Certain commercial custard products also contain rennin to help give them their finished form.

As the shorter amino-acid chains, called *peptides,* reach the first portion of the small intestine, more enzymes, especially from the pancreas and the intestinal-wall cells, break them further. Each enzyme is structured so that it can break a specific kind of linkage in the chain. Eventually, the individual amino acids are separated out and can be absorbed through the intestine and into the bloodstream.

This absorption is a complex process, in some ways still mysterious. Such factors as vitamin B-6 are needed, to help the amino acids through the intestinal wall. Also, there is a puzzling system in which certain amino acids get priority for passage. Why should there be a priority system? It appears to be based upon the needs of the cells for different amounts of the different amino acids—the amounts specifically determined by the formulae for the particular proteins being made by the cells.

The amino acids which have been separated from food proteins, and which have crossed the intestinal wall into the bloodstream, now form a kind of central pool from which each cell must draw its raw materials. But unlike the sugars which enter the blood from carbohydrate, each amino acid must retain its identity—in order to make the varied sequences and structures of human proteins.

So unlike the need for carbohydrate, which ultimately is a single, total requirement for one sugar, the need for protein is actually a composite of some twenty different needs for some twenty different nutrients, the amino acids. And these needs are not equal, either in quantity or in importance.

Amino Acids and the Differences in Protein Quality

Earlier, we saw that nutrition information labels on foods assigned three different levels of protein quality. These quality differences are based on the ability of foods to supply amino acids in something like the proportions of the body's needs. And the primary determinant of that quality of a food is how well it supplies one group of amino acids, those which are described as *essential.* *

At first glance, this may seem like a contradiction in terms. For we have just suggested that the body must have *all* amino acids to do its

---

*An alternate terminology has been proposed by Dr. Alfred Harper—that of *indispensable* and *dispensable* amino acids—which describes these relationships well.

work of making proteins. And we have seen earlier that *all* must be present at one time. Why, then, are some amino acids so special?

The answer is quite simple. It is that some amino acids can be made by the body, as long as the body has enough of the chemical element nitrogen, the presence of which characterizes proteins. In other words, these *non-essential* amino acids are available to the cells as long as a sufficient quantity of protein is consumed, no matter what its origin and amino acid composition.

But another group of amino acids cannot be made by the body. These must be present in foods in adequate amounts. If we do not eat foods with enough of these *essential* amino acids, the inevitable result will be that the body cannot produce the proteins it requires. Adequate intakes of essential amino acids are in this way similar to the more familiar requirements for specific vitamins and minerals. The essential amino acids are:

Isoleucine	Phenylalanine
Leucine	Threonine
Lysine	Tryptophan
Methionine	Valine
	Histidine

This classification is for adults only. For children, since they are growing, need another amino acid which, for them, is essential, even though adults need not be concerned about it. This is Arginine.

To complete the list, the non-essential amino acids which the body can make are:

Alanine	Hydroxyproline
Aspartic Acid	Proline
Cystine	Serine
Glutamic Acid	Tyrosine
Glycine	

We must now note, however, that the chemistry of life is not quite as simple as we might like it to be; and two of the "non-essential" amino acids might really be classified in a special way.

Why? The essential amino acid *methionine* is usually listed as being needed to the extent of 1.1 grams per day. But if enough *cystine,* usually called "non-essential," is present in the diet, the need for methionine drops some 80 percent, to only about 0.2 grams daily. The relationship between these two derives from the fact that both of these amino acids are partly composed of certain sulfur-containing groups. Similarly, there is much less of the supposedly essential *phenylalanine* needed when enough *tryosine* is available in the food. For both incorporate special chemical structures which cause them to be grouped as aromatic amino acids.

The essentiality of some amino acids has led to a popular misnomer. For it is common to describe proteins which contain adequate proportions of all the essential amino acids as "complete," and those which do not as "incomplete." This, however, is inexact, and it can mislead. For in reality, the vast majority of foods contain some amount of all the amino acids. The critical difference rests with whether the quantity of each essential amino acid is sufficient.

The classic example is that wheat protein is somewhat low in *lysine* (though it has some), while beans are low in *methionine*. In a dietary in which the principal protein source is either of these foods, the shortage of the particular low-level amino acid may cause some problems. On the other hand, if the single food is eaten in sufficient quantity, there are few problems. For then there is enough of even the low-level amino acid. For example, even though wheat might be called an "incomplete" protein source, a diet which includes enough wheat can supply enough lysine. This was demonstrated recently when Mickelsen fed volunteers a diet which depended for most of its protein on eight slices of bread at each meal. Within a few weeks it could be shown that the volunteers were receiving adequate amino acids, even though by much conventional theory their main protein source was deficient in lysine.*

In a mixed diet, low-level amino acids can be compensated for by the correct combination of "incomplete" protein sources. For example, if one eats both wheat *and* beans, the two protein sources make up for one another's amino-acid deficiencies. So grains and legumes are spoken of as being *complementary* in terms of protein. That is, each protein source makes up for the amino-acid shortages of the other. In general, however, the nutritional rule of thumb is that animal-source foods provide adequate amounts of essential amino acids, while vegetable sources are usually somewhat lacking. So nutritionists consider that the easiest short-cut to amino-acid safety is to include a modest amount of animal-source foods in the dietary—not including some, however, such as butter or sour cream, which contain little total protein.

While modern nutritional terminology no longer refers to animal-

---

*Actually, it now appears that wheat has enough lysine to offer a high-quality protein for the *adult* human. For most amino-acid research has been done with *growing-age* rats, which prove to have much more need for lysine, proportionately, than do grown humans.)

source proteins as "complete," it describes them as being of "higher quality." And conversely, vegetable-source proteins are spoken of as being "lower quality."

It was this simplified concept of two protein qualities which FDA adopted for labeling; it then took cognizance of a third quality (such as the protein of gelatin), which is too poor to support life. But most nutritionists accepted this simplification with some misgivings. For while the plan was entirely safe for those who consumed "higher quality" protein foods, there is wide variation in the proteins of fruits, vegetables, and grains. In this grouping, soy protein becomes equated in value to that of apples and plums, yet it is really quite close to the quality of much meat. In the end, however, certain realities of protein and food led nearly all nutritionists to agree, if with some reluctance, to the FDA plan.

To understand why the plan works, we must know something of just how the body uses amino acids, once they have been separated from food proteins and absorbed. Moreover, this understanding can enable us to choose this most costly part of our food with wisdom, with economy, and with realistic knowledge of how these foods can support good health—or how, improperly used, they can harm us.

REFERENCES

1. Deutsch, R. *Nutrition 1-2-3,* lecture at Amer. Dietetic Assn., Phila., 1974, unpub.
2. Hale, W. et al. *Illustrated History of Eating and Drinking through the Ages,* Vol. I, Horizon Cookbook, Amer. Heritage, New York, 1968. p. 316.
3. Tannahill, R. *Food in History, Stein and Day, New York, 1973, p. 300.*
4. McHenry, E. *From Lavoisier to Beaumont and Hopkins,* in *Human Nutrition Historic and Scientific,* N.Y. Acad. Med., 1960.

General References

7. Jones, W. *Philosophy and Medicine in Ancient Greece,* Johns Hopkins Press, Baltimore, 1946.
8. Petronius, *The Satyricon,* Modern Library, New York.
9. Simon, A. *Food,* Burke, London, 1949.
10. Stewart, G. and Amerine, M. *Introduction to Food Science and Technology,* Academic Press, New York, 1973—See "Evolution of Food Processing," pp. 1—27.
11. Pyke, M. *Food and Society,* Murray, London, 1968.
12. Jacob, H. *Six Thousand Years of Bread,* Doubleday, NY, 1944.
13. Lowenberg, M. et al. *Early Times Through Roman Times* and *Medieval Times through the 19th Century,* in *Food and Man,* Wiley, New York, 1974, pp. 1–116.
14. Clark, J. and Goldblith, S. *Processing of foods in Ancient Rome,* Food Tech. Jan. 1976, p. 30.
15. Pariser, E. *Foods in Ancient Egypt and Classical Greece,* Food Tech., Jan. 1976, p. 23.
16. *Historical Statistics of the U.S.: Colonial Times to 1957,* U.S. Dept. of Commerce, Washington, 1960.

17. *The Protein Gap,* AIF Bur. for Tech. Assistance, Wash., 1970.
18. *National Food Situation* (quarterly) Economic Res. Service, USDA, Washington (passim, 1961—74).
19. Handbook of Agricultural Statistics, Part IV, Food Consumption in Canada, 1926—55, Dominion Bureau of Statistics and Dept. of Agriculture, Ottawa.
20. Shute, D. and Yaukowsky, Z. *Trends in per capita food consumption in Canada,* Canadian Farm Economics, 8:25—31, 1973.
21. Miller, G. and Lachance, P. *Protein: Chemistry and nutrition,* Food Prod. Devel., Dec. 1973.
22. Lawrie, R. ed. *Proteins as Human Foods,* Avi, Westport, Conn., 1970.
23. Lewis, H. *Fifty years of study of the role of protein in nutrition,* JADA, 28:701—6, 1952.
24. Albanese, A. and Orto, L. *The Proteins and Amino Acids,* in Modern Nutrition in Health and Disease, Lea & Febiger, Phila. 1973.

Additional General References—see chapter 9

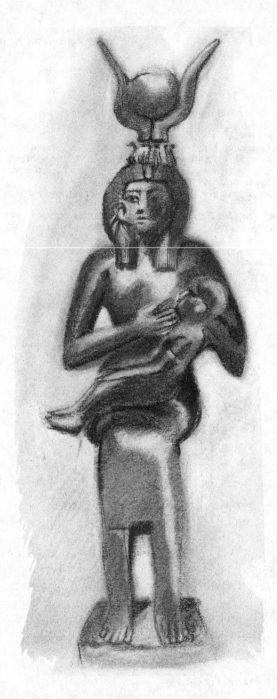

The amino acids of proteins are the raw materials of heredity, the keys to life chemistry, handed from generation to generation. *Isis and Horus as Mother and Child. Egyptian bronze, fourth to second century, B.C.*

chapter 9

PUTTING AMINO ACIDS TO WORK

How can we test the reality of claims that eating more protein is the answer to many of our nutrition problems, and that it can prevent or cure many medical problems as well?

If such ideas are true, then one of two other propositions must also be true. One possibility is that we are not getting enough protein to meet our needs—in which case the result would range from retarded growth and intellect to early death. The other possibility is that we aren't really living up to our full health potential—that extra amounts of protein would somehow enable our bodies to function better.

PROTEINS ARE MADE TO ORDER

To test these ideas, we must understand how heredity dictates the chemistry of our bodies. For the heredity which shapes our lives expresses itself by providing each cell with instructions for making proteins from amino acids.

These instructions must be precise. For a small change in amino-acid sequence or structure can make a protein unusable—or even lethal.

The method by which the trillions of cells in a human body encode this information and use it has been known for scarcely a generation. It was only in 1962 that the Nobel Prize went to Watson, Crick, and Wilkins for discerning this secret of life, probably the most important scientific discovery of our century. These three young men demonstrated how the instructions for making every one of the more than 100,000 proteins of the body were carried in every cell, in a tiny amount of DNA.

DNA (*deoxyribonucleic acid)* is a chain of molecules, similar to the sugar chains which form starches and the amino-acid chains which form proteins. DNA is a chain of substances called *nucleotides.* Each of these is made of a sugar, a phosphate (a combination of phosphorus and oxygen), and a base (a nitrogen-bearing chemical which looks like a second cousin to an amino acid). It is the sequencing of the nucleotides in DNA which shows the cells how to make proteins.

DNA AND THE PROTEIN BLUEPRINTS

In each microscopic human cell is a tiny inner chamber—the nucleus. And it is in the nucleus that we find DNA. The strands of DNA, each an extremely long chain of small molecules, occur in pairs. And each human cell nucleus holds 23 pairs.

The nucleotides which make the DNA chain are grouped in threes, and each threesome is known as a *triplet.* Understanding the meaning of the triplets, and the way in which they do their work, was the key to breaking the genetic code. That key is essentially simple. Each triplet represents the code signal for a particular amino acid. Thus a sequence of triplets becomes the code for a chain of amino acids—for a protein. Each strand of DNA holds a long series of triplet sequences—hence a long series of formulas for proteins.

Just how the system operates in a cell is not yet known fully. But the outlines are clear. In general, a blueprint from the DNA is sent out of the nucleus into the main body of the cell, the *cytoplasm.* In that cytoplasm there circulate free amino acids and other chemicals.

These are assembled according to the number and order dictated by the blueprint transmitted from the nucleus.

Part of the wonder of this process is its astonishing smallness. For except for a relatively few cells which are extremely small or large, typical body cells are on the order of 20 to 30 microns in diameter: A line of 1,000 of them would be about an inch long. The nucleus, of course, is much smaller. And the 23 pairs of tiny DNA strands in each nucleus are estimated to hold some two billion sets of protein-making instructions.

Each DNA pair is a *chromosome.* The two strands of DNA are twined about each other in a spiral—the *double helix.* And the strands are linked together at each nucleotide. So under the electron microscope, a chromosome looks something like an extremely long railroad track which has been twisted into a spiral, with the links between the nucleotides being the ties.

How the cell understands what proteins must be made, and how it then signals the chromosomes in the nucleus that a protein is needed, remains a mystery. But when a certain protein is required, the spiral opens up, and the two DNA strands separate for a length. That length is the part of the strand which holds the code for the needed protein.

Floating free in the nucleus are some nucleotides which are slightly different from those which make up the DNA triplets. The difference is in a special sugar. DNA nucleotides are partly made from a sugar called *deoxyribose,* from which DNA takes its name. The free-floating nucleotides are made with the sugar *ribose;* the chains which *they* eventually make up are known as *ribonucleic acids,* or RNA.

Each nucleotide in the DNA has the power to attract an RNA nucleotide which matches it, and no other. As soon as the DNA spiral opens up, the nucleotides which have been exposed attract matching RNA nucleotides. These RNA nucleotides link together to form a complementary sequence, a replica of the sequence which was exposed when the DNA spiral opened.

In effect the DNA molecule transfers to the RNA molecule an image of the code for the needed protein—not unlike the negative of a photograph: indeed very like a photo of a master blueprint.

When the new RNA chain is complete, it pulls free, and the DNA spiral closes again. This molecular copy of the DNA blueprint is known as *RNA messenger,* for it now takes the blueprint out of the nucleus and into the cytoplasm of the cell. Here the RNA messenger attaches itself to a very tiny body inside the cell, a *ribosome,* probably about a thousandth of the size of the cell itself. The ribosome becomes the workshop where the new protein will be made.

Remember, the RNA holds a series of code triplets which call for amino acids, in perfect sequence. So these amino acids must now be brought to the RNA and assembled into the needed protein. This job of delivering the amino acids to the ribosome is done by triplets of another kind of ribonucleic acids, appropriately called *transfer RNA.* The triplets of transfer RNA are loose in the cytoplasm. Each picks up the amino acid its code calls for and carries it to the ribosome. Following the blueprint which the messenger RNA has brought from the nucleus, the transfer RNA triplets put their amino acids into their appropriate places, much as one would lay out parts on a pattern.

Once the amino acids are arranged in proper sequence, linkages are made between them, and *protein synthesis* has been accomplished. (However, how the *shape* of the new protein molecule is determined still puzzles researchers.)

DNA AND SOME FACTS ABOUT NUTRITION

On first look, the way in which heredity operates by controlling the synthesis of proteins may seem a matter of mainly theoretical interest. But from this information, we can make a number of practical deductions which allow us to test some popular nutrition ideas.

Most basically, we can now see that it is the constituent amino acids which are important, since it is they, rather than whole proteins, that the cells require from food. For we can see that, because the triplets of transfer RNA are each coded for specific amino acids, they cannot make use of anything else as they gather up the raw materials for the making of the new protein. If this were not an extremely specific system, the cells could not follow the very precise instructions of heredity. In a broad sense, we may say the central rule of the system is "no substitutions."

Do We Need to Eat Sunflower Seeds?

This knowledge calls into question the claims of some "health food" enthusiasts that certain special foods have extraordinary properties as protein sources. Many seeds and sprouts, for example, are sold with this implication.

But because RNA relentlessly seeks out only amino acids, and because we know that all molecules of any one amino acid are completely interchangeable, we can conclude that, for protein synthesis, the food source of the amino acids does not matter. If the amino acid *lysine* is what the DNA blueprint calls for, the transfer RNA will seek lysine and nothing else—without concern for whether that lysine molecule came from hot dogs, canned tuna, sunflower seeds, or soy sprouts. Nor could the lysine from one source be different from any other; if it were, it could not be used.

Don't Allergies Prove that Proteins Differ for Health?

As was pointed out earlier, there is no question that different arrangements of amino acids make different proteins. But, contrary to some implications of health-fooders, this does not affect the way in which the cells use the amino acids from these proteins.

True, allergies are considered to be reactions to proteins. It is also true that, unlike carbohydrates—which cannot be absorbed into the bloodstream until they have been broken into single sugars—some whole proteins can be carried through the intestinal wall and into the circulation. This is the basis of one concept of food allergies, which holds that the allergic reaction results from the absorption of whole proteins, which in turn are perceived by the body as foreign substances, so that they are then attacked by the immune systems.

The mechanisms of this process are not yet entirely known. We do not fully understand why some whole proteins get through to the bloodstream. But we do know that this happens. And we know that usually, at the site of an allergic reaction, there are large numbers of *eosinophils*, white blood cells which are involved in our immune defenses. So treatment depends upon identifying the foods which send problem proteins into the blood of an individual, eliminating these from the diet for a time, and then gradually reintroducing them.

But all of this has no bearing on the basic use of amino acids by the cells. For with our understanding of how the cells use amino acids, we can see that *whole* proteins cannot be used in this way. So nutritionally, our only concern is to choose foods which meet our amino-acid needs.

Do Pure Amino Acids Make Good Meals?

Logic would suggest that eating pure amino acids (not connected in protein chains) would be the best way to make sure that all our needs are met. But we really do much better when the amino acids come from foods. For apparently, the complicated mechanisms of absorbing amino acids from the intestine require that some amino-acid chains be present. In some attempts to maintain the nutrition of the ill, especially those (such as certain post-surgical patients) who have digestive problems, it has been found that pure amino acids taken by mouth are not well absorbed. When liquid foods which are used for these patients are formulated with a mix of some pure amino acids and some short chains, there seems to be better absorption.

This information is not solely of interest to the physician. For it raises some questions about the usefulness of certain protein-supplement capsules and powders which are made of "pure amino acids"; ordinary food can supply the same amino acids much more cheaply, and with other needed nutrients to boot.*

Do We Need to Eat DNA?

Recently, an interesting new diet has been propounded by a Dr. Benjamin Frank—in a book, and in two lay journals, *Family Circle* and the *Enquirer,* which were quick to hurry the news to their readers. In what he calls the "no-aging diet," Dr. Frank rightly explains the importance of DNA and RNA in our lives. For good health, he then says, "Foods high in DNA and RNA—nucleic acids—are the key." Saying that we don't eat enough of such foods, Dr. Frank reports that his patients do, "and look younger by being healthy." Their appearances of age, he adds, regress by as much as 15 years.

Frank maintains that the quality of our RNA and DNA goes down as we age. So the older we get, the more important it is for us to get new RNA and DNA, and he gives us instructions on how to do so through our diets.

There is, of course, no question that we do get these chromosomal strands in our foods. For all life forms depend upon them for the hereditary blueprints which their cells follow; the humblest carrot

---

*However, we shall see that there are some important uses of single amino acids to fortify lower-quality proteins, so that, for example, grain products can support life and growth.

and the simplest onion do so as much as we. After all, without such hereditary determination, a radish could just as well become a turnip.

The real question, however, is whether our own cells can restore their RNA and DNA from what we eat. As we have seen, the genius of heredity is replication, the making of exactly the same chemicals over and over again. We do not need an electron microscope to see this. As a carrot grows, it simply makes more carrot.

This happens not only because DNA dictates the making of specific proteins; it also occurs because, as we learn in biology, the whole cell divides, yielding two cells where one was before, each with the same heredity. So it is that cells replace themselves, many every few days. So it is that the fertilized egg cell in the human mother divides and multiplies and grows. With each division, although the cells gradually change and become specialized groups for different body parts, the DNA in the cell nucleus separates. Each DNA strand makes a kind of mirror image of itself, until each has a new spiraling partner, until where there were two twining strands to make a chromosome there are now four, enough to make two double strands, for two identical cells.

According to Dr. Frank's thesis, we can make up for defects (aging effects) in this replication by taking in new DNA from food. Is this a realistic possibility? More than 10 million readers have been led to believe that it is.

If it is, then we must consider the consequences. Dr. Frank recommends such foods as sardines, salmon, and the organs of the cow, as DNA-rich. Recalling the extreme specificity of DNA, if we could make use of the DNA of other life forms in the manner Dr. Frank suggests, we would begin to make protein according to the blue-prints of the chromosomal strands of these organisms. We would form the structures and chemicals suitable to fins, horns, and tails. One might expect photographs of Dr. Frank's rejuvenated patients to be interesting in the extreme.

Fasting—Does It Matter When We Get Our Amino Acids?

We have already mentioned that all amino acids need to be present in the bloodstream at one time, in order for the making of proteins to go ahead smoothly. Knowing the way RNA calls for the appropriate amino acids to assemble particular proteins helps to make this clearer. For what can the messenger RNA do when there is a blank where an amino acid ought to be? Plainly, it simply cannot make the needed protein.

In practice, we know that the RNA must release the other amino acids back into the cytoplasm, to wait for the missing molecules. We also know that RNA does not have very much time to find the amino acids it needs, a matter of a few minutes perhaps. This, of course, is one of the reasons why nutritionists are concerned about the skipping of breakfast, the eating of badly unbalanced breakfasts low in essential amino acids, and certainly about a current belief that fasting for several days will cure illness by "cleaning out the blood."

Because the body processes continue as long as life continues, cells continue to die and break down, chemical processes go on, and the wastes and residues are carried away by the blood. These processes must continue just as the burning of fuel must not stop. So all that is being cleaned out of the blood of meal-skippers and fasters are the nutrients needed to replace the chemicals and structures which have been used. While fuel can be replaced from the body's reserve storage of fat, the shortage of amino acids may or may not be made up (either by using nitrogen wastes, or by breaking down body cells). If essential amino acids are missing, the protein synthesis for repair and replacement is stopped. Such shortages are particularly harmful in times of growth, such as childhood and pregnancy.

These realities of amino-acid use suggest some commonsense rules for eating protein. But just how to choose foods to provide the cells with a complete pool of amino acids is easier to understand if we learn a little more of how proteins are made and taken apart.

HOW TO MAKE OR BREAK A PROTEIN

The amino acids which compose proteins look like this in their general design:

$$AMINO\ GROUP$$
$$|$$
$$RADICAL-C-ACID\ GROUP$$
$$|$$
$$H$$

In this picture, the "C" is carbon and the "H" is hydrogen. The *amino group* is just an atom of nitrogen holding two atoms of hydrogen (NH_2). It is really ammonia, which has lost one atom of hydrogen, and this is why early researchers observed that proteins gave off ammonia if treated in certain ways. The *acid group* is an atom of carbon which holds two atoms of oxygen and one of hydrogen (COOH). So this much of an amino acid is quite simple (although a few are somewhat more complicated, having two amino and acid groups).

The main difference among amino acids is in the *radical*. This can be as simple as a single hydrogen atom, or it can be quite a fancy structure. It is in the radical that we may find some other elements, too, such as sulfur, phosphorus, or iodine.

Now let us apply this pattern to the simplest of amino acids, glycine. It can be shown like this:

(amino group)

NH_2

|

(radical) H—C—COOH (acid)

|

H

If you look at some more complicated amino acids, you will see that if you identify the component parts—aminos, acids, and radicals—the pattern will remain relatively simple.

One of the important qualities of an amino acid is its ability to combine with other amino acids. And to make long chains, it must be able to join others at two points—just as people making a human chain must link up with *both* hands.

Chemically, this ability for double linkage (the quality of being *amphoteric*) rests with the combining potential of both the amino group and the acid group. The amino of one molecule can join with the acid of another, and so on. Again comparing to our human chain, if a number of us line up side by side, we can link by joining our right hand to our neighbor's left, and our left to his right.

Let us see the pattern as two glycines join. To make matters clearer, we will rotate one glycine a little. And we will also expand our picture of the groups which are joining, to show each atom separately (NH_2 becomes H—N—H, etc.)

```
H—N—H                        H      H
  |                          |      |
H—C—C—OH                     N      C—H
  |   ||                     |      |
  H   O          →           H      COOH
Glycine I          H₂0  ←           Glycine II
```

Under the influence of an enzyme, a small part is now broken from each of the glycine molecules. On the left, we see that it is the OH broken from the acid group. And in glycine molecule II it is one of the H's bonded to the N of the amino group.

Looking more closely at the area of reaction, we see something like this.

$$\underset{O}{\overset{\displaystyle C-OH}{\|}} \qquad \overset{\displaystyle -N-}{\underset{H}{|}}$$
$$H-O-H$$

Notice that four chemical bonds are now open. The two fragments broken from the two amino acids can join together to make one stable compound. It is H_2O—water.

In the acid group of the first glycine, the carbon is left open, and in the amino group of the second glycine, the nitrogen is left open. The carbon and nitrogen snap together, and the two amino acids have joined.

We have witnessed some basic phenomena of biochemistry. First, to open up chemical bonds on each of the amino acids, the H and OH atoms were broken off and formed water. This is essentially the same process we saw when glucose molecules broke apart or joined together. It is *hydrolysis.* Moreover, as with carbohydrates, hydrolysis is also the method by which proteins are broken apart. A molecule of water must be added, to supply two hydrogen atoms and one of oxygen.

Why is this addition necessary? Let us look again at the amino acids we saw joined. First, we see that neither is really an amino acid any longer, for each has given up a small part of itself, and for this reason is called an amino acid *residue.* So while it is common to say that a protein is a chain of amino acids, it is not fully accurate. Remember, too, that in the protein chain, nearly all the amino acids have given up not just one portion to join together, but two, since nearly all have taken two partners, as in our example of people joining hands.

The combining portion of an amino acid thus satisfies the charges of its open chemical bonds by joining with others, in what is known as a *peptide linkage.* Whenever it is separated from the others, it is left again with unsatisfied chemical bonds. To be a stable compound on its own, the charges of those bonds must be satisfied, and the hydrogen and oxygen atoms from water do this job.

WHERE WE GET OUR AMINO ACIDS

We have already seen that it is the rare American who is lacking in protein intake and that almost all of us get far more than we need. As one Federal staff report concludes: "although the precise number of persons with insufficient protein intake is unknown, the aggregate figures of the major nutrition surveys indicate that protein deficiency is probably the least common of all major nutrient deficiencies in the United States."

Elsewhere in this same report, it is stated that: "Even those young and middle age adult males at the lowest income level in our society are still consuming some 230% of the average requirement for protein." The HANES study (Health and Nutrition Examination Survey, United States) recently reviewed the average protein consumption of some 10,000 people between one and seventy-four years of age and found that it was almost 200 percent of the average need *of adult males* (who generally need the most protein).

But how can we say how much is enough?

Not All Our Amino Acids Must Come From Food.

It is popularly assumed that all the amino acids we need must come from our food each day. If this were true, no one could have survived starvation on a life raft or the low-protein diets of the Vietnamese prison camps. For the body's stores of free amino acids are very small, and the needs are constant. Estimates are that a typical adult male's cells synthesize some 90 grams of proteins daily. True, in the U.S., his intake of food protein is at least this high. But the RDA set by the Food and Nutrition Board, including a liberal safety margin, is only 56 grams a day.

How is this seeming discrepancy accounted for? The fact is that most of the amino acids we need can come from tissue proteins and other body chemicals which have broken down. The body is thrifty and tends to conserve these useful materials. In fact, it appears that the body conserves still more when protein intake is at low levels.

Remember that the amino acids we take in from food are not "new," but were part of other lives. In general,* those in a steak once

---

*There is some oversimplification here; for instance, some amino acids may be synthesized in the course of the food chain.

served a cow, and before the cow, the grain in the cow's feed. In a sense, these amino acids may be compared to the sound bricks in a worn-out building. Indeed, theoretically, the amino acids used by human cells could go on being parts of one life or another indefinitely. We get a graphic example from animals in the jungle, who cycle amino acids from species to species.

This recycling of amino acids within the body becomes a key factor in determining how much we need to ingest. So for a moment, let us look more closely at how amino acids are used.

What Happens to Amino Acids We Eat?

Since there is a steady loss of protein from the body, despite some recycling, obviously some of our food amino acids are first used by the cells to synthesize replacements for what is lost. A very small amount of excess can remain as a reserve in the liver, blood, and muscles. The rest are broken apart, and serve either as fuel or as raw materials.

In breaking down an amino acid, first the amino group (the nitrogen-bearing part) is removed, a process called *deamination*. This leaves a structure of mainly carbon, hydrogen and oxygen, which looks much like a carbohydrate. In fact, this residue (called a *keto-acid*) can be burned as a fuel through the same final metabolic pathway that carbohydrate uses, the *Krebs cycle.*

So if one eats excess protein and too little carbohydrate for fuel, much of the protein will merely burn up. In effect, one will have paid meat prices for carbohydrate, and even so, the protein is not as efficient a fuel. This is what happens in low-carbohydrate reducing diets.

On the other hand, if one has plenty of calories in food without burning protein residue, the amino-acid residues are converted to fat and stored in the adipose cells. This process is nicely efficient. Excess amino acids are just as good fat-makers as carbohydrates.

What happens to the amino groups which we said were broken off? These can be used to make nitrogen-using chemicals of several kinds. Since the amino groups of amino acids are always the same, and the radicals of amino acids are the key differences, the body can juggle these parts around, like pieces of an erector set. The majority of this use is the making of non-essential and semi-essential amino acids. The body can make the radicals of non-essential amino acids which it needs; then it tacks on available amino groups. This exchanging of amino groups is known as *transamination*.

If the amino groups are not needed for such work, they are either changed into ammonia (from NH_2 to NH_3) by adding one atom of hydrogen or into other nitrogenous compounds such as *urea*. Such chemicals are not tolerated well in large amounts, so the body disposes of them. While some nitrogen wastes are excreted in the stools, most of such wastes in the blood are removed by the kidneys and flushed away with water, in the urine. This is one reason why people on "high protein" reducing diets urinate a lot, and one reason for the deceptive short-term weight loss of dehydration.

Because nitrogen is a part of the excreted protein wastes, the amount of nitrogen can, as we shall see, serve as a measure of the amount of protein given up by the body.

MEASURING OUR PROTEIN USE AND NEED

Clearly, to choose foods well, we must know something about (1) How much total protein loss we must replace with food, (2) What kinds of essential amino acids must be replaced, and roughly in what proportions, and (3) What different foods supply in the way of both amino acid quantity and quality.

Many tests can be applied to answer these questions. But to get the general idea of how protein need and use is assessed, let us look at just three concepts. Each will show us how one of the above questions is answered.

1. Nitrogen Balance—a Measure for Total Protein.

If the amount of protein we eat just supplies the amount our body is losing, this is the state of *equilibrium*. We can use as a gauge the relative gains and losses of nitrogen—the *nitrogen balance*. This is not as fine a balance as it might seem, for the body seems to adjust to rather wide variations.

To check nitrogen balance, one compares the nitrogen content of urine, feces, skin and other secretion losses to the nitrogen content of the food taken in. In general, nitrogen makes up some 16 percent of protein, so for every gram of nitrogen going in or out of the body, one can assume that roughly 6.25 grams of protein were involved as the source.

Nitrogen balance studies are painstaking and costly, so they are usually done only for research purposes. But they have taught nutrition scientists much. *Positive nitrogen balance* occurs if we are taking in and keeping more protein than we lose. This means that growth is occurring, as in childhood or pregnancy.

Negative nitrogen balance generally means that we are losing more nitrogen in wastes than we are taking in. This can mean that we are not getting enough protein—our losses are not being replaced from food.

From such studies of several kinds, the RDA Committee estimated that its reference man, of 154 pounds, loses about 23 grams of protein daily, which need to be replaced. This adds up to about .32 grams of protein for each kilogram of body weight (or about .15 grams for each pound).

However, because not all foods supply protein which is easily digestible, because efficiency of absorption seems to decrease as we near our intake needs, the Committee arrived at a true protein requirement of perhaps .47 grams of protein for each kilogram of body weight, or about 33 grams a day for a reference male adult.

Then, to be safe, to provide for disease stresses and other possible problems, the Committee ended by recommending .80 grams of protein for each kilogram of weight, or 56 grams a day as the RDA for the reference man. This compares with the 23 grams a day which he probably really needs.

Special protein needs, as for children and pregnant women, will be looked at later. But if you multiply your own weight in kilograms by .8 (or multiply your weight in pounds by .36), you will get an idea of how much protein you need, in grams. (A rough shortcut is to divide your weight in pounds by three.) Now let us get a quick idea of how much protein you probably eat.

To feed his 154 pounds, our reference male adult eats some 2,500 calories daily. Since his diet averages about 15 percent protein, this means some 375 calories come from this nutrient. And since protein provides about four calories per gram, we can conclude that he gets about 94 grams of protein a day to replace a probable daily loss of 23 grams.

Draw your own conclusions. On this basis, do you agree with

Adelle Davis, with Dr. Atkins, and with some protein-supplement manufacturers that we should all increase our protein intake? What possible reason could there be?

2. The Quality of Protein—Its Value for Life.

Since we know that the real key to our needs for protein is the cells' need for amino acids, however, we also know that measuring *total* protein is not enough. The RDA Committee, in making its recommendations, assumed the typical American mixed diet as the source. As we look at our amino-acid needs, and how foods supply them, we shall see that this was a sound assumption.

But for the food shopper, FDA concluded, labels should tell more about the biological values of proteins, since higher quality proteins tend to have higher price tags. To show such values, FDA chose one of a number of possible biological criteria for protein—the PER, or *Protein Efficiency Ratio.* This method of assessment derives, in essence, from the first experiments which taught us that proteins differed in their usefulness to the body, that some amino acids were essential, and that the presence or absence of essential amino acids could mean life or death.

In these experiments—conducted by such pioneers as Osborne, Mendel, and Rose—animals were fed on individual proteins, such as those of corn, wheat, or milk. When single-source proteins proved inadequate and the animals sickened or failed to grow, the researchers knew that something was missing. By isolating and comparing the amino acids in the different proteins, the experimenters were able to learn which amino acids were essential and how much of each was needed.

In modern PER experiments to test the nutritive value of protein in a food, special diets are fed for four weeks to very young rats. All the other needed nutrients are present in this diet, but the sole source of protein is the test food.

Regularly during the experiment and at the end of the four weeks, the animals are weighed. The extent of their growth shows how well the test protein met their amino-acid needs. For example, in tests of the protein which FDA uses as its standard for high quality, the *casein* of milk, for each two grams of protein fed, there are five grams of weight gain. Thus, for each gram of protein, there are 2.5 grams of gain (five divided by two). So the PER of casein—found by dividing the amount of protein fed into the weight gain—is 2.5.

Foods which show as good nutritive value for protein as milk, or better, are classified as high in protein quality. So their U.S. RDA for protein is set at 45 grams. Foods which show lower nutritive values for protein, less than the PER of milk protein, are classified accordingly. The percentage of U.S. RDA supplied by a serving is based upon an assumed daily allowance of 65 grams. Foods for which the protein PER is less than 20 percent of those of casein (e.g., gelatin) may not be labeled as contributing to daily protein needs.

3. Chemical Scores for Proteins.

While the FDA method for showing protein quality works fairly well, it has weaknesses, as we saw at the end of Chapter Eight. The root of these weaknesses is that a person using the system to choose protein foods could get 100 percent of U.S. RDA but might not get enough of all essential amino acids.*

How much is enough? The RDA Committee of the Food and Nutrition Board reviewed the research on this question and came to the conclusion that our essential amino acid needs can be met by a rather small portion of our total protein intake: "For adult man it appears that only 20 percent of the total nitrogen requirement need be supplied from the indispensable amino acids, assuming they are in a well-balanced pattern."

In real terms, using the protein RDAs, we find that this 20 percent figure means that only some 12 grams of essential amino acids, or less than half an ounce, will meet the daily needs of most of us nicely. How well does a small serving of steak do in meeting this need? If we take some 3.5 ounces of meat cut from a T-bone steak, and add up the content of just its essential amino acids, we get a total of more than 9.5 grams. In other words, some 3.5 ounces of cooked steak yields much better than three-fourths of the essential amino acids for the day. Barely three ounces of cooked hamburger does almost as well—almost 9 grams.

A glass of milk, supplying about four more grams of essential amino acids, or a slice of cheese, offering a little less, would, when

---

*Nor does PER permit the quality of mixed proteins to be predicted.

added to the small meat serving, satisfy our daily need for these nutrients. This does not take into account any of the essential amino acids which are found liberally in grains or even vegetables.

Remember that, while plant-source foods do not have adequate proportions of *all* essential amino acids, many of them have most. So a U.N. (F.A.O.) method* for evaluating proteins, in order to suggest their contribution of essential amino acids, looks at those essential amino acids which are low in a food as *limiting.* In this way, the U.N. assigns a "chemical score" to such proteins, which is determined by the one most limiting essential amino acid. For example, wheat has only some 30 percent of the lysine it should have to make a well-balanced protein food. So wheat is given a chemical score of 30 percent. In practical terms, this means that, if you are going to get all your protein from wheat, you will need a little more than three times the total recommended total daily protein in order to get sufficient lysine.

So if you want to survive on wheat, you can see from food-composition tables that it will take a little more than three cups of wheat flour a day to do so.** In practical terms, of course, other foods would probably contribute, and it is unlikely that wheat would supply all your protein.

Do We Get Enough Essential Amino Acids?

By implication, this question has already been answered in more than one way; as a nation we certainly do. But to pin the answer down more closely, and to suggest how we can use tables of amino-acid content to judge diets, let us try another exercise. Let us compare the RDA figures for essential amino acids needed by a reference adult male with two other numbers—Phipard's calculations in 1950 of typical per capita amino-acid intake, and the amount of each essential amino acid contained in 3.5 ounces of medium-grade cooked hamburger. (If anything, the typical intake figures are higher than the ones we use, since meat consumption has increased.)

---

*Actually a method used by others, and at least as early as 1940.

**The baking of the flour would actually change the nutrient contributions; in particular, lysine contribution would be lowered a little.

Table 9-1.

Amino Acid	Adult Male Need	Supplied by 3.5 oz of Hamburger	Typical Per Capita Intake
Isoeucine	.84 grams	1.3 grams	5.2 grams
Leucine	1.12 grams	2.0 grams	8.0 grams
Lysine	.84 grams	2.2 grams	6.1 grams
Methionine	.70 grams	.62 grams	3.4 grams
Phenylalanine	1.12 grams	1.0 grams	4.6 grams
Threonine	.56 grams	1.1 grams	3.9 grams
Tyrptophan	.21 grams	.29 grams	1.2 grams
Valine	.96 grams	1.4 grams	5.5 grams
Histidine*	(unknown)		(unknown)

Keep in mind that a hamburger bun would add more protein, as would even the most highly processed french fries. And also note that this is only one serving of one rather cheap food. A less fatty meat serving would have provided more amino acids. Yet except for only two of the essential amino acids, the requirements are more than met.

The two essential amino acids not fully supplied by the hamburger patty are methionine and phenylalanine. If we look back to the preceding chapter, we will recall that these are the two amino acids which can be "spared" by non-essential amino acids—that in the presence of cystine and tyrosine, much less is needed of these two essentials.

So the fact is that a hamburger patty just about does it all, as far as essential amino acids are concerned. Add a slice of cheese to the burger, and all the requirements are exceeded for the entire day. These are adult male requirements, too, the largest requirements of any group, except for pregnant and lactating women.** And they include ample safety margins; one could probably survive well on less. There seems little question that an ordinary American diet easily meets amino acid requirements.

---

*The fact that histidine, previously thought to be essential only for children, is really also essential for adults, has only recently been learned. But since histidine appears to be liberal in most good protein sources, it may be assumed to be plentiful in normal diets.

**However, we should always keep in mind that larger people have somewhat larger needs.

Comparing Proteins for Quality.

Despite the fact the average American has no amino-acid shortage in his diet, the reality is that some Americans are not average. For example, some people have unusual tastes or beliefs which can lead them into amino-acid trouble.

As we have seen, not all good sources of protein are good sources of all necessary amino acids. Also the presence of proteins or of specific amino acids in a chemical analysis need not mean that the body is able to use all of them; by and large, animal-source foods supply protein in a form which is almost entirely usable, but as much as a third of the protein from some plant sources may be lost to waste, upon digestion.

Let us see how these factors may apply—if we compare our hamburger to the egg (considered to have the highest biological value of any common food protein), to dried beans, and to brown rice, which we may remember was almost the sole protein source of the Macrobiotic diet. We will compare for 100-gram (3.5 ounce) portions, in each case giving amino acid quantities in grams.

Table 9-2.

Amino Acids	Hamburger	Egg	Dried Bean (Cooked)	Brown Rice (Cooked)
Isoleucine	1.3	.85	.45	.12
Leucine	2.0	1.1	.67	.22
Lysine	2.2	.82	.58	.10
Methionine	.62	.40	.08	.05
Phenylalanine	1.0	.75	.43	.13
Threonine	1.1	.64	.34	.10
Tryptophan	.56	.21	.07	.03
Valine	.29	.95	.48	.18
Histidine	(unknown, but not of concern generally)			
Total Essential Amino Acids	9.91*	5.7*	3.1*	1.83*
Total Protein	25.	12.9	7.8	2.55
Calories in 100 grams	(257)	(162)	(118)	(119)

*Plus histidine values.

Plants Can Supply Protein, But . . .

We must remember that neither beans nor rice will, on digestion, yield *all* their protein to the body. For example, only some 80 percent of the bean protein would be used. So the apparent 7.8 grams of total protein will in reality be only about 6.2 grams in terms of true nutritive value.

We must also remember that we are comparing weights of the cooked food. Both beans and rice are much diluted with water in the cooking. We can see this on food labels and also in our table: the beans and rice in the 100-gram portions provide only about 120 calories. The hamburger is more than twice as caloric. Plant-source foods are bulky.

From these two facts, we learn a key principle of protein nutrition—that relatively large amounts of plant-source foods must be consumed to match the protein obtained from animal-sources. For example, 100 grams of brown rice is two-thirds of a cup in the cooked form. 100 grams of white beans make half a cup when cooked. So for the beans to supply the total protein of the hamburger would take approximately two full cups; for the rice it would take well over seven cups. (This is after the digestibility factor is taken into account.)

Much the same would be true if the computation were limited to just the essential amino acids, except that some of these are limited in the two vegetable foods. Note in the beans, for example, that there are only .08 grams of methionine in a 100-gram serving, against the adult need for .70 grams a day, or against the burger content of .62. So it would take almost five cups of beans to supply the RDA for methionine. Of course this amount can be eaten, but the eater had better be fond of beans, and, as we saw, the indigestible carbohydrate will give the intestinal bacteria a busy day.

In real terms, large amounts of these individual plant-source foods can supply adequate amino acids, but may not make for a very interesting diet—and may be susceptible to some of the other problems of nutrition. Consider the beans. The required amount would fill 1¼ quart jars and would add up to 1,100 calories.

Rice, because of its most limiting amino acid, lysine, would theoretically require more than five and one half cups. If we take into account incomplete protein digestibility, the amount grows larger. Our lysine need would require some seven cups, almost enough to fill two one-quart milk cartons, and would represent 1,250 calories.

Combining plant-source protein foods can reduce the amounts needed, but the rules of thumb for combination do not always work well. For example, it is common to group grains and legumes to relieve one another's amino-acid limitations. But in the case of beans and rice, we see that the limiting methionine of the beans is really not all that plentiful in rice. A high volume of the two is still needed.

Some Guides to Amino-Acid Limitations

Because it is not all that easy to analyze the amino-acid profiles of foods, here are some general cautions about the kinds of limited amino acids found in vegetable protein sources:

Table 9-3

Food	Limiting Amino Acids
Cereal grains and millets	Lysine and Threonine
Legumes (peas and beans)	Methionine, Tryptophan
Soybeans, Rice	Methionine
Sesame, Sunflower seeds	Lysine
Peanuts	Methionine, lysine, threonine
Green leafy vegetables	Methionine

Plainly, the hard-to-get amino acids follow a pattern, usually related to three key essentials, methionine, lysine, and tryptophan. So it is that, in the making of vegetable proteins (such as soy-based meat extenders or milks), or in seeking combinations of vegetable protein sources (as for those in the world who are short of protein), these three amino acids are the ones which receive most of the attention.

Technology has made possible the adding of such amino acids, rather cheaply, to such foods as the soy proteins and wheat. For example, a serious problem of protein malnutrition among the children of Hong Kong was alleviated by the addition of methionine to a soy "milk." A large segment of the population of Tunisia is receiving wheat which has been supplemented with lysine. And some of our own "high-protein" breakfast cereals are also supplemented with lysine.

Which Foods Have Most Essential Amino Acids?

The proportions of essential amino acids in foods have little meaning if the foods are not relatively rich sources of these nutrients. It may be worthwhile to glance at some representative foods which hold a goodly proportion of essential amino acids. Again, nitrogen serves as a gauge, through measurement of what part of the food's nitrogen derives from essentials. Note that this fraction rarely goes over one third.

Over 35 percent of total nitrogen from EAAs
Eggs and milk

Over 30 percent of total nitrogen from EAAs
Meat, fish, beans, peas, soybeans, sweet potato, spinach

Over 25 percent of total nitrogen from EAAs
Lentils, oats, cornmeal, cottonseed meal,
sesame seed meal, white potato, rice, cashews

Over 20 percent of total nitrogen from EAAs
Barley, wheat flour, peanuts, almonds

Bear in mind that these figures are meaningless unless we take into account what they are percentages of; that is, how much total protein we get from the food. For example, spinach fits into the over-thirty-percent group. A pound of spinach, raw, offers 14.5 grams of protein. This is really not a high concentration of protein. But the contribution of foods such as spinach can be important.

A pound of spinach is a lot. A cup of it weighs a little less than two ounces, so it would take eight cups of raw spinach to supply those 14.5 grams of protein, or about 31 cups to give us our daily adult male protein RDA. On the other hand, if we eat a generous serving of cooked spinach, one cup, we get over 5 grams of protein. And the quality is not all that bad. For our reference woman, that cup of spinach represents some 10 percent of her total daily protein. And it is because of such protein supplies in so many foods, each contributing a part of the daily need, if we eat a varied diet, that we need not overburden ourselves with expensive meats.

One 5.5 inch stalk of broccoli can give us some 3.6 grams of protein; nine brussels sprouts supply almost five; three-fourths of a cup of kale, cooked, gives us over four grams; five large mushrooms give us over three grams; a small baked potato gives us some four grams; a large tomato gives us a couple of grams. Important sources of protein? Not at all, if we eat just one of these. But if we follow all the other dietary injunctions for variety and balance in what we eat, it is easy to see that these "extra" foods as a group can be important contributors of protein.

It is also easy to see why vegetarians who eat liberally and variously from the vegetable and grain world survive and thrive. A cursory glance at the "protein" foods they consume may tell us that they are doomed to malnutrition. But a closer inspection, with careful attention to protein values, shows us that a full variety of foods from the vegetable world, with each food contributing its own profile of amino-acids, can easily keep us in good nitrogen balance.

Can Vegetarians Survive?

Of course they can. They simply need a little more knowledge than the carnivores. For the meat-eater, life is very simple in terms of getting adequate protein, as we have seen in our analysis of one rather modest beef burger. Since most of us thoroughly enjoy our meat, and since it does supply not only a full assurance of adequate protein, but like all food groups, its own particular coterie of other valuable nutrients, the safest shortcut recommendation for a good protein diet in a rich land is to eat meat, fish, and poultry.

On the other hand, the vegetarian must be careful to avoid nutrition faddism. Since he depends for his protein on an intermingling of foods, he at once becomes vulnerable if he narrows his diet overmuch. Among other things, the complete vegetarian (or *vegan*) must understand that meats are protein shortcuts; therefore, he cannot substitute any *single* food (possibly except for amino-acid supplemented vegetable proteins) for the meat portion of meals, unless he is prepared to do so in bulk quantities much greater than those common for servings of meats. He must think of protein as coming from his whole dietary, not just from one or two sources.

Unhappily, quite a few vegans do not understand this. They assign magical protein values to such foods as brown rice. (We have seen the quantities of rice needed to furnish essential amino acids—some 5.5 cups daily.) In this way, they walk a kind of protein tightrope. The narrow margin for error in such cases shows up in pregnancy, for example. A vegan woman, of reference size, needs some 48 grams of protein daily. Pregnant, her RDA jumps to 78 grams. Imagine how much more brown rice she would need to meet this new RDA.

There is little trouble, however, for the sensible *lacto-ovo* vegetarian, one who eats dairy products and eggs. For smallish amounts of these foods can close the amino-acid gaps. Two large eggs, for instance, can furnish the *whole* daily lysine RDA. Three glasses of fortified skim milk can meet the whole RDA for methionine. A little cheese, some textured vegetable protein, such as is now available in any supermarket, and the vegetarian protein problem is solved. It is commonly fortified with limiting amino acids and bolstered with the vitamin B-12 which in nature must be taken from some sort of animal food.

Proteins and Economics for Meat Eaters.

Since protein is the most expensive macronutrient, it offers a particularly important key to sensible consumerism. On the most obvious level, the person who believes that his health or the development of his muscles depend upon a one-pound T-bone for dinner, will pay dearly for his nutritional ignorance. As a related source of economic waste, it is common to find unwarranted enthusiasm for the prominent listing of proteins on food labels: the public overconcern with getting enough has led certain food marketers to manipulate advertising, labels, and package instructions to create some protein illusions.

Cheese provides a good example. It is correctly associated with protein in the public mind. A little goes a long way—though it may not go far enough in certain products which actually do not contain much of it. Let us look at two examples, lifted almost at random from a frozen-food display. One is a *cauliflower in cheese sauce,* costing 62 cents. Its label shows 10 percent of protein U.S. RDA per serving. (One of the virtues of cheese for the labeler is that it is a high-quality protein source, so that U.S. RDA is only 45 grams.)

At a glance, this food seems like a nice protein booster for the meal. But closer inspection shows that the nutrition information is based upon a serving of one cup, which is eight ounces. The whole package is only ten ounces.

So it would take three packages, costing $1.86, to supply a person with a third of protein U.S. RDA, an absolute minimum for dinner. For this amount of money one could buy enough meat for three or four people, able to supply each with the bulk of his essential amino acids for the day.

The same company offers a rice and peas combination, shown in a large bowl on the package, but labeled in smaller print as a "side dish." The label shows that a serving contains 6 percent of U.S. RDA for protein. But the small print shows that this package holds only "one and three-eighths servings." Is this what the consumer really expects? Is a serving, as actually used, going to supply a significant part of a day's needed protein?

Undoubtedly, the consumer is paying for the adding of a few frozen peas and some seasoning to a little rice, just as he pays for the cheese sauce in the first example. The flavor may be worthwhile, though it is hard to imagine to whom. But from a nutritional point of view, such packaging and labeling warrant real caution.

The same principles apply to many a convenience main dish—as was suggested in the earlier discussion of "helpers" and packaged macaroni and cheese.

Of Low Incomes and Hot Dogs.

When meat prices shot up not long ago, many families reported that they were forced to depend upon "cheaper" meats for protein, while filling in with "starches" such as beans, peas, potatoes and noodles. The cheaper meats were hot dogs and bologna, sausages, and such hammy preparations as *Spam.* Let us examine these bargains in terms of protein nutrition.

A typical frankfurter (ten to a pound) at $1.19 per package costs about 12 cents. It provides some 5.6 grams of protein, so each gram of protein costs about 2.1 cents. Now look at a roast of beef, the sort of meat which poor Americans feel they can no longer afford to serve. Assume that this roast sells for $1.69 per pound. Using USDA's figure for the weight of cooked meat provided by each raw and boned pound (11.7 ounces), one computes that each of those cooked ounces costs 14.4 cents.

USDAs handbook of food composition shows that this amount of cooked roast provides 78.1 grams of high quality protein. Thus each ounce provides 6.7 grams of protein; each gram of protein costs 14.4 cents (the cost per ounce) divided by 6.7 grams, or 2.1 cents, just about the same as the cost of the protein in a hot dog. Looking at the two protein sources from a slightly different point of view, about a quarter-pound serving of roast costs some 50 cents and offers some 23.5 grams of protein. To get the same protein takes 4.2 hot dogs.

But though these two foods have some equivalence as protein sources, they differ in other respects. Consider calories. A cooked pound of roast supplies about 1,150 calories, or some 98 calories per ounce, and our 3.5 ounce serving offers about 350 calories with its protein. Each frankfurter provides some 140 calories in its 1.6 ounces. And since it takes 4.2 frankfurters to furnish the 23.5 grams of protein in our serving of roast, they give us almost 600 calories. Why so much more? Because the franks hold so much more fat, in common with bologna and most other "luncheon meats."

The conclusion of the practical nutritionist? Frankfurters are a bargain—in fats and calories, not in protein.

This bargain, according to one study by a manufacturer of sausage casings, is served in 95 percent of all U.S. homes. The "heavy user" is defined as a household that eats 20 or more hot dogs a month. Heaviest users are "child-oriented mothers representing 32 percent of all American households and buying 41 percent of the hot dogs." One group of these heavy users is of below average income with little interest in cooking. But another is the "young, fairly well-educated urban mother who shops carefully," and the third is the "family-centered suburbanite, well-educated, with above-average income and a casual approach to life."

Some Protein Rules of Thumb

Since protein of high quality is the most expensive item on the household food budget, it pays to look closely at the *amounts* we really need. And it pays to look closely at how much apparent bargain sources provide. In general, that close look will tell us that the real bargains in nutritional terms can be the tastiest of meats—if one recognizes that small servings will do for health.

To repeat, the protein recommendations of the Food and Nutrition Board do not establish *minimals,* but rather generous safety margins. The most liberal nutritionists commend to us a diet in which 40 to 50 percent of the protein RDA ought to be of high quality proteins. In most cases, one *small* serving of meat and a glass of milk or a slice of cheese will meet those liberal suggestions. The rest is provided by common foods which are not usually thought of as protein sources.

Will extra protein mean extra health? We have no reason to believe so. The wide safety margins of RDAs include plenty for growth and for muscle building. The actual consumption of high-quality protein is so great, we shall see, that even the average pregnant woman in the U.S. is already consuming enough to take care of her special needs.* As we have seen, our needs for protein (actually the amino-acid demands of the cells as determined by our chromosomes) are basically dictated by needs for tissue building and repair, and are not related to physical activity. The RDA Committee flatly states that, in looking at RDAs, "no increment" need be added for work.

Recently, however, in what is sadly a typical brochure of nutrition information for consumers, *Citibank* observed: "Your body's need for protein cannot be overestimated." It certainly can be. As just one example, probably the primary reason why our RDAs for calcium are now set at *twice* those of most of the world is that we consume so much protein. The exaggeration of any nutrient in our diet has an impact on the diet as a whole; eat more protein and you need more calcium. (Protein wastes are excreted, carrying calcium along.)

There are other effects as well. For much of the time, when we reach out for more protein, thinking to benefit, we lard our food with fat. In our hot dog, as an example, each one provides, along with its 5.6 grams of protein, 112 calories of fat. Through the ages the rich man's diet has been a diet rich in fat.

Being among the nutritionally rich of the world, we need to understand that we are fat eaters, too. We must know something of the possible penalties for this characteristic. In the process we shall see that if the food-rich and the food-poor of the world could share their traditional meals, both might be better fitted to survive.

---

*Note that this is an average. The HANES survey shows some shortage among very low-income women. Pregnancy calls for a kind of dietary check-up on the food habits of all women.

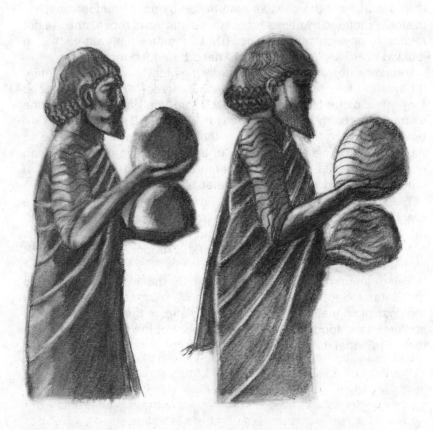

Fats supply much of the richness and flavor of food and so have been highly prized from earliest time. *Bringing Tributes of Butter to King Xerxes, Persian relief, fifth century, B.C.*

chapter 10

MYSTERIES AND SIMPLICITIES OF FATS

The oldtimers of the Hudson's Bay Company, who knew the vagaries of the far Arctic north very well, called it "rabbit starvation." And anthropologist-explorer Vilhjalmur Stefansson, who left Harvard in 1906 to live and hunt with Arctic tribes, explained that this name was used " . . . because it was commonest among rabbit hunters, though it could occur . . . in a caribou country when the game was lean."[1]

But Stefansson himself described the problem as "fat hunger." He tells us that, "After the last scrap of fat is gone from the diet of a hunting people, headache and diarrhea will start. Fur traders believed that death from fat starvation would come in from four to eight weeks . . . When traders heard of rabbit starvation among a group of Athapascans, they tried to remedy it, usually by sending them some bacon or lard."

Stefansson also reports that, while this problem was common

among the Athapascans (a widespread group of Indian tribes who shared common language roots), it was rare among the inland Eskimos. Why? Because " . . . inlanders bought pokes of seal oil from the coastal people which they carried with them in case of shortage." He elaborates that the Eskimo families began the winters with 200-pound sealskin bags, filled with white whale oil, seal oil, ". . . and also a little polar bear fat."

The true nature of the condition of the "fat hungry" Indians is obscure. But in speculating about them, we can observe some basic principles of fats in nutrition.

FAT IS NOT EVIL

In recent years, *lipids*—the appropriate scientific name for the whole family of fatty substances—have fallen into poor repute. In this book we have repeatedly noted the higher caloric value of fats, the relationship of those calories to obesity and to the rising fat content of the Western diet, and we have implied that most of our diets contain too much lipid.

Medicine warns the public of the possible relationship between dietary fat and disease. For example, a recent American Heart Association summary to physicians,[2] a large pamphlet with each page boldly bordered in black, cites a statement (rendered jointly by the AMA's Council on Foods and Nutrition and the Food and Nutrition Board) to the effect that: "The average level of the plasma lipids of most American men and women is undesirably high, and that reasonable means must be adopted to reduce the conditions that contribute to coronary heart disease."[3] In similar fashion, the cardiologists urge that we reduce our consumption of dietary fats, especially those of certain special kinds.

We see here the genesis of a public attitude. And for the unwary it can be misleading. For any evils which may be associated with dietary fats are related to excessive use, not to harm in the nutrients themselves. And lipids should be seen first as essential nutrients.

Indian Hunger and EFAs

We really cannot say whether the Athapascan Indians whose game grew scarce and lean actually suffered from fat starvation. But we shall see, first of all, that a certain amount of "essential fatty acids"

(EFAs) are indispensable to life, and that, like essential amino acids, these must be included in our food.

While the role of essential fatty acids in nutrition is very basic—they are needed for such jobs as the building of the membranes of cells and as constituents of many fundamental chemicals—our total need for them is small. The Food and Nutrition Board recommends that EFAs supply about one to two percent of our total calories. This suggests a need for only some three to six grams per day.

EFAs are scarce in most meats. A three-ounce piece of cooked rump roast contains only 0.5 grams of EFA, compared to 23.2 grams of total fat, EFAs representing about a fiftieth of the fat total. Beef, being a domesticated-animal meat, tends to be fatter than game. Hungry game has still less fat. So perhaps the Athapascans, with little access to plant foods in hard times, did suffer from some sort of fat shortage.

The whale, seal, and fish oils of the Eskimos would indeed have been able to supply some EFA. Fish, sought by the Eskimos, have a much higher proportion of EFA than do meats. For example, a piece of herring weighing less than two ounces (50 grams), provides 1.4 grams of EFA with its 7.6 grams of total fat, about a fifth of the fat total. A quarter to half a pound of fairly oily fish would probably have met the EFA daily need.

The richest source of these essential fatty acids, however, are most vegetable oils.

Fats Carry Vitamins, Too

Another speculation about the Athapascan illness stems from the fact that when the game were short of feed, plant foods would have been scarce for the Indians as well. This could indicate a shortage of some micronutrients.

But even without this assumption, it is possible that the Indians had been cut off from some vitamins. For vitamins A, D, E and K are "fat-soluble." That is, they accompany fats in foods. (Vitamin A can be obtained from low-fat foods, but this, we shall see, is a special circumstance which is due to the fact that the body is able to convert another chemical into vitamin A.) The Eskimo oils would be good sources of fat-soluble vitamins. Polar bear liver, for example, is one of the richest known sources in all the food world. But these Indians thought the livers of the animals they hunted were fit only for their dogs.

So while we have no sure answers about the Athapascan malady, they serve to suggest some of the ways in which fats play a broad nutritional role. And we have seen a little of why the realistic nutritionist does not regard them necessarily as dietary villains.

But the Indian malnutrition can symbolize our view of fats in still another important way. For just as we seem to have as many questions as answers in trying to explain the Athapascan deaths, so do we lack firm knowledge about much of the role of lipids in our own nutrition and health.

WHAT IS A FAT?

Fats—or we should really remember that the scientific classification is lipids—are a group of chemical compounds which do not dissolve in water, but do dissolve in organic solvents (solvents which have a chemical backbone of carbon), such as ether or chloroform. To put it simply, fats added to water break up into globules, as on the surface of chicken soup, leading to the classic statement that oil and water do not mix. Similarly, if one dribbles gravy on one's clothing when the airplane bumps, water will not sponge it away. Instead one must use cleaning fluid, or an organic solvent, or at the very least, some alcoholic beverage (don't try wine).

Chemically, lipids are structures which may remind us of carbohydrates. For they are made of carbon, hydrogen and oxygen. But the lipid looks as if almost all the oxygen is missing.

This missing oxygen is a necessary component for life. For recall that the burning of fuel is a process of oxidation. In a sense, fats are less oxidized than are sugars, which therefore have a lesser potential for "burning" as fuel. Witness the crude oil lamps used in so many cultures for millennia, really nothing much more than dishes of oil with some sort of wick. From Aladdin, to the Roman catacombs, to Colonial America, these were the basic lighting utensils. It is hard to imagine lamps filled with sugar.

The lipid family is a large one, with some of the same capability for variation which is characteristic of both proteins and carbohydrates. But the lipids in foods nearly all (perhaps 98 percent) belong to the same sub-family of chemicals, called the *triglycerides.* The name derives from the common basic structure of these compounds. For they are each composed of a molecule of *glycerol,* which is linked to three *fatty acids.*

Glycerol is a fairly familiar substance, which has the household name of *glycerine.* Indeed, it is probably more familiar to most consumers than they suspect, since glycerol is one of the most basic ingredients of the creams and greases which are rubbed into so many hands and faces, mixed with colors and spread on the lips, or worked into hair for "styling."

Chemically, glycerol looks like the top half of an ordinary glucose molecule:

```
       Glycerol                        Glucose
          H                               H
          |                               |
      H—C—OH                          H—C—OH
          |                               |
      H—C—OH                          H—C—OH
          |                               |
      H—C—OH                          H—C—OH
          |                               |
          H                          HO—C—H
                                          |
                                      H—C—OH
                                          |
                                      H—C—
                                          ‖
                                          O
```

This similarity is nutritionally significant in several ways.

First, we can see that glycerol is the part of a fat which the body can break off and use as carbohydrate for energy. And since glycerol is quite a small part of the total fat molecule, we can get an idea of why, on the average, only some 10 percent of food fats can be used in this way.

The second significance suggests the origin of fats—in plants. Just by looking at the structure of glycerol one can imagine how it can be made by a plant in much the same way sugars are made. Finally, it is clear that glycerol (like glucose) is not a compact fuel. The quality of compact energy in fats is due to the three fatty acids which the glycerol holds.

Let us make a comparison between glucose and *caproic acid,* a simple fatty acid found in butter and coconut oil:

<pre>
        Caproic acid   Glucose
        (a fatty acid)

             H   H
             | |
          H—C—H   H—C—OH
             | |
          H—C—H   H—C—OH
             | |
          H—C—H   H—C—OH
             | |
          H—C—H   HO—C—H
             | |
          H—C—H   H—C—OH
             | |
         HO—C   H—C
             ‖   ‖
             O   O
</pre>

Notice that the glucose molecule contains five more oxygen atoms, suggesting at once the greater "burnability" of the fatty acid. And as a final bit of chemistry, for the moment, notice also the COOH group at the bottom of the fatty acid. This is the structure which allows a fatty acid to be linked to glycerol, or broken away.

A Chemical Recipe for Fats.

The COOH group at the bottom of the drawing of the fatty acid is the same as the acid group which we found in amino acids, and it provides the combining point of the fatty acid. The process looks like this, with our fatty acid turned on its side to make the joining clearer:

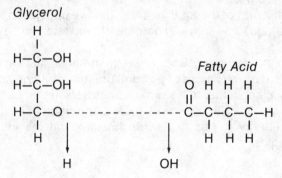

The OH is broken from the fatty acid at the same time that an H is broken from the glycerol. Of course, we get HOH, or water. Once again, *hydrolysis* is the key, this time to making or breaking *triglycerides.*

To make triglycerides, we simply add two more fatty acids to the glycerol, by the same process, each time freeing a new molecule of water. To take triglycerides apart, in digestion for example, we simply put the molecules of water back, and then the glycerol and the fatty acids are able to stand separately.

Not All Lipids Are Triglycerides

Triglycerides are examples of *simple lipids.* That is, they are made of a combination of fatty acids and an alcohol (glycerol). When certain other alcohols are substituted for the glycerol, we get *waxes,* which are better for making drawers slide than for eating. Some tiny amounts of waxes are, however, found in the world of edible vegetables.

One can also guess that, among the simple lipids, if there are *tri*-glycerides, there may also be combinations of glycerol with just one or two fatty acids, instead of three. Indeed there are; we will see that they abound during fat digestion. They are also familiar names on food packages, as the *mono-* and *di-glycerides.* They are used as additives (emulsifiers), for purposes such as enhancing texture in bakery goods, and are no more threatening in a cake mix than they are in our own intestines, where they are plentiful as a part of the natural digestive process after every meal.

Not All Lipids Are Fats

While there can be a tendency to think of lipids as just so much fuel, the fact is that they, like proteins and carbohydrates, are also involved in the more exotic chemistry of life. This leads us to two more classes of lipids.

The first class is produced when simple lipids combine with other chemicals, to make *compound lipids.* Only small amounts of these compounds are found in our food. But large numbers of them are made in the body and used in important ways. Generally they are named for the chemicals which join the simple lipids; *glycolipids* are combinations with carbohydrates; *lipoproteins* are made with proteins; *phospholipids* are made with phosphorus compounds. We shall see more of these.

The other class is made up of *derived lipids*. As the name implies, these are chemicals which are made from the simple and compound lipids, usually when they are broken down by hydrolysis. To get some idea of what potent factors these derived lipids can be in life, consider just one group of them, deriving from *sterols.*

One lipid in this group is *7-dehydrocholesterol.* This is the stuff found in the fat beneath our skin, which when irradiated by sunlight produces vitamin D-3*. Another is *cholesterol,* the great dietary concern of so many who suffer from heart disease. And to draw the picture just a little more broadly, we should know that cholesterol plays important roles in the brain, the nervous system, sexual secretions, and in digestion. Sterol-derived chemicals also take part in the all-important hormones produced by the adrenal glands.

We can see that lipids, like the other macronutrients, enter into the whole chemical breadth of life, that they are as vital building blocks as are the amino acids.

HOW MUCH FAT SHOULD WE EAT?

The fact that we require only tiny amounts of essential fatty acids does not mean that we should limit our total intake to anything like this quantity. As we have already suggested, the basic fuel from food is largely some mix of carbohydrate and fat. And the proportions of each are largely determined by the popular eating habits, and the affluence, of each culture.

Some simple mathematics, coupled with some basic knowledge of food composition, can help us to analyze the balance of fat, protein, and carbohydrate in our diets. Let us assume that a day's food provides about 2,500 calories, with an RDA for protein at about 60 grams. (These numbers are a little high for people under about 150 pounds, and a little low for bigger people.) At four calories per gram, about 10 percent of the diet, or about 240 calories, will have to come from protein.

---

*This is the form of vitamin D which we make ourselves. When we see vitamin D on labels, it may be shown as coming from "irradiated ergosterol," a chemical derived from plants.

Low-fat Eating

Nutritionists frequently refer to the fact that many Orientals and Africans get 80 percent of their diets in carbohydrates and only about 10 percent in fats, and that these people seem to get along nutritionally very well. One might wonder whether we should also try to stay within similar limits, restricting fat intake to 10 percent of our daily 2,500 calories (for the RDA reference man). But let us see how this squares with the realities of our own food tastes and habits.

If 250 calories are left for fats, and if fats offer some 9 calories to the gram, then such a diet would have less than 28 grams of fat. Two small hot dogs supply 23 grams of fat, as does a cooked, moderately lean 4-oz hamburger. A 10-oz T-bone steak gives us 149 grams of fat. A tablespoon of peanut butter has more than 8 grams. A tablespoon of mayonnaise provides over 11 grams, a tablespoon of french dressing almost 10 grams—and you might try limiting yourself to a tablespoon of dressing in your next salad. A cup of whole milk is 8.5 grams of fat—even the "low-fat" has about 5 grams. A very small pat of butter, less than a fifth of an ounce, gives you some 5 grams (and you might try this amount, one level *tea*spoon, on your next slice of thick French bread.) One chicken thigh, scarcely more than two ounces, has about 7 grams of fat, and a single egg has almost 6 grams.

Ten-percent-fat diets are used therapeutically, but they are not consumed with much joy. (On the other hand, if they are followed, they are very effective for weight reduction.)

Now You See Fat—Now You Don't

We thus see how common fats are in the American diet—without any mention of the deep-fat fryer, or such traditions as cookies, pies, frozen creams, and chocolate coatings—and we can learn a basic concept about fats and foods. It is that, in general, only some 40-50 percent of our dietary fat is visible.

There is a tendency to think "fat" only as one adds oil to salad dressing, butters bread, puts sour cream onto a baked potato, trims the chop on one's plate, or notices the greasy residue on last night's dishes. The vast bulk of our dietary fat is concealed, or semi-concealed, as in the nice marbling of the roast. And in truth, it can take quite a sensitive palate to distinguish appreciable differences of hidden fat among different servings of meat, cookies, cheese and crackers, and so forth.

One of the virtues of labeling is that it can identify those differences. Comparing fat contents, gram for gram, can be extremely helpful in making food choices.

The tabulation below, derived from an FDA publication, groups foods by fat content. Keep in mind that the percentages shown are based on *weight*, not calories, of fat. The caloric percentage is higher, of course, because each gram of fat offers more energy than the same weight of other nutrients. (Remember, too, that much of the weight of many foods is in water.)

More than 90 percent fat
Salad and cooking oils and fats, or lard.

More than 80 percent fat
Butter and margarine.

More than 70 percent fat
Mayonnaise, macadamia nuts and pecans.

More than 50 percent fat
Walnuts, dried unsweetened coconut, almonds,
bacon, and baking chocolate.

More than 30 percent fat
Broiled loin steaks, spareribs, broiled pork
chops, cheddar and cream cheeses, potato chips,
french dressing, and chocolate candy.

More than 20 percent fat
Pot roast, lamb chops, frankfurters, lean ground
beef, most cookies.

More than 10 percent fat
Most broiled fish and chicken, crabmeat, cottage
cheese, beef liver, creamed soups, sherbet.

A Fat American Day

To see how fats can add up, especially from hidden sources, let us hypothesize a day's eating for an American man with a taste for fatty foods. It might go like this:

Breakfast

Food Portion	*Fat in Grams*
A half a cup of orange juice	0.3
Two scrambled eggs	16.6
Three slices of broiled bacon (medium thick)	11.7
Two homemade biscuits, 2 in. in diameter	9.6
One tablespoon of butter or margarine	11.5
Two cups of coffee, with one Tbsp. cream (half and half)	1.4
Breakfast Total	51.5

Morning Snack

Two cake doughnuts (about 2 oz. each)	21.6
Two cups of coffee with half and half	1.4
Snack total	23.0

Lunch

Fast-food "quarter-pound (raw) burger	25.0
Hamburger bun	2.2
One tablespoon of 1000-island dressing	8.0
French fries (about 2 oz.)	2.3
Two cups of commercial chocolate drink (made with ice milk)	27.0
Lunch total	64.5

Afternoon break

Cola drink	—
Four cookies (two-inch sandwich-type)	9.0
Afternoon break total	9.0

Dinner

Pre-dinner snack with cocktail	
Two ounces cashew nuts, 28 kernels	26.0
Twenty potato chips	16.0
Salad with 3 Tbsp. blue cheese dressing	23.5
Chuck roast, 6 oz. piece	32.6
Two Tbsp. brown gravy	7.0
Top-of-the-stove stuffing (instead of potatoes)	10.0
Frozen green peas	.5
Slice of pecan pie	31.6
with 4 oz. vanilla ice cream	7.0
One cup of coffee with half and half	1.8
1 cloverleaf commercial roll, (one oz.)	3.0
1 level teaspoon of butter	3.8
Dinner total	162.8
Total of fats for the day	310.4 grams

Is this intake exaggerated? Judge for yourself. At nine calories per gram, the *fats alone* yield 2,794 calories, rather a lot of fuel—and the total calories in the listed food, when those from protein and carbohydrate are included, are much higher. For a large, very active person this could provide about the right amount of energy.* The question is whether he is wise to get so many of the calories in fat.

The Temperate Fat-Eater's Diet

While our sample diet provides far more total calories than most of us eat, close examination, especially of each meal as a separate entity, shows us that the general pattern of food consumption tends to be characteristic of our society. There are both cultural and economic reasons for this. For one thing, fat content is closely related to flavor. Even the flavoring chemicals in fruits and vegetables are commonly contained in droplets of oils. Fats tend to take up and absorb flavors. The smokey barbecue savor is largely the result of the burning of fat and the absorption of some of the smoke into the remaining fat.

There are other factors which favor fats: They are still relatively cheap in our economy; they are particularly satisfying; and cooking in fat is fast. These are particularly important matters in the "fast food" world. As a nation, we eat a third of our meals in commercial establishments, where every penny of cost and every minute of time count far more than they do in home cooking. Saving a cent on a burger means little to you and me, but much to McDonald's.

In nutritional terms, this high-fat pattern is extremely meaningful. Our fatty day does not hold an enormous *bulk* of food. We confront again the caloric compactness of fats. The one-ounce cloverleaf roll in the meal plan has *twice* the fat of the one-ounce slice of bread, and hence more calories.

This *caloric density* in fatty foods helps to circumvent bodily mechanisms which would limit our energy intake. How? Remember that, as far as we know, these mechanisms work partly by reacting to changes in blood values. Since fats leave the stomach slowly, have relatively little bulk for filling up the stomach (another warning signal to the appetite mechanism), and cannot get into the circulation until

*The dinner is analyzed in detail, for other nutrients, in Chapter Twelve.

they reach the small intestine, we can take in a lot of fat calories before our body tells us to stop.

If you doubt this, think about nuts. A handful of peanuts, even if you do not have a very big hand, can easily be two tablespoons, or more than 160 calories. And this does not seem like much food if you are at a party and waiting until nine o'clock for dinner to be served. The macadamia nut provides an even more impressive example. Though no bigger than a couple of peanuts, the average macadamia nut contains almost two grams of fat—a mere dozen amount to some 220 calories, but weigh only an ounce.

Now compare this to a relatively fat-free food, such as mustard greens. (A somewhat ludicrous comparison can help illustrate a principle.) 220 calories of mustard greens are more than seven half-cup servings, cooked, weighing 25 times as much as the dozen nuts. Think of how much more aware you would be of three and a half cups of cooked mustard greens as a before-dinner snack.

Like most nuts, macadamias are quite good sources of iron, and our 12 nuts give us 0.6 mg. of this mineral. But the same caloric value of mustard greens provided 12.6 mg. The nuts have 16 mg. of calcium; the greens have almost 1,000. Nuts are pretty good protein sources, and our 12 give us 2.8 grams. But while greens are not normally thought of for protein, the huge amount represented by 220 calories gives us 15.4 grams of protein—along with a slather of B vitamins, enough vitamin C to meet adult male RDAs for seven and a half days, and enough vitamin A for ten days.

The comparison is hardly realistic. But when we deal in realistic quantities, the nutritive contribution is still impressive (and the relative values of the two foods become even clearer). For the normal serving of the greens, half a cup, obviously makes genuinely important contributions of important nutrients—for example, our vitamin A for the day and some to spare. Yet by removing two rather small macadamias from the day's menu we make room for the half cup (31 calories) of the greens.

When one stops to think about it, the moral is rather appalling. So little fat-laden food can displace such an abundance of nutritionally-rich food. Assuming that our intake of calories tends to be fairly constant, such items as the two small nuts will often take the caloric place of the greens—as will many, many other fatty foods, such as less than a teaspoon of salad dressing, or an extra teaspoon of butter or margarine.

Excessive fats, repeatedly chosen for the day's food, can have very real and very great negative impact on the nutritive qualities of our dietary. And often these choices are not even consciously made. We reach for a little more flavor and get a little more fat.

It takes only a little knowledge and a little thought to moderate this pattern. The temperate fat-eater gets a better diet as a rule. So it is that in recent years nutritionists have begun to advocate a modest reduction in fats. In a moment, we shall see some simple ways this is done. But let us first look at another possible reason for doing it.

Fats and the Healthy Heart

One of the deepest, and also one of the most confused, popular nutritional concerns of our day is the possible relationship between the fats we eat and diseases of the heart and blood vessels. While there are many unanswered questions about this relationship, there are some practical matters of food choice which are quite clear. The first involves the effect of high fat consumption on *atherosclerosis,* the roughening and thickening of the blood vessels, complicated by deposits of fatty substances in these vital canals.

Well over 800,000 Americans are killed every year by heart attacks, strokes, and related disorders. Actually, far more deaths are probably involved, because of the endless deleterious effects of circulatory problems upon so many body systems. Millions more survive but are handicapped to some extent. The yearly medical bill is in the tens of billions; the human costs, of course, cannot be measured. What, for example, is a case of premature senility worth?

Atherosclerosis is the precursor of this plague. Narrowing vessels not only force the heart to work harder at its pumping, but they can shut down supplies of oxygen and nutrients carried in the blood. Clot formation can close the pinched passageways entirely. When this happens in one of the main vessels which feed the heart, we have the dramatic conclusion of the heart attack. But many other less dramatic events in the circulation can also lead to suffering, crippling, and death.

What causes atherosclerosis? No one really knows. In part, it may be a natural concomitant of aging. But in some people, it is as though their aging were speeded up.

Why do some people's blood vessels deteriorate in this more rapid way? There are many factors, and again, heredity appears to be foremost. Each of these factors (carefully elicited from population studies, such as the classic Framingham, Massachusetts Study) implies a greater risk of accelerated atherosclerosis and heart attack. The risk grows if one is male, aging, has ancestors who had early heart attacks or strokes, if one smokes, has high blood pressure, gets little exercise, has a competitive kind of personality and lives with pressure, is obese, or has diabetes. Put a pattern of these together, and the risk rises dramatically.

For more than a generation, dietary fat intake, and the ways in which one's body deals with this fat, have been considered by many thoughtful scientists to be other factors. The evidence is extremely complex, as is the physiology involved. The arguments, of which we shall see a little, rage back and forth. We do not yet have a certain answer.

Then why do so many press so hard for dietary change? In part, the answer is, because elevated levels of fatty substances in the blood have been found to be a risk factor—and because diet is one of the few things we can really change.

The plea for reduction of total fat intake is related to the fact that atherosclerotic vessels and clots are fatty, and the high fat consumption sends high levels of fat through the blood. It is also related in an obvious way to obesity, which in turn is related to high blood pressure and the progress of diabetes, as well as to patterns of physical exercise.

How Much Should We Reduce Fats?

Considering the other nutritional problems which are definitely involved in excessive fat consumption, the Heart Association urgings for reduced total fats seem reasonable indeed to most nutritionists. And that reduction is not as great as many think. In its "prudent diet" concept—which, as the name implies, is based on the idea that although much information is still lacking, the prudent person would use some caution—the Heart Association recommends that fat intake be limited to 35 percent of our calories, with a corresponding increase in carbohydrate.

How painful is such restriction? Assume that a reference man consumes 2,500 calories, and that, rather typically, about 45 percent of this is from fat. That is 1,125 calories of fat, or 125 grams a day. 35 percent would be 875 fat calories daily, or a little less than 100 grams. The difference is less than an ounce, 28 grams, or 250 calories of daily fat.

Look back at our fat day again. One ounce of cashew nuts instead of two before dinner would have saved 9 grams, and one ounce of potato chips would have saved 8 grams. Hold back about a third of the salad dressing, and the deed is about done. It can be even simpler. Instead of six ounces of the roast, three would supply plenty of protein and save 31 grams of fat. Fish for dinner would have done the job handsomely.

Bread instead of biscuits, a lower-fat coffee cake instead of doughnuts, milk instead of cream in the coffee, a little more restraint in butter or margarine, the wider use of fruits and vegetables, a fruit pie instead of the pecan, low-fat or skim milk instead of the chocolate beverage, a cheese sandwich instead of the burger (or perhaps chicken salad, or tuna, bacon and tomato or turkey), potatoes instead of the fatty convenience stuffing—these sorts of changes, in modest combinations, would have brought the fat content down, and also paved the way for the inclusion of some missing nutrients.

To reduce fats to a nutritionally desirable level means removing the equivalent of about two tablespoons of oil from the typical daily diet, leaving perhaps eight tablespoons. We really do not have to sacrifice our favorite foods. We merely have to become a little fat-wise and fat-conscious.

If these fat calories are eased from the diet, moreover, and replaced with complex carbohydrate foods in variety—grains, fruits and vegetables—there are some automatic benefits. The diet becomes much bulkier, and total calories are likely to fall. Such a bulky diet, somewhat limited in fats, is a great aid to weight control. And as we shall see in detail, this shift in dietary balance tends automatically to give us more of those vitamins and minerals which are most commonly lacking in our society.

UNDERSTANDING THE FATS IN FOODS

When you stop to think about it, you realize that you can tell a good deal about food fats by their appearance. For example, cooking oil looks quite different from pork fat, and such differences count in cooking. We observe that the fat of bacon, taken from the refrigerator, is white and firm between the lean streaks. As we cook the bacon, pools of clear liquid appear. We pour some off into a container, and because the fat holds the smoky bacon flavor so well, we may elect to fry an egg in the rest. By the time we have eaten the egg, we look into the container and see that the clear liquid is once again a firm white solid. We have made some important observations which help to explain the chemistry of fats, of how they are made, digested, absorbed, and used.

Fat and Some Simplicities of Saturation

Before we can understand the digestive fate of fats, we must know a little about the chemistry of saturation. For our purposes we can assume that virtually all food fats are triglycerides, made of glycerol and three fatty acids. Because glycerol is always the same, differences between triglycerides are accounted for by differences among the fatty acids.

One simplicity of fats, long a relief to chemistry students, is that they do not get their variety, as carbohydrates and proteins do, by chaining and unchaining into long skeins. Triglyceride molecules tend to stay rather small and discreet. Look back at our illustrated model of caproic acid (p. 216) and note that this fatty acid has a skeleton only six carbons long. For the most part, the fatty acids in foods rarely average more than 20 carbons. Yet through small changes in form, and through different combinations of three different fatty acids with each glycerol, triglycerides can be chemical chameleons. The fat in cow's milk, for example, has been estimated to be capable of offering some 125,000 different triglycerides.

This extreme variability in small molecules begins to explain why we probably know less of the chemistry of fat than of other macronutrients—especially since, everywhere we look in life, we tend to find these jumbled mixtures.

We can, however, observe that, at room temperature, certain fats are liquid and others are solid. And this reflects a basic difference in fatty acids. The solid fats, as in bacon, are predominantly *saturated fatty acids;* the liquid fats, such as salad oil, are predominantly *unsaturated fatty acids.*

Of course, every shopper knows about unsaturated fatty acids—or was it *poly*unsaturated?—and that there is something good—or was it bad?—and more expensive about them. Aren't they why we buy the corn oil margarine—or was it safflower—if we really love our families? Anyway, they have something to do with the natural peanut butter— or with whether it is hydrogenated—so that it doesn't separate—or does it? And the ad said that is better for you, or was it worse?

Happily, the essential chemistry of all this is really less complicated than the simplistic advertising. A saturated fatty acid is one in which all the positions for hydrogen (H) are filled, as in *stearic* acid, common in meats:

```
    H   H   H   H   H   H   H   H   H   H   H   H   H   H   H   H   H  OH
    |   |   |   |   |   |   |   |   |   |   |   |   |   |   |   |   |   |
H — C — C — C — C — C — C — C — C — C — C — C — C — C — C — C — C — C — C
    |   |   |   |   |   |   |   |   |   |   |   |   |   |   |   |   |   ||
    H   H   H   H   H   H   H   H   H   H   H   H   H   H   H   H   H   O
```

An unsaturated fatty acid is one in which two or more of the carbons do not hold all the possible hydrogen, as in the case of *oleic acid,* common in oils such as olive oil:

```
    H   H   H   H   H   H   H   H   H   H   H   H   H   H   H   H   H  OH
    |   |   |   |   |   |   |   |   |   |   |   |   |   |   |   |   |   |
H — C — C — C — C — C — C — C — C — C = C — C — C — C — C — C — C — C — C
    |   |   |   |   |   |   |   |   |               |   |   |   |   |   ||
    H   H   H   H   H   H   H   H                   H   H   H   H   H   O
```

Let us look at these two structures carefully, First, the saturated stearic acid with all its hydrogens (that is, fully hydrogenated) is part of a solid. The unsaturated oleic acid, missing two hydrogens, is part of a liquid oil. Both molecules have 18 carbons, and in most other ways are exactly alike. They are considered *long-chain fatty acids.* Many fatty acids are shorter, but the important ones tend to be long-chain.

The oleic acid is *mono-unsaturated,* although we see that *two* hydrogens are missing. For in eliminating a hydrogen, a carbon must satisfy its empty bond by using it with its neighboring carbon, which in turn must then also have a bond free. For the two to join together, *both* must do without a hydrogen atom. Thus, it is the *double bond* between two carbons which is counted in classifying with the prefix, *mono.*

A *polyunsaturated fatty acid* (PUFA) is one with more than one double bond. Using another 18-carbon molecule, the difference looks like this:

```
    H   H   H   H   H   H   H   H   H   H   H   H   H   H   H   H   H  OH
    |   |   |   |   |   |   |   |   |   |   |   |   |   |   |   |   |   |
H – C – C – C – C – C – C = C – C – C = C – C – C – C – C – C – C – C – C
    |   |   |   |   |       |           |   |   |   |   |   |   |   |   ||
    H   H   H   H   H       H           H   H   H   H   H   H   H   H   O
```

This is *linoleic* acid, the truly essential fatty acid. Two others (linolenic and arachidonic) are essential in a way, but the body can make them if it has *linoleic* acid. The body can make many fatty acids, building them up in pairs of carbons with their accompanying hydrogens. But among other things, the position of the double bond is crucial, and the body cannot assemble the particular structure of linoleic acid.

Breaking and Building Fatty Acids

The ability of the body to assemble these carbon pairs and to take them apart is most important. For example, it is fundamental in making storage fat from extra carbohydrate—and also from protein once the amino group is removed. Similarly, the breaking apart of both our own stored fats and the fats in food is part of the process by which fats are used in the energy cycle. These processes proceed, again, by hydrolysis.

(As a footnote, this breaking down of fats for energy does not go well unless there is some carbohydrate available, leading to an old physiological slogan that "Fat burns in the flame of carbohydrate." Again we see why a diet without carbohydrate is not desirable. If at least some 10 percent of the dietary calories are not carbohydrate, some fats break down just so far and no further; half-way products—acids and ketones—accumulate in the blood, and the kidneys try to remove them with water in the urine. The acids and ketones account for some of the undesirable side effects of extremely low-carbohydrate eating.)

What kind of fats does the body store and make? Quite logically, saturated fats. There are some chemical reasons, due to greater simplicities of structure among these. But there is also a practical reason, which can help us to keep the difference in mind. It is the low melting point of *un*saturated fats. The body is at 98.6 degrees, well above the melting point of unsaturated fatty acids. If the body used these for storage, when we stood up, all of our subcutaneous stores of fat would run down to our feet.

SATURATED FATS, CHOLESTEROL AND DIETARY REALITY

Since most of the fat which our bodies deposit in tissue is of the saturated variety, it is not surprising that the unwanted fatty deposits in blood vessels are largely of this type. This suggests why researchers began to look at saturated fats in seeking some causes of heart disease.

On the other hand, remember that the body *makes* saturated fat—from such diverse materials as proteins, carbohydrates and even polyunsaturated fats. The essential question for the heart is, why are the fat deposits laid down? And the essential question for the nutritionist is, what effect does food have?

There are no certain answers to either of these questions, and this is why there is great controversy. The confusion is added to by makers and sellers of foods containing the various kinds of fat, who emphasize evidence in one direction or the other. There is an enormous body of that evidence now. Some populations, but not all, which consume much saturated fat seem to have more heart disease. Some animal experiments, but not all, are very suggestive of a relationship between the type of fat eaten and the condition of blood vessels and the heart.

One critical area of discussion centers about the now established fact that people who have higher levels of the lipid substance *cholesterol,* which we will examine shortly, also have greater risk of heart attacks and related ills. Moreover, for reasons which are still unknown, it appears that diets rich in saturated fats lead to higher cholesterol levels in the blood and that diets lower in saturated fats and higher in polyunsaturated fats can reduce the serum cholesterol.

Does this mean we should all reduce our saturated fats? Not necessarily all of us. It appears that about a third of U.S. men and somewhat more women have "normal" levels of cholesterol. The rest of us average toward undesirably higher levels. There are many factors other than just diet which influence cholesterol levels—and the risk of heart attack. Our heredity, habits of exercise, smoking, stressful living, blood pressure, obesity, and disease states such as diabetes, all are involved in this extremely complex problem.

In their 1972 joint statement, the Food and Nutrition Board and the Council on Foods and Nutrition of the AMA observed that we should stop "temporizing with this major national health problem." They recommended that all of us have regular blood tests, first to try and determine if we have tendencies toward the indicated risk patterns of atherosclerosis, and then to keep watch on cholesterol and other indicative blood substances. They urged the maintaining of proper weight and exercise levels. For those people who proved to be in high risk categories, the two groups urged dietary restriction to reduce cholesterol in the blood and keep it low.

The question remains, however, what blanket changes, if any, ought to be recommended for the dietary patterns of the country as a whole. Here much controversy boils. The Heart Association, for example, urges that its "prudent diet" is prudent for all of us. Other well-documented arguments are more moderate. While it seems clear that a reduction in total fat consumption would represent better nutrition for most of us, what of saturated fats and cholesterol in the diet?

In its labeling regulations, FDA states that it is "not taking a position in the debate over the role of fats . . . in cardiovascular disease; it is merely allowing such information about food to appear on the label." When grams of saturated and polyunsaturated fat are shown, they must be accompanied by the disclaimer: "Information on fat content is provided for individuals who on the advice of a physician are modifying their total dietary intake of fat." Essentially the same disclaimer is required for statements of cholesterol content. This should not be interpreted as a rejection of the cardiologists' position. It is only that the Government believes that it should not imply that a final scientific decision has been reached when it has not.

If one fits a pattern with a high risk of atherosclerosis, the decision about dietary changes in saturated-fat and cholesterol intake is a medical one. If one does not fit such a pattern, the decision is more a personal one. Let us see what is involved in such changes.

LOOKING AT FOODS AND FATTY ACIDS

Contrary to the popular image, fat-containing foods are actually fatty acid mixtures. Meat fat is not totally saturated, nor is oil totally polyunsaturated. Rather, we can only speak of preponderances of fatty acid types. Less than half the fat of butter or beef or pork is saturated. Conversely, little more than a third of fatty acids in a special corn-oil margarine are polyunsaturated; 40 percent are saturated or monounsaturated.

It is important to remember that we are dealing with mixtures, when we look at Heart Association recommendations, for otherwise they will seem more restrictive than they are. They call for less than 10 percent of total calories to come from saturated fatty acids, and up to 10 percent of total calories to come from polyunsaturated fatty acids, with the remainder from monounsaturated forms.

This means, for the person consuming 2,500 calories a day: saturated fatty acids (SFA) less than 250 calories; polyunsaturated fatty acids (PUFA) up to 250 calories; and up to 375 calories from monounsaturated fatty acids (MUFA). The SFA is the hard part for most Americans.

Going back to our four-ounce moderately lean burger, it has some 24 grams of total fat, of which 11.5 grams are SFA. And we have now used over 100 of our 250-calorie allowance (9×11.5). Our serving of chuck roast, which supplied over 60 grams of fat in six ounces, is not so forbidding if we trim away every bit of excess fat and eat a three-ounce serving. It then gives us only 6 grams, or 54 calories of SFA, about the same as a two-inch cube of devil's food cake.

Using the abbreviated table in the Appendix, we find that the Heart Association plan does not require meals which are really much more restrictive than our plan for simply cutting back on total fats a bit. For much of our hidden fat proves to be of the saturated kind.

Some of the tempting foods shown in our fatty day food diary—those including plant foods or using vegetable oils—have considerable polyunsaturated fatty acid. The peanuts are 14 percent PUFA and only 9 percent SFA, out of the total fat content of 50 percent. Our doughnuts are fried in vegetable oil. Our salad dressing is mostly made with oil.

It takes a little experimenting to learn to put the fat content of food in perspective—to sort out calories and fat percents and grams of fat—but it is instructive. For rule-of-thumb interpretation, the percentages of fatty acids in fats give us an easy idea of some proportions, as in this sampler.*

---

*Values from USDA Handbook No. 456. The totals do not add to 100 percent due to presence of unlisted lipids.

Table 10–1.

Food	Sat. %	Mono-Unsat.	Poly-Unsat.
Safflower oil	8	15	72
Corn oil	10	28	53
Cottonseed (usually labeled as "vegetable")	25	21	50
Soy oil	15	20	52
Peanut oil	18	47	29
Olive oil	11	76	7
Regular-type margarine (stick)	18	51	27
Soft-type margarine (tub)	19	37	39
Ground beef (21% fat)	48	44	2
Butter	55	33	3
Eggs	32	44	8
Tuna (canned, drained)	27	21	21

Averages of fat content in meats vary widely, even within one category, such as beef. But the fat in beef, lamb, or pork is about 45 percent each of saturated and monounsaturated fatty acids, with only from 2 to 6 percent polyunsaturated. Poultry tends to have some 30 percent of its fat in saturated form, some 40 percent in monounsaturated, and about 20 percent of polyunsaturates.

Most fish has little fat, and a large part of that is usually polyunsaturated. Egg fats are similar to those of meat, though somewhat more unsaturated. Vegetables, fruits, and grains have so little fat as to be unimportant sources.

Note in table 10-1 above the effect of hydrogenation of vegetable oil to make a more butter-like margarine (the "stick" type in the table). In this process, designed to keep fats in foods from separating, and to give them a more solid form, processors are actually converting the form of some fatty acids. They can either fill in all the possible places for hydrogen atoms, or, in "partial hydrogenation," just fill in some. If we compare cottonseed oil and partially hydrogenated margarine which is made from it, we see that before processing the oil had 50 percent PUFA and that afterward it had only 27 percent—and that monounsaturates rose sharply from 21 percent to 51 percent.

This exercise also tells us how to read *ingredients* labels for more information on saturation, by looking for "hydrogenated vegetable oils" and noting their order in the ingredients—especially in crackers, cakes, pie crusts, and the like. Nutrition information labels may give us exact values for different types of fat.

To understand some of the differences between SFA and PUFA, and how they relate to cholesterol, it helps to know a little more about how the body uses them. So let us take a closer look at how these nutrients fare when we eat them.

When We Swallow a Fat

A basic problem for the body, in trying to break down fats and use them for fuel and the body's needed chemicals, is that the body is essentially a watery system. And fats don't dissolve in water. This may be one reason why fats got a reputation as being hard to digest. The digestive systems of infants and some elderly people may have a little more difficulty in dealing with fats, but by and large they can handle them.

As we have seen, fats do slow down digestion, however. So if one overeats *and* consumes a high fat meal—a likely combination, since so many of our luxury foods are fatty and are popular when we feast— one may experience the discomfort of overeating for a longer period of time. (We might also keep in mind that overheated fats seem able to irritate the intestines of some otherwise normal people.)

As we chew and swallow fats, we break them apart physically, but not chemically. We also warm them up, melting them a bit. The first object of digestion is to get fats into tiny particles, so that they will make an *emulsion* with the watery body fluids in which they will not actually dissolve. The aim is to expose as much fat surface as possible to digestive enzymes. Foods which are already emulsified when we eat them may have their fats broken apart to some extent in the stomach, through a *lipase* (fat-splitting enzyme). To see such an emulsion, shake a bottle of salad dressing and watch the oil emulsify with the vinegar.

But the bulk of the fat is emulsified and broken down in the small intestine. Bile, made in the liver and stored in the gall bladder, is the emulsifying agent. It is bitter-tasting stuff, as one notes on regurgitation after a fatty meal, and the "gall" bladder gets its name from this bitterness. The presence of fat in the intestine sends a hormone to the gall bladder, which makes it contract and send out its emulsifier. The proper name for the gall bladder is the *cholecyst, chole* meaning bile and *cyst* referring to a sac. Thus the word *chole*sterol means a sterol of bile, and we shall soon see the significance of this.

Once the fats are emulsified, *lipases* from the pancreas and intestinal cells attack. Fatty acids are broken away from the glycerols, sometimes completely and sometimes only partially, producing separate glycerol, monoglycerides, diglycerides, and free fatty acids.

The glycerol and the shorter-chain free fatty acids—those which are only 12 carbons or less in length—can go through the intestinal wall and on into the bloodstream, then on to the liver through the portal vein. But to travel through the blood these short-chain fatty acids must combine with small amounts of protein. These protein-fat combinations, *lipoproteins,* are the body's basic method for transporting lipids through the blood. This is a way of dealing with the insolubility of fatty substances in water.

The longer-chain fatty acids cannot follow this route, however. (These are the fatty acids which are 14 carbons or more in length.) The longer-chain fatty acids, together with certain monoglycerides and diglycerides, take another path. Bile salts help to divide the particles of lipid in which these occur very finely, to about one-hundredth the size they were on entering the intestine. Helped to stay in this fine-particle form by the bile salts, the resulting emulsion is able to enter the intestinal wall at certain points.

Once the intestinal wall was seen merely as a gateway for the lipids. But now it is understood that the cells of the wall carry out a very subtle operation. Here the larger lipid particles are combined with cholesterol, phospholipids, and some protein, to make tiny complex bodies called *chylomicrons.* For this process, the vast majority of mono- and di-glycerides and fatty acids are recombined as new triglycerides before being joined to the other chemicals. Only about one percent of the chylomicrons are composed of free fatty acids by the time the job is done.

What is the purpose of each of these chemicals and of all the intricate modification? No one really knows yet. These are the sort of difficult problems which must be resolved before we truly understand how fats are used by the body.

The chylomicrons now move toward the liver. But unlike other nutrients, which travel through the portal vein, the chylomicrons take another route. They pass from the intestinal wall into the *lymph* system. This is a very poorly understood circulation network, which picks up fluids from various tissues. It is in this slow-moving stream that the chylomicrons travel to the left subclavian vein. There they enter the blood and finally go to the liver.

The liver forms new lipoproteins from the lipid materials, and in this form the lipids are carried in the blood to all the tissues of the body. It is in the different types of lipoproteins that we find most of the cholesterol in the body.

Why Is Cholesterol Found in Lipoproteins?

While popular thinking might lead us to believe that we would be better off without cholesterol, this idea is specious. The fact is that cholesterol is an important body chemical which plays many valuable roles. It is found in every body cell in the cell membranes, and is also an important part of some key hormones, of bile acids, and the chemistry of vitamin D and reproductive substances.

Indeed, if we ate no cholesterol at all, we would still have plenty—and might even show excesses—because the majority of our cholesterol is made by the body, by the liver and the intestinal cells, to the tune of between one and two *grams* a day. Once this cholesterol is made, it has to be sent out to the cells, and apparently the lipoproteins are the best vehicles for distributing this higher alcohol through the body.

What the exact role of cholesterol is in atherosclerosis no one yet knows, except that important amounts of it are found in the fatty deposits of atherosclerotic arteries. Its presence in the blood, moreover, beyond the "normal" levels of 150-250 milligrams percent, is an indicator of unusual risk of heart attack. The excessive presence of cholesterol long enough after a meal, when lipoproteins should have cleared somewhat from the bloodstream, suggests that higher-than-desirable levels of fatty substances tend to remain in the blood. For the cholesterol is a kind of traveling companion of these substances.

(The most precise information about how well we deal with lipids in the blood comes from an assessment of the lipoproteins themselves. From the blood's content of different types of lipoproteins, the informed physician can learn more, for example, about what kinds of dietary modifications are necessary. For some people who deal with fats abnormally do not show elevated levels of cholesterol, but have high levels of other lipids, such as triglycerides.)

When the amount of cholesterol in the blood is very high, the correlation with the risk of heart disease is great. But when cholesterol is only slightly elevated, these correlations are not always very convincing. One noted heart surgeon, Dr. Michael DeBakey, reports that 80 percent of his patients with "severe occlusive coronary artery disease" had cholesterol levels much like those of normals. Others have made similar findings.

Should We Eat Less Cholesterol?

USDA estimates average daily cholesterol intake at from 600 to 900 mg. For most people this is less than their own bodies make. The American Heart Association urges that we reduce this intake to 300 mg. daily.

In simple terms, cholesterol is a good indicator of how we deal with some lipids. It apparently also indicates how much we consume of these lipids. There is no question that restriction of total fats, saturated fats, and cholesterol in the diet will lower cholesterol levels in the blood. The important question is whether this lowering has any real effect on health. We aren't sure.

Why are the diets of heart patients routinely modified for lower intake of fat and cholesterol? To improve the odds. Much of the treatment of the heart patient is aimed at reducing all the factors which increase his risk. Blood lipids are among those factors.

But what should healthy people do about the fats and cholesterols in their diets?

The Personal Decision about Lipids

As we can see, at this stage of scientific knowledge, there are no guarantees about dietary changes and heart disease. So the decision about dietary fat, for the person who does not now show signs of high risk, remains a personal and individual one.

But here we must add a caution. For the experts who counsel dietary modifications to stave off possible heart disease, caution that the earlier one begins, the better is one's chance of being effective. Some, for example, are in favor of saturated-fat and cholesterol restriction from birth. In 1972, however, the American Academy of Pediatrics rejected this idea for infants as unjustified, except in some special cases. The cases for universally agreed upon restriction are those in which a strong inborn tendency is shown for unusually high blood lipids. These cases can show actual symptoms of progressing disease even in childhood.

But what if a medical examination reveals no symptoms or sign of high risk, such as high blood lipids, high blood pressure, or diabetes? In that case, there are some further questions to explore, such as:

Is there much early heart or blood-vessel disease among your close relatives?

Do you smoke?

Do you get very little exercise?

Are you quite overweight?

Are you male?

Do you tend to live in a stressful, competitive way?

Each *yes* answer means greater risk and more reason to try to protect yourself by dietary means. Of course the questions themselves suggest some protective changes of lifestyle: You could, after all, stop smoking, get more exercise, reduce, and so forth. The consideration of the other risk factors is most important. For together they seem to have far more effect than does control of serum cholesterol by itself.

But if additional risk factors do appear in your own personal profile, or if judgment inclines you to follow the prudent diet recommended by the Heart Association, let us take a look at how difficult the dietary changes will be. We might view them in three phases.

Phase one is the reduction of total fat intake to 35 percent or less of total calories. We have already considered this change and seen that it is a basic and reasonable fundamental of better nutrition. We have also seen that there is room in the 35-percent-fat diet for a free choice of good-tasting food.

Phase two requires some closer restriction. For we must now hold saturated fats to only 10 percent of calories, keep polyunsaturated fats up to another 10 percent, and use monounsaturated fats for the remainder (no more than another 15 percent of calories). The difficulty of this phase is really a matter of one's personal tastes. As we have seen in our look at how different foods supply different types of fatty acids, the beef-and-butter eater may have to make some sharp changes. The person who really loves fish and poultry should have little problem.

The consumption of the recommended PUFAs is a burden for very few people, except those who despise salads (and so cannot consume salad oils easily) and dislike the taste of margarines. And the final restriction on monounsaturated fats is generally a logical consequence of the other fat changes and limitations. (Remember, too, that these recommendations for fat balance are not really intended as mathematically rigid rules; they are merely guidelines for reference.)

One suggestion made by some nutritionists is that we approach these modifications in stages—to first try shifting the general balance of the diet toward less fat (phase one), and then examine our food habits in this new mode to see how much of each fat type we are consuming. For in making the basic reduction, we tend to cut down our saturated fat intake almost automatically, as we start to avoid the most fat-rich foods.* In other words, if we try the modifications of phase one, chances are that we have already moved much closer to the recommendations of phase two, and may even have met them, depending on our particular food tastes.

Phase three requires limiting dietary cholesterol to 300 mg. a day. Many Americans find this step uncomfortably confining, although reports from some heart patients suggest that they do not find the diet unpleasant once they get used to it.

To see why the restriction is hard for some, look at the table of cholesterol content in foods set out in Appendix G. It may be worthwhile to check your own diet for the last 24 hours, to get some idea of how much cholesterol you are consuming now and how your diet would have to change to ingest only 300 mg. a day.

The table can be a little deceiving. We may note that beef or pork or turkey have only 75 mg. (a fourth of the recommended daily total) in a serving. But have we noticed that this serving is three ounces? Is a

---

*As an example, Friedman and Yanochik persuaded a number of Arizona families to limit their *protein* intake to RDA levels. There was a resulting reduction of animal-source foods, and of fats and particularly saturated fats, which brought diets to roughly "prudent" levels. There were also general reductions in weight and in levels of fat content in the blood.

three-ounce steak enough? A ten-ounce steak, which is what many people eat, may provide more like 250 mg., almost the day's allowance.

Some foods must be virtually denied—organ meats at 230 to 680 mg. in a small serving, eggs at 250 mg., or brains at up to 1,700 mg. The Heart Association diet allows three "visible" eggs a week, apparently as a concession to the general nutrient quality and the popularity of eggs.

Even without this particular restriction on cholesterol intake, lowering intake of total fats tends to lower cholesterol consumption considerably, and emphasis on reducing the amount of saturated fats will bring it down even further. Is it worthwhile to invoke special prohibitions on a few special foods? Is it necessary? There is no sure answer.

It may be helpful to know that, in their joint 1972 statement, the AMA and the Food and Nutrition Board did not espouse the Heart Association's plan, for everyone—only for those who were advised by their physicians to lower blood cholesterol levels and keep them at a reduced level. One reason for this decision is that the plan is not easy for some people to follow. Another reason is that some people have problems with blood lipids which are not helped, and could even be worsened, by the self-prescription of a cholesterol-lowering dietary (especially those people with hypertriglyceridemia).

As we look at the vitamins and minerals in the next chapter, we will see further confirmation that a reduction of total fats is helpful, if not necessary, for most of us, in order to get all of the nutrients our bodies are known to need. Beyond this, however, unless we are given medical instructions, the choice of how much attention we give to dietary lipids is a personal matter, for which there is not yet conclusive proof.

REFERENCES

1. Stefansson, V., *Food and Food Habits in Alaska and Northern Canada,* in Human Nutrition, Historic and Scientific, N.Y. Acad. of Med., International Universities Press, New York, 1960.

General References

2. Alfin-Slater, R. and Aftergood, L., *Fats and Other Lipids,* in Modern Nutrition in Health and Disease, Lea & Febiger, Phila., 1973, pp. 117—141.
3. Levy, R. and Ernst, N. *Diet, Hyperlipidemia and Atherosclerosis,* in Modern Nutrition in Health and Disease, Lea & Febiger, Phila, 1973.
4. Stare, F., Alfin-Slater, R. et al. *Atherosclerosis,* Medcom, New York, 1974.
5. Stamler, J., Epstein, F., *Coronary heart disease,* Prev. Med., 1:27, 1972.

6. Keys, A., *Coronary heart disease in seven countries,* Circulation, 41—42 (supplement), 1970.
7. Alfin-Slater, R. and Aftergood, L., *Physiological functions of essential fatty acids,* Progr. Biochem. Pharmacol. 6:214, 1971.
8. Levy, R. and Stone, N., *Atherosclerosis: Role of Lipoproteins in the Pathogenesis of Atherosclerosis,* Williams & Wilkins, Baltimore, 1972.
10. Fredrickson, D., *A physician's guide to hyperlipidemia,* Mod. Concepts Cardiovasc. Disease 41:7, 1972.
11. Macdonald, I., *Relationship between dietary carbohydrates and fats in their influence on serum lipid concentrations,* Clin. Sci. 43:265, 1972.
13. Committee on Nutrition, *Childhood diet and coronary heart disease,* Pediatrics, 49:305, 1972.
14. Dayton, S. and Pearce, M. *Cholesterol, atherosclerosis, ischemic heart disease and stroke,* Ann. Intern. Med., 72:97, 1970.
15. *Diet and coronary heart disease,* (a report), Nutrition Today, Jan/Feb., 1975, p. 16.
16. Symposium: *Dairy lipids and lipid metabolism,* Dairy Council Digest, 40:1.
17. *Fats in Food and Diet,* USDA Information Bulletin No. 361.
18. *Current research on dietary fatty acids,* Dairy Council Digest, May/June 1970.
19. Feeley, R. et al. *Cholesterol content of foods,* JADA, Vol. 61, No. 2, August, 1972, p. 134.
20. *Diet and Coronary Heart Disease,* statement of Amer. Heart Assn., New York, 1973.
21. AMA/Food and Nutrition Board, *Diet and coronary heart disease, A joint policy statement,* JAMA 222:267—94, 1972.
22. Doyle, J. and Kannel, W., *Coronary Risk Factors: 10-year finding in 8600 Americans,* Paper presented to the VI World Congress of Cardiology, London, Sep. 1970.
23. Gordon, T. and Kannel, W. *Premature mortality from coronary heart disease: The Framingham Study,* JAMA, 215:1617—25, 1971.
24. Reiser, R. *Saturated fat in the diet and serum cholesterol concentration: A critical examination of the literature.* Amer. J. Clin. Nutrition, May, 1973, pp. 524–55.

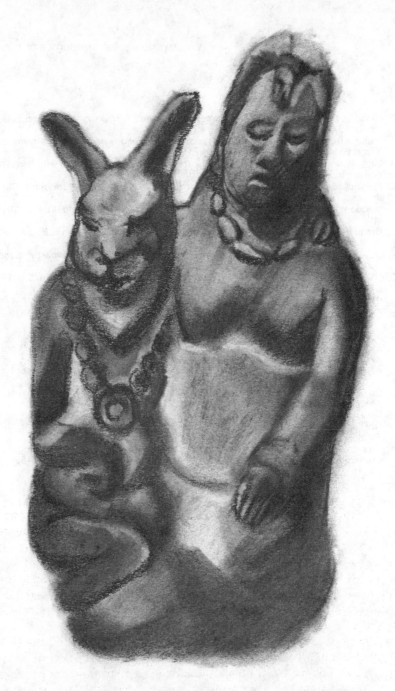

For moderns, the vitamins and minerals seem to symbolize the health-giving properties of foods, much as spirits represented them in primitive societies. *Ixchel and the
Rabbit Spirit. Mayan figurine of the early goddess of medicine and fertility is joined
with an animal food symbol. Yucatan, Mexico.*

chapter 11

VITAMINS AND MINERALS, FROM A TO ZINC

In 1915, at least 200,000 Southerners were suffering, and in many cases dying, from *pellagra*. The name came from Italy, where it meant "rough skin," and referred to the fact that the first signs were rashes on exposed parts of the body, which fissured and developed into sores. As the disease progressed, the sores and cracks spread to the mouth. Then diarrhea began, with back pains and general exhaustion. Victims became sleepless and irritable, and in the end there was dementia and death.

In 1913 Dr. Joseph Goldberger was sent to the South by the U.S. Public Health Service, to seek the cause and cure of pellagra. Most physicians believed that he should look for a microbe—that pellagra was an infection. But after preliminary research, Goldberger began to look for something else.

By May 7, 1915, he thought he had an answer. First he had to lay to rest the belief that pellagra was a contagious disease. So on that day

243

at the U.S. Pellagra Hospital in Spartanburg, South Carolina, Goldberger, his wife Mary, and four assistants took the risk. Into a little
flour, they stirred some intestinal wastes from a patient sick with
pellagra. Then they added some scalings from the skin sores of other
patients. Each of the six swallowed some of this noxious mixture.
Then, for good measure, they injected one another with the blood of
a pellagrous woman.

For Goldberger was sure that pellagra was not contagious, but
rather a nutritional deficiency problem. And soon he proved that,
with dietary changes, he could cure the disease.

WHAT IS A VITAMIN?

It is hard for many people to realize that when the first guns of
World War I were fired, and Goldberger was patiently asking questions through the orphanages of Georgia and Mississippi, the scientific concepts of vitamins were just beginning to take shape.

A decade before, Hopkins had said that there was something more
to nutrition than protein and carbohydrate and fat, some sort of tiny
essence needed for life. Until that time, scientists had merely sought
the correct proportions of the three macronutrients. When Hopkins
fed only these nutrients in rather pure form to rats, they sickened.
When he added small amounts of certain foods—a teaspoon of milk,
for example—they thrived.

In 1913, when Casimir Funk, working in London, found a substance that would cure *beriberi* in pigeons, he was sure that it was *the*
missing chemical. He knew that the stuff was an *amine,* and that it
was essential to life (in Latin, *vita*). So he called it the *vita-amine.*

Beriberi had been known for thousands of years, from the time
when the Chinese learned to polish rice to a pleasing whiteness. It
still mystified the Dutch when they took over Indonesia in the 1880s,
and the disease appeared in the lands they held (where they had set
up mills to provide people with the nicest quality of rice). For some
reason, it did not occur among the rebels, who did not have the
advantage of modern milling.

Dr. Christian Eijkman was sent to Java to find the microbes which
were thought to cause the outbreak of beriberi (which means "I
cannot"—the name signifies the weakness, lassitude, and degeneration which characterize the disease.) When Eijkman fed an experi-

mental colony of chickens polished rice being given to hospital patients, they too developed beriberi. Eijkman thought the chickens had been infected. But when a thrifty caretaker merely put the flock on cheaper, unpolished native rice, they got well. When Eijkman returned to the Netherlands, he wrote a paper called "The Truth Need Not Necessarily Be Simple." But he did not really have an answer. Later, Funk also worked on beriberi, using pigeons. He found that they could be cured by feeding them sweepings from the floor of a grain mill. Then he made an extract of the grain hulls, gave it to the pigeons, and within hours they were on their feet.

This story caught the imagination of the world. It was the *vita-amine*—nutrition's missing link.

Of Vitamin Deficiencies and Narrow Diets

But by 1916, the Americans, McCollum and Kennedy, had opined that there must be not one *vitamine,* but two—one soluble in water and one in fats.

Goldberger and his team did not suspect that the cause of pellagra was an absent "vitamine." They were sure that the cause was related to a protein deficiency. True, their disease, like beriberi, resulted from a narrow diet. But they found that they could overcome pellagra by giving patients more protein to eat.

The Southern pellagra victims often had enough food, but it was limited mainly to corn. Added to the corn were greens and rice, gravy and sweet syrup, and sweet potatoes. In one orphanage Goldberger used Federal funds to improve the diets of the pellagrous group. The babies had been all right; they got milk. And the youngsters of 12 or more were not ill; they did work, and so for strength, they got some beans and meat. It was the children in between who got only what little was left over, and many were sick with pellagra. Goldberger made sure that they ate meat four times a week, peas and beans all winter, and an egg a day. And the pellagra disappeared.

By 1921 Goldberger's team had found that they could cure pellagra with a single amino acid, *tryptophan,* in its pure form. And they had seen that the principal foods eaten by those with pellagra were low in tryptophan.

Then came a blow—evidence that others had cured pellagra with an extract of yeast, an extract that contained no nitrogen from amino acids. The puzzle became bewildering. For if pellagra could be cured by this yeast extract, how could the cause of the disease be a shortage of an amino acid? And why should tryptophan cure pellagra? All that the scientists knew for sure was that there was something wrong with a diet composed mainly of corn.

The solution? The main protein of corn is *zein.* Zein is a limited protein, limited chiefly in two amino acids, *lysine* and *tryptophan.* The missing nutrient which led to pellagra was not lysine or tryptophan, however; it was the vitamin *niacin* (which was not to be isolated until 1937). The yeast extract which had cured pellagra had contained niacin.

Then why should tryptophan have cured pellagra, too? Because the body can convert tryptophan to niacin. Each 60 extra milligrams of tryptophan can furnish a milligram of niacin. And high-quality proteins have considerable tryptophan.

When Is a Vitamin Supplement Necessary?

If we look at the realities of niacin, we can see why deficiencies of this vitamin are practically nonexistent in America today, and why special supplements are pointless.

First, look at the best sources of niacin. Usually these are also the richest sources of protein—foods such as meats, poultry, fish, eggs, and legumes. And the same foods which are good sources of niacin tend also to be good sources of the amino acid (tryptophan) which can be converted to the vitamin. So among a high-protein-eating people, a niacin shortage is hard to imagine.

We have seen that the U.S. per capita consumption of tryptophan is some 1,200 mg. a day. The need for this amino acid is about 200 mg. So almost 1,000 mg. are left over to yield niacin. At the 60-to-1 conversion rate, (60 mg. of tryptophan yielding 1 mg. of niacin), we can each get an average of some 17 milligrams of converted niacin from our food each day. This happens to equal the U.S. RDA. This then would supply our needs, even without allowing for the fact that the foods which contain generous amounts of tryptophan also supply much pure niacin.

It seems plain from this information—and from recent surveys which show no significant deficiencies of niacin in the U.S.—that adding extra niacin to our intake is pointless. According to the Food and Nutrition Board, Americans get between 50 and 300 percent more niacin than the U.S. RDA. (And remember that the U.S. RDA is based upon the RDA, with its safety margins, and that the U.S. RDA is usually based on the highest recommendation for a normal adult, generally for the typical adult male.)

However, most breakfast cereals contain (mainly through additives) 25 percent of U.S. RDA for niacin. And most popular one-every-morning vitamin pills have large amounts of niacin, usually 100 percent of U.S. RDA. Niacin is even an ingredient of enriched flour, cornmeal, and the like.

How Do We Know How Much of a Vitamin We Need?

In general, the basic understanding of vitamin needs comes from observations of deficiency signs. The minimal need is that which prevents deficiency symptoms. But the bare minimum is not used as the standard; one does not put health on a tightrope. To understand something of how science determines a healthful intake of a vitamin, we must know a little more about what vitamins do.

We have seen repeatedly how the body breaks foods down into simple chemical building materials or fuels. We have seen how proteins from foods are separated into their constituent amino acids, and how new proteins are built. We have seen carbohydrates broken down into simple sugars, the sugars converted into glucose, and then burned or stored. We have seen how hydrolysis takes fats apart and puts them together again.

How did these reactions take place? In almost every case, *enzymes* did the work. The cells, with the blueprints provided by DNA, make the protein portion of these enzymes (the *apoenzymes*); but often, to function properly, enzymes require *coenzymes.*

The situation is a little like trying to open a tightly sealed jar with one hand. Apply all the force you like with one hand by itself, addressing the force to the lid, and nothing happens; the jar turns with it. We need two hands to open the jar, one turning the lid and the other holding the jar. In effect, the coenzyme acts like a second hand, which holds the jar while the first hand turns the lid.

The role of coenzyme is the chief function of most vitamins, especially of the water-soluble vitamins in the B complex. The vitamin does not necessarily undertake this role alone; it generally acts as the essential active part of a larger total coenzyme. For example, niacin is a key part of two coenzymes.

We have also seen that similar basic chemical reactions, such as hydrolysis, are repeated in many different body processes. So it is not surprising to learn that the coenzymes as a group have chemical functions which can be used in a number of processes. In a sense, we might see them as tools with special capabilities, like certain sizes and shapes of wrench or screwdriver. Just as a specific wrench might be used for various jobs in the building of a house—here by a carpenter and there by an electrician or plumber—so vitamins may take part in a variety of jobs. Niacin's coenzymes, as examples, are important in breaking down carbohydrate for energy; they are crucial to the synthesis of triglycerides by the body; and they are essential in the supplying of oxygen to many tissues. In light of the wide variety of such work, it is not hard to see why a pellagra victim, short of niacin, feels weak, particularly when one remembers that glucose is the efficient fuel for the brain and nervous system.

This all suggests some other ways in which we can determine when vitamins are adequately supplied. For when we have enough of a vitamin which serves in a coenzyme, the chemical reactions which it fosters produce specific products. When the vitamin is in short supply, the reactions may not take place, or may take place only partially, and there will be less of the particular products. Commonly, the chemical products of complete or incomplete reactions can be identified in the blood or the body wastes. And this can indicate the adequacy of vitamin intake. For example, much of what we know about niacin needs was first learned by Dr. Grace Goldsmith and her colleagues, who found that up to a certain point, increasing tryptophan and niacin intake yielded more products of niacin-linked reactions in the urine.

Information about vitamin intakes can be gained in some cases by checking how much of the vitamin spills over into the urine because there is an excess—as in the case of vitamin C. Or certain levels of vitamin in the blood, as in the case of vitamin A, may indicate that more is available than the body can use.

Do Extra Vitamins Offer Extra Health?

Again, let us look at niacin as an example. There is a popular belief that a kind of "super nutrition" is possible through the gulping of extra-large doses of vitamins. Consider niacin's role in making energy available from glucose. So far as science knows, no more can be helpful than the amount needed to deal with the available glucose.

It is partly because of this relationship of niacin to energy use that the need for niacin is related to the number of calories we take in. The RDA Committee, including its usual safety margins, recommends that we get 6.6 mg. of niacin for each 1,000 calories we eat. Is it sensible then, to do as many people do, and consume pills containing 50 mg. of niacin a day? Only if they are eating 7,570 calories a day, a reasonable intake for a 473-pound (or an extremely active) man. (And of course this assumes that among the 7,570 calories of food, there is no niacin, and no protein which contains any tryptophan.)

This example suggests why nutritionists say that rarely are supplemental nutrients needed by normal people who consume good, varied diets. In considering micronutrients, we should remember that the plan of life is awesomely well integrated. The chemicals which we need to make use of food are either produced by the body or available in our food. If human existence depends on a health-food store full of pills, how has mankind survived?

But, if niacin helps to supply the needed energy of our brains and nerves, can't we improve their function with more niacin? No more than supplying a machine with more and more fuel would make it run faster and faster without limit. If this were true, we could outfit the family station wagon with a very large gas tank and a huge fuel pump and enter it at Indianapolis. Obviously the design of the system sets a ceiling on how much fuel can be used.

When Will Vitamins Cure Disease?

Not long ago, an issue of *Glamour* magazine offered its readers an article on "Vitamins—Do They Really Cure Everything from Colds to Menstrual Cramps to Schizophrenia?"[1]

A feature of the article was a two-page chart, entitled, "Therapy Claims of Vitamin Enthusiasts." In the lefthand column of the chart was a long list of ailments. To the right were five columns for vitamins, with testimonials from the late Adelle Davis and others which had said they would prevent or relieve the ailments. Niacin, for example, was claimed as a preventative and cure for anxiety and schizophrenia, as well as skin problems.

Where did the enthusiasts get the idea that the vitamins would cure these illnesses? Simple. If one looks through the catalog of deficiency symptoms for various nutrients, one finds that virtually every organ of the body can be involved in *some* deficiency state. One also finds that when the deficient nutrient is restored to the diet, the symptoms are likely to abate. With niacin, for example, there are skin, brain and nerve symptoms of deficiency, and if niacin is replaced in time, these ills will go away.

It is thus easy to see how some enthusiasts began to believe in curative links between particular vitamins and particular organs. If a shortage of the vitamin can injure the organ, they assumed, then whenever that organ is in trouble, vitamins will make it better. But as we see with niacin, vitamins are related less to organs than to chemical reactions. When a vitamin is missing, a whole spectrum of symptoms appears, ranging over the whole body, a fact enthusiasts often forget.

Seeing a tendency of the gums to bleed, certain dentists think of scurvy and prescribe vitamin C, forgetting that the bleeding gums are only one sign of the total bodily problem of scurvy. (There is also tenderness of the extremities and muscle weakness, hemorrhages under the skin, in the nose, and throughout the body, often quite painful; there is delayed healing of wounds and high risk of infection.) When one understands the well documented fact that scurvy is now practically unknown in the U.S., it is not logical to prescribe vitamin C for every bleeding gum.

In extra doses, used essentially as medicines, vitamins and minerals cure scarcely anything except deficiencies of vitamins and minerals.

Not long ago, Dr. Alfred Harper, then chairman of the RDA Committee, wrote to Senator William Proxmire (relative to possible legislation regulating large doses of micronutrients). Said Harper: "When a nutrient is used to treat a disease that is NOT caused by an inadequate intake of that nutrient, the use is no longer nutritional, it is pharmaceutical. The nutrient is being used as a drug."[2]

There are a few situations, although very few, in which nutrients are responsibly used as drugs. For example, Harper cites the use of vitamin C to treat certain bladder infections, by making the urine more acid. But note that in this use, vitamin C is not intended to function as a vitamin. It is being used primarily because it is a mild acid, because excesses of ascorbic acid are cleared by the kidneys and quickly dumped into the bladder, and because it is relatively nontoxic in the amounts needed to make the urine sufficiently acid.

On the other hand, there are some healers who become fascinated by the deficiency-symptom relationship, and prescribe massive doses of a vitamin. An example is the "orthomolecular psychiatrist," who gives "megavitamin" doses of niacin to people with schizophrenia—because niacin stops the dementia of pellagra.

One of the old names for a type of schizophrenia was *dementia,* especially *dementia praecox,* the lamentably common schizophrenia which emerges at the border of adolescence and adulthood. The origin of the disorder has not been explained, no reliable cure has been found, and there is often a spontaneous remission—characteristics which make it fertile ground for vitamin "cures."

An expert panel of the American Psychiatric Association reviewed the uses of megavitamin therapy, and concluded, " . . . The results and claims of the advocates of megavitamin therapy have not been confirmed . . . their credibility is further diminished by a consistent refusal over the past decade to perform controlled experiments and to report their results in a scientifically acceptable fashion . . . Under these circumstances this (panel) considers the massive publicity which they promulgate via radio, the lay press and popular books . . . to be deplorable."[3]

Nevertheless, the orthomolecular enthusiasts continue to treat virtually every variety of serious emotional illness with megavitamins, particularly with niacin. One popular book describes the supposed nutritional science behind such treatment, illustrating with the case of a girl called Joan, who supposedly took diet pills and ate very little for about a month.[4] "In the space of a month," write the authors, "the strain on her nutritional reserves was so severe that she developed pellagra—but apparently only the mental symptoms of the deficiency disease. This is confirmation of the theory behind 'orthomolecular psychiatry.' " (The theory of Dr. Linus Pauling.) Norman Cousins, editor of the *Saturday Review,* is reported to have been so impressed with Joan's story that he wrote an article about her pellagra of just the brain and nerves. Science, of course, knows that pellagra is an illness of the whole body.

How much niacin (among other things) is such a patient given? Dosages are commonly between 3,000 and 4,000 mg. daily—or the RDA for some 230 days at the highest level. At 6.6 mg. of niacin per 1,000 calories, we may compute that a megavitamin patient was being equipped to deal with some 600,000 calories of food a day. As a comparable example, we might note that Pauling's dosage of vitamin C for the common cold, 1,000 mg. per hour, would supply in about 12 hours the RDA of vitamin C for some nine months,[5] an amount which has no possible relation to vitamin function.

The chemical and physiologic thinking behind such doses is obscure to most scientists. But the hazards are often clear. We have noted examples even with water-soluble vitamins, where most of an excess is simply urinated away (but where injury can be caused in the process). But the hazards are especially notable in the case of fat-soluble vitamins, such as vitamin A, in which long-term doses of only five to ten times the U.S. RDA have had toxic effects. Yet in a recent issue of one health-food magazine, a columnist responds to a reader's letter by recommending 100,000 units daily, 20 times the U.S. RDA, and saying: "Any toxicity found from A and D vitamins has always been caused by the synthetic forms. The natural forms . . . can be taken with impunity."[6] This idea is quite untrue.

Defining Vitamins—"Natural" and Synthetic

Are "natural" and synthetic forms of vitamins really different from one another? To answer this question, we ought first to define our terms. Because the family of vitamins is so large and various, any useful definition tends to be broad. An example of a definition for vitamins is:

Vitamins are organic substances in foods which are essential in small amounts for body processes.

This definition distinguishes vitamins from other nutrients in several ways. First, the fact that they are organic (made with a skeleton of carbons) separates them from minerals. Second, the fact that they are needed in very small amounts sets them apart from other organic nutrients—fats, proteins, carbohydrates. Third, they are food essentials, meaning that they must originate outside our cells. (We have seen that some vitamins are made by bacteria in our intestines; however, they are thus still nutrients which originate outside our cells, although we may not be ingesting them in food.) Fourth, the fact that they are necessary for body processes tells us that the processes will be interfered with when vitamin supplies are inadequate, and will usually be restored when deficiencies are made up.

Both "natural" vitamins—those which are extracted from foods—and synthetic vitamins made by the chemist, who assembles the proper atoms in the proper form, meet the tests of this definition. If synthetic vitamins (the term derives from the Greek for "put together") are given, no deficiency occurs; and if there are deficiency symptoms, they are relieved equally well by the man-made forms.

Those who market "natural" vitamins often maintain or imply that something extra comes with them. Obviously, this is true only if the vitamins come in foods (the "extra" being other ingredients of the foods), not if pure vitamin extracts are taken. If we look at our friend niacin chemically, we can see that it is not difficult for the modern chemist to make it (probably one reason why it is used so liberally as a "fortifier"). There are two slightly different forms of this vitamin—niacin, or *nicotinic acid,* the form found whole in foods, and the form which occurs when the vitamin is made from the amino acid tryptophan (*nicotinamide* or *nicotinic acid amide*).

Nicotinic Acid	*Nicotinic Acid Amide*
(Niacin)	(Niacinamide)

$$
\begin{array}{cc}
\text{N} & \text{N} \\
\diagup \ \diagdown\!\!\!\!= & \diagup \ \diagdown\!\!\!\!= \\
\text{H--C} \quad \text{CH} & \text{H--C} \quad \text{CH} \\
\| \qquad | & \| \qquad | \\
\text{H--C} \quad \text{C--COOH} & \text{H--C} \quad \text{C--CONH}_2 \\
\diagdown\ \diagup\!\!= & \diagdown\ \diagup\!\!= \\
\text{C} & \text{C} \\
| & | \\
\text{H} & \text{H}
\end{array}
$$

These two molecules are identical, except for a difference at the lower righthand corner. Here niacin has an acid group, COOH, like that in amino acids, whereas the niacinamide has $CONH_2$. The NH_2 is of course the amino group, not surprising to find in a molecule formed from an amino acid.

The chemist can synthesize either form. Why do many people become suspicious of a man-made vitamin? Possibly because the word synthetic is often slightly misused. *Synthetic* rubber, for example, is not a reproduction of rubber made from trees; it is something that merely looks and acts similarly. The term synthetic tends to be used loosely by some industry, but not in nutrition, where it means an exact reproduction of the molecule.

One particularly meaningless idea is that the source from which the vitamin was refined makes a difference. For example, "natural vitamin C from rose hips" is only vitamin C.* Milligram for milligram it is the same as the vitamin C from oranges, potatoes, or cabbage. However, it is not surprising that special "kinds" of vitamins are bought at premium prices, in a land where people regularly pay more for sucrose refined from cane than for sucrose refined from beets. Sugar cane and beets are quite different; oranges and potatoes are different. But sucrose is sucrose and vitamin C is vitamin C.

No attempt will be made to provide an exhaustive catalog of the vitamins, the origins of their discovery, their biological function, clinical aspects of deficiency and excess, etc. Such information is readily available, but is often of little use to any but the scientist or the physician. Keeping in mind the realities of useful nutrition information, here are some of the basic simplicities of the micronutrients.

Thiamin (vitamin B-1)

The absence of this vitamin was the cause of the ancient plague of beriberi; its deficiency symptoms are related to the fact that it plays a key role as a coenzyme in our use of carbohydrates. One does not see beriberi in our society, for thiamin is widely distributed in our foods.

When there is inadequacy of thiamin intake it is apt to result from the fact that it is one of the vitamins that is spread rather thin; few foods supply very much of it. For example, the U.S. RDA is 1.5 mg. And there are few foods which supply even 10 percent of this amount. Pork is, among the common foods, perhaps the best thiamin source, offering about a third of the U.S. RDA in a three-ounce serving. But other reputedly good sources, such as a cup of cooked oatmeal or a half-cup serving of peas or lima beans, or a modest serving of liver, provide only about 10 percent of U.S. RDA.

What may we infer from this? First, that it takes many sources of thiamin to supply a day's recommendation. If the average food we eat has from five to ten percent of U.S. RDA, we can see that it will require some ten to twenty servings of such foods daily to do the job.**

---

*In actual commerce, much of the vitamin C value in such products has sometimes been found to come from pure ascorbic acid powder which has never been near a rose.

**In rare instances, thiamin deficiency can result from eating food which contains an enzyme that destroys this vitamin. For example, raw tuna has such an antivitamin. Since enzymes are inactivated by cooking, however, cooked tuna is perfectly safe.

This characteristic of thiamin is one of the causes of the concern which practical nutritionists feel about excessive dilution of the diet with pure fat or sugar; it leaves less room in the diet for the food variety needed to supply adequate thiamin. The problem is compounded somewhat by the fact that thiamin is destroyed by heat and is easily dissolved away in cooking water. Unless thiamin sources are carefully cooked, for a minimal time in a minimal amount of water, they may not provide the amount of vitamin shown in food tables.

It should not surprise us, considering these facts (and also some special considerations for certain population groups, which will be discussed later), that thiamin intake runs fairly close to the margin of U.S. RDAs. On the other hand, the allowances for this vitamin are based on the needs of teen-aged boys, who need more thiamin than others. For thiamin needs are related to calories consumed. The RDA Committee estimates a very safe level of 0.5 mg. for each 1,000 calories of food. So the U.S. RDA of 1.5 mg. should take care of 3,000 calories a day. An average adult or preadolescent child does not consume 3,000 calories worth of food daily.

(Keep in mind—not only for thiamin, but also for other vitamins—that dietary "deficiencies" which show up in surveys may mean intakes below recommended levels. These are not necessarily intakes which will produce true *nutritional deficiencies,* with their attendant clinical symptoms. They may be only departures from a reference value.)

Because thiamin intakes are not liberal, flours are usually enriched with this vitamin; so is rice. The shortest cooking time tends to be best for preserving thiamin in green vegetables, noodles, and the like. And soda should not be added to green vegetables to make them greener; it makes thiamin less stable.

Despite the fact that there is no one sufficient source, a varied diet should make thiamin supplements unnecessary. Breakfast cereals, which are commonly fortified with 25 percent of the U.S. RDA for thiamin, are one easy way to get thiamin insurance. The small amounts sprinkled through foods should close any gap for most Americans, if the diet is well varied. Daily intake is important, because very little of the vitamin can be stored.

Riboflavin (vitamin B—2)

Riboflavin provides one of the nutritional question marks for Americans. Modern surveys suggest that intakes may be low among many people. Again, however, there is the question of whether the reported deficiencies are more statistical than real, in the sense of deficiency symptoms. But there is enough of a question to warrant some special attention to this vitamin.

Riboflavin forms an important coenzyme for energy use, for protein metabolism, and for the respiration of tissues. So requirements for it are also related to caloric intake, at 0.6 mg. per 1,000 calories. The U.S. RDA (1.7 mg.) will liberally take care of some 3,000 calories of food, so modest departures from the U.S. RDA should not be of great concern for most people.

The marginal consumption of riboflavin seems related to two main factors. One is that, like thiamin, riboflavin is found widely, but in small amounts, in a variety of foods; and even fewer sources of riboflavin are rich. Secondly, our eating patterns have tended to shift away from some of the best sources. Milk is perhaps the best common source, with about 5 percent of the U.S. RDA in a cup. And we have been drinking less milk. Liver can give us more than two days' supply, but one does not often eat liver. And while cheese is a good replacement for milk as a calcium source, it is not as good a replacement for riboflavin.

Lowered intakes of green vegetables, wheat, eggs, and starchier vegetables have also cut into our intake of riboflavin. 100-gram meat servings, among the better sources, offer only about 13 or 14 percent of the U.S. RDA. Most fruits offer only about 5 percent. Mushrooms are among the few rich vegetable sources.

The identified deficiency symptoms tend to be rather minor, such as mouth sores and cracks. Lethal deficiencies have not been discerned in man. This leads to some speculation that the vitamin might be produced to some extent by intestinal bacteria.

Riboflavin is found in every body cell, and it is commonly bound to proteins in foods (which helps protect it from cooking losses). But it is sensitive to ultraviolet light, a reason not to buy milk in clear containers, and also a reason to keep bread out of the light.

Riboflavin is frequently found in foods in which rather proportional amounts of calcium are also present. So attention to getting enough of one is likely to provide for the other.

Niacin.

There is little of everyday importance that we have not already said about this vitamin (in the past sometimes referred to as B—3). We might summarize that, since it is furnished both by foods which Americans usually eat in quantity, and also by conversion from tryptophan (also plentiful in our diets) it is seldom of dietary concern. An exception might be for the vegan kind of vegetarian, who shuns dairy and egg products. Pellagra has virtually disappeared from the U.S.

Folacin, or Folic Acid

While these terms are often used interchangeably, *folacin* is the general word for a group of chemicals which have the activity of folic acid. One of the most recently discovered vitamins,folacin has been called by a variety of names, some of which one may still encounter occasionally (from vitamin M to vitamin B—10 or B$_c$). But while the vitamin fits into the B complex, nutritionists seem to like the name folacin—perhaps because it derives from the Latin word for *leaf,* and green, leafy vegetables are among the best sources. It was first isolated from spinach leaves.

While folic acid is needed in very tiny amounts (the U.S. RDA is only 400 *micro*grams—abbreviated as mcg.—or 0.4 mg.), it forms co-enzymes for some most important chemistry—for example, the making of the nucleic acids for the blueprinting of heredity. A deficiency of folacin can lead to extremely serious anemia (*macrocytic anemia,* a distortion in the size, number, and oxygen-carrying capacity of the red blood cells).

Folacin may well be the hardest to get of the vitamins. It is scarce in most foods; ample servings of green, leafy vegetables, which are among the best sources, usually provide no more than 60 to 70 of the 400 recommended micrograms. Liver, wheat germ, and brewer's yeast are among the few excellent sources, with the first two supplying some three-fourths of U.S. RDA in 100 grams. Servings of most kinds of beans supply about a third of the U.S. RDA.

But most of the common foods supply rather minor amounts of this vitamin—milk, 1.5 mcg.; beef, about 10 mcg. per 100 grams; bread, 3 to 7 mcg. per slice; breakfast cereals, from 1 to 30 mcg. (the more bran, the more folacin); most nuts, fewer than 10 mcg. per ounce; most fruits, about 1 to 7 mcg.; potatoes, about 12 mcg. per small serving. Clearly, one could consume quite a good diet, eat one leafy vegetable a day, yet miss the high-level folacin foods. So it is not surprising that our folacin intake is thought to be marginal.

To make matters worse, folacin is quite heat-sensitive. It is especially so in an acid medium, so the habit in some areas of adding some vinegar to greens while cooking compounds the problem. The vinegar can be added after cooking, with little adverse effect.

It is not hard to see how in times of rapid cell-division, as in pregnancy or cases of premature infants, there would be a sharp rise in the need for folacin, because the production of nucleic acids must then be rapid. One can also understand how folacin intake could be compromised when total food intake is diminished, for instance, in reducing diets or alcoholism; this is the case with many B vitamins, but especially folacin.

Supplements are limited for this vitamin, because it can mask the signs of certain anemias when taken in large quantities. But limited supplements, since they are in an especially usable form, go a long way toward meeting needs.

Actually, the RDA Committee feels that we probably need only 50 mcg. of true folic acid. But the RDA is set much higher, because the vitamin is easily lost in cooking and storage, and because the folacin in many foods is bound to a non-essential amino acid (glutamic acid), which makes questionable the amount actually absorbed. Some experts believe, however, that some folacin may be synthesized by intestinal bacteria. In general, our questions about folacin, and our understanding of its importance, have brought a special new interest to the nutritionist's oft-heard plea to eat our vegetables.

Vitamin B—6

The coenzyme activities of B—6, many of them understood in just the last generation and some still probably unknown, are many and various. The vitamin is found in three forms, *pyridoxine, pyridoxal* and *pyridoxamine,* all of which seem able to function nicely in the many tasks the coenzyme is called upon to perform. In its coenzyme role, it is involved in the removal and transfer of amino groups in protein metabolism; it moves sulfurs around in certain amino acids, helps convert tryptophan to niacin, participates in the absorption of amino acids from the intestine, and takes part in the chemical reactions of the blood and brain, as well as the chemistry of essential fatty acids. Predictably, the penalties of deficiency may be severe and wide-ranging.

The classic B—6 deficiency story involves a batch of commercial infant formula, which was heated intensely, destroying much of the vitamin. The babies began to have convulsions, which disappeared as soon as they were given supplements of B—6.

B—6 deficiencies are rare in most conventional diets. (Observe that an infant is on a very narrow diet indeed, often with little chance to supplement any weakness of his one basic food source: the nipple or bottle.) However, B—6 can be a problem for many young women who take contraceptive pills. And the extra needs for B—6 in pregnancy may not be met.

One protective factor is that the need for this vitamin tends to increase proportionately with protein consumption, and good sources of protein, especially animal sources, are commonly good sources of B—6. The U.S. RDA of 2 mg., is set high enough to take care of very high protein intakes. Most meats provide about a sixth to a fifth of the RDA in a modest 100-gram serving. Some fish, such as salmon and mackerel, offer double the B—6 of meat. On the other hand, grains and some dairy products are not very good sources. Two slices of bread have only 1–2 percent of B—6 RDA.*

While a milk serving has about a third of the amount of B—6 in a meat serving, it also has only about a third of the protein. But when cheeses are made from the milk, even cottage cheese, the B—6 becomes quite low compared to the protein. And an egg, while giving us more than 10 percent of the U.S. RDA for protein, provides only 3 percent of our U.S. RDA for B—6.

There is reason for vegetarians to be alert to B—6, since the vitamin is not plentiful in grains, peas and beans, or in supplemental foods such as eggs and dairy products. Thinking green can help these people, and others with special needs for B—6. For most very green foods have a high B—6 content. Avocados, for example, have more than meat, and spinach is quite high.

But rules of thumb have limited value, and it is best to look through the composition tables. For example, potatoes are a good source—a large baked potato can supply a fourth of the RDA, and even french fries have quite a bit. Rice has more than most grains, and to some extent so does sweet corn. Conversely, luncheon meats and sausages are very low in the vitamin.

The B—6 story is a case in point for dietary balance. Consider as a contrasting example the popular "high protein" diets. For although

---

*An average, of course, that may vary with the content of milk powder, etc.

meat is rather protective as a B—6 source, it still takes some six servings a day to supply *all* our needs. Relatively few calories of such foods as rice, potatoes and corn—foods often thought of as "starchy" and "fattening"—can make substantial contributions to close the gap. Certainly it takes few calories of greens (foods also banned in extreme low-carbohydrate diets) to add a lot of B—6. We will see more examples of the importance of this pattern for nutritional balance.

Vitamin B—12 (Cobalamin)

This vitamin, the last to be discovered (in 1948), takes on important coenzyme roles, and seems to be involved in the metabolism of proteins, fats, and carbohydrates, in numerous special aspects of body chemistry. Fortunately it is plentiful in animal-source foods, and deficiencies in the U.S. are very rare, generally confined to people who reject animal foods.

Partly because the knowledge of B—12 is so recent, the RDA Committee set its recommendations quite high in 1968, then cut them sharply in its 1974 revision, to 3.0 micrograms. The U.S. RDA still uses the 1968 figure (not on the basis of scientific evidence, but simply because FDA established its standards for the U.S. RDA before the 1974 revision). So the U.S. RDA at this writing is 6.0 mcg. Commenting on this, the Labeling Committee of the National Nutrition Consortium observed that: "The U.S. RDA for vitamin B—12 is set very high, at perhaps ten times levels needed as a minimum by most people."

The fact that B—12 is found almost exclusively in animal cells has led to some concern about excessive use of *unfortified* soy proteins. The buyer of these proteins, who uses them as meat substitutes, should choose products with added B—12. Such fortification is almost universal, except in the case of "natural" food sources. The need for B—12 furnishes a persuasive argument for including milk and eggs, and if possible fish, in a vegetarian diet. The vegan definitely needs B—12 supplementation, aiming at 3 mcg. daily, although there is little reason to worry if he misses this by half. He might also note that many breakfast cereals are fortified with B—12.

A few people are not able to absorb B—12 normally. This results in a condition called *pernicious anemia* and requires a lifetime of injections of the vitamin.

Pantothenic Acid

This vitamin forms part of one of the master enzymes of the body, *coenzyme A,* which stands at a kind of metabolic crossroads. Its pivotal role in so many protein, fat, and carbohydrate reactions, and its presence in almost every body tissue, are of great scientific interest. But in terms of practical nutritional choice, pantothenic acid is virtually unavoidable. Not only is it present in our own tissues, but in those of almost all other living things, plant and animal. Its very name is derived from a Greek word which means something like "from everywhere."

While some pantothenic acid can be lost in food preparation, both at home and in industry, such losses have been taken into account in the setting of the U.S. RDA at 10 mg. But even the narrowest and sparsest of diets do not seem to lead to pantothenic acid deficiency.

Earlier (in Chapter Five, p. 108) we saw how the U.S. RDA for pantothenic acid was determined, and saw that there are apparently sources of the vitamin in addition to the food supply—probably intestinal bacteria. In sum, pantothenic acid need not be a dietary concern.

Biotin

This is another essential vitamin in the world of coenzymes. As with pantothenic acid, no RDA has been chosen, though there is a U.S. RDA of 0.3 mg. Again, there is no need for dietary concern about biotin.

We have observed that biotin is liberally made by the microorganisms of the intestines, and the only known deficiencies have been those artificially induced in volunteers, by the feeding of an antivitamin and careful elimination of biotin-rich foods. As a matter of curiosity, but of no practical import, the antivitamin, *avidin,* is found in the *raw* white of eggs. To produce deficiency took the equivalent of the avidin in two dozen raw egg whites a day.

The U.S. diet is generally ample to meet the U.S. RDA; and it is supplemented by the substantial amounts produced by our indwelling microbes.

Vitamin C (Ascorbic Acid)

Almost everyone knows that in the 1750s a British doctor cured shipboard scurvy with citrus fruit, and that thereafter limes were carried on British ships to prevent this lethal deficiency disease (leading to calling the British "limeys"). Without meaning to detract from the historical reputation of Dr. James Lind, Captain in the Royal Navy, the story is a little misleading and encourages the myth that citrus is essential if we are to be spared a deficiency of vitamin C.

Scurvy had been known for some 3,000 years before 1750. Here and there throughout history, its sufferers have been cured by eating something. For example, in 1535 Cartier's men, exploring Canada, fell ill of scurvy and began to die. An Indian told Cartier that he had been healed by the juice of the leaves of a tree. In eight days Cartier's men were well again, cured by this juice.

What was the tree? It could have been sassafras, hemlock, willow, or any number of evergreens, or almost any edible green food, so widely is vitamin C distributed. In 1617, John Woodall prescribed lemons to ward off scurvy on long voyages. And when Lind did publish his *Treatise of the Scurvy,* the Royal Navy did nothing about it for fifty years. A hundred years later, the westering American pioneers were still dying of scurvy by the thousands, leading to the planting of citrus in California. In World War I, thousands of troops died of scurvy.

The point is, historically, that until the isolation of vitamin C in 1932, scurvy was not truly understood, and was not eradicated. But there are any number of adequate sources of vitamin C, and if citrus were wholly lost from our food supply, we might fall below our RDAs for vitamin C, but we would not become scorbutic (affected with scurvy).

Why? Partly because in the average normal person, only 10 mg. of vitamin C a day will prevent scurvy, less than a fourth of the RDA for the adult male, and a sixth of the U.S. RDA.* What would it take to supply this minimal amount of vitamin C?—a fifth of a cup of raw

*However, to maintain the desired body pool of vitamin C, 30 mg. a day seem to be needed.

cabbage, one Brussels sprout, a fifteenth of a cup of broccoli, a small ear of corn, two large leaves of the greener lettuce, half a serving of liver, an ounce of canteloupe, a tablespoon of green pepper, 30 potato chips, a third of a cup of sauerkraut, half an ounce of strawberries, two ounces of tomato juice, or, if all else fails, your ration of Kool-Aid.

Vitamin C has an extremely broad metabolic function in the body— in the formation of connective tissue and the matrix of bone, the body's use of calcium and iron, the prevention of infant anemias, the integrity of the capillaries and the prevention of hemorrhage, the making of key hormones, and a host of other bodily work. As we have seen repeatedly, such urgently needed nutrients tend to be plentiful in the balanced scheme of life.

Most life forms have some use for vitamin C (keep in mind that plants do not make vitamins just for us), and nearly all of them can make it from the simple sugar glucose. Only a few lamentable species cannot make it: monkeys, guinea pigs, a bird called the red-vented bulbul, an obscure Indian fruit bat—and one other, man.

The U.S. RDA for vitamin C is 60 mg., but only because it does not take into consideration the 1974 RDA, of 45 mg. for the adult male. This allowance which is 50 percent higher than the standards of Canada, Britain, or the U.N., is easy to get; it is generally satisfied in America.

Probably no vitamin is more popular today, more acclaimed as a cure for more diseases. But the National Nutrition Consortium's Labeling Committee stated: "Various enthusiasts say that vitamin C will prevent or cure everything from hepatitis to high blood pressure, from kidney disease to prostate infection, heart disease, fat, tumors, colds, varicose veins, and even schizophrenia. Science finds such claims to be largely or entirely unsubstantiated."[7]

One really needs to make no special effort to be safe from vitamin C deficiency, certainly less than is warranted to insure adequate amounts of such marginally-consumed nutrients as B—6 and ribo-flavin. A sensible consumption of fruits and vegetables guarantees adequate C, unless these foods are boiled mercilessly and/or chopped up into tiny pieces. Vitamin C is susceptible to heat and air and to dissolving in cooking water. The vitamin C in foods is protected when the food is acid, not overcooked, and stored in covered containers.

One cannot possibly get the huge amounts recommended to cure so many diseases, except from supplements. And there is no clear evidence of nutritional value for amounts beyond those easily obtained in foods.* The RDA Committee deals with the question of "megadoses" of vitamin C as follows: "Although vitamin C in large amounts may have some pharmacologic or drug-like effects, these are not related to the normal functioning of the vitamin at nutritional levels . . . The Food and Nutrition Board feels that many of these claims are not sufficiently substantiated, or the effects are not of sufficient magnitude, and that routine consumption of large amounts of ascorbic acid is not advisable without medical advice."

THE FAT-SOLUBLE VITAMINS

In any health-food store nowadays, one can buy quantities of "Vitamin F" rather cheaply. The main thing wrong with doing so—in the hope of new vitality, better hair growth, beautiful skin, and whatever other promises the particular clerk may make—is that there is no such thing as vitamin F. The compound is really one of essential fatty acids. It is a most unusual American who does not get the small needed amount of essential fatty acids from food, mainly vegetable oils. And in any case, they are not vitamins.

Healthy people have little need for supplements of the fat-soluble nutrients which *are* vitamins. Only one of these appears to be short in our national dietary. That shortage is easily repaired, as we shall see, by some minor changes which can take care of the vitamin and mineral needs of the vast majority of us.

Vitamin A (Retinol)

Vitamin A does not meet RDA levels for many modern Americans. And it is easy to see why, when one thinks about the common dietary patterns of the day.

True vitamin A, *retinol,* is found only in animal-source foods associated with fats and oils, as in liver or in fish oils. Since it is

---

*As for the most commonly believed *drug* value, there is no good evidence that vitamin C will prevent colds. Some work does suggest a modest decrease in cold *severity* may result from modestly higher intake, with about 250 mg. per day having maximal effect.

colorless, why do we associate a yellow color with vitamin A? Because the yellow pigments, the *carotenoids,* mainly *beta-carotene,* can serve as precursors, or *provitamins,* of vitamin A. That is, the body can break apart carotene from plants to make true vitamin A. Thus it is that the yellow of carrots, pumpkin, winter squash, yams, or canteloupe all denote rich sources of provitamin A.

But all that is yellow is not vitamin A. The yellow pigments of corn and egg yolks, for example, do not indicate vitamin A. On the other hand, the deep greens of vegetables usually do. So spinach and kale, watercress, the greener lettuce, mustard greens, and broccoli are also good vitamin A sources. So are green peas, green peppers, endive, asparagus, and so forth.

Milk, butter, and margarine are good vitamin A sources; but on the other hand, except for livers, meats are not, generally offering less than one percent of the U.S. RDA of 5,000 international units. The American avoidance of green and yellow vegetables, the reduction in our milk consumption, and our disinterest in fruits (with the exception of oranges for breakfast, offering only perhaps six percent of the U.S. RDA) help to explain why vitamin A has become an American nutrient problem. In the Ten State Survey, at least a third of the children had low blood-serum levels of vitamin A.

As we consider the vitamin A content of foods, we note that these values, like those of other fat-soluble vitamins, are not expressed in milligrams, but in *units* of one kind or another. Why the difference? It is because these vitamins occur in different forms, and the several forms have different degrees of biological effect. For example, pure vitamin A has about twice the biological value of the beta-carotene found in vegetables. *International units* (I.U.) are the measure most often found in tables, serving as a single measure to cut across differing values of vitamin compounds.

In an attempt to be even more accurate, a United Nations Committee (FAO/WHO) decided a few years ago to list vitamin A in terms of *retinol equivalents,* retinol being the pure form of the vitamin. The RDAs are now shown in both the retinol values (*REs*) and in I.U. The mathematics of converting various vitamin A forms to REs can be handled quite simply. To get REs, divide I.U.s by five. (So the RDA of 5,000 I.U. of vitamin A becomes 1,000 REs.) The international units have been retained as the basis of the U.S. RDAs for vitamin A. The fact that the conversion of provitamin A into retinol is not very efficient (about 15 to 35 percent) should be no cause for concern.

The true vitamin value is revealed in the I.U.s or REs shown in the tables.

Perhaps the most striking sign of vitamin A deficiency is visual. Night vision drops off, and eventually blindness can ensue. For retinol gets its very name from its role in vision. Xerophthalmia and keratomalacia, due to lack of vitamin A, are almost unknown in the U.S., but are major causes of blindness in parts of Asia and the Middle East. More than a million cases of vitamin A deficiency blindness are believed to occur in these areas every year. Fortunately, our own vitamin A shortages are not severe enough to cause such problems.

Other results of vitamin A deficiency include problems of the skin and the body's mucous membranes, in the latter case, leaving certain tissues more susceptible to infection. Growth and reproduction can also be impeded, as may be the development of tooth enamel.

It is commonly said that, in the U.S. *hypervitaminosis A,* an overdosage of the vitamin, may be more of a medical problem than shortage. Such excess can cause blurred vision, lost appetite, high irritability, skin problems, hair loss, headaches, diarrhea, nausea, drowsiness, even brain damage.

Because vitamin A, like the other fat-soluble vitamins, can be stored in the liver, our consumption of them need not be quite so constant as with water-soluble vitamins. For example, eat a fairly good-sized carrot (some 10,000 I.U.), and your vitamin A allowance is met for two days.

The regular use of much carrot juice, or the similar use of juices from other high vitamin A sources, presents a possible hazard. Fortunately, when the source of the excess vitamin is carotenoids, there is an early warning from the coloring chemicals; the skin begins to turn yellow.

How can one regulate vitamin A intake to desirable levels? The foods which could supply our missing vitamin A are also those which furnish good quantities of B—6 and folacin. Make sure to get enough green and yellow vegetables, and the odds are that you will get all the often missing vitamins in one package. The green foods with A also are likely to contain B—6, folacin, vitamin C, and some other B vitamins, including meaningful amounts of riboflavin.

This association is not mere coincidence. If vitamin shortages have developed because of certain changes in food-consumption patterns, it stands to reason that most of the missing vitamins will be absent because we have disdained the same foods—especially starchy vegetables, grains, and fruits. Restoring these foods in a balanced way will restore the lost micronutrients.

Vitamin D

Once rickets—with its twisted and deformed joints and bones—was commonplace in northern Europe. The disorder became common in the 1700s, as the Industrial Revolution brought slum crowding in the cities, and the smoke poured into the air to block the sun.

For rickets is a deficiency disease, caused by lack of vitamin D. Few foods other than liver supply much D. Nature seems to have relied to a large extent on the sun, which irradiates the skin, causing sterols beneath the skin to form vitamin D—3. (D—3 is the form more often found in liver, eggs, and fatty fish.) The D vitamins are essential to the absorption and utilization of calcium to build bone.*

If the sun is cut off, by a northerly geography, fog, smog, or a life indoors, vitamin D must somehow be ingested. As insurance against vitamin D deficiency in infants, who are after all building bone much faster than adults, most U.S. milk is fortified with 400 units of vitamin D per quart. Except in unusual circumstances, however, it would appear that most adults have no need for vitamin D beyond that generated by sunlight.

Since excess vitamin D can be quite toxic—with such afflictions as weight loss, vomiting, irritability, and the depositing of calcium into such soft tissues as those of the lungs and kidneys—self-prescription of extra vitamin D is a poor idea (beyond the amounts found in fortified foods). British experience has shown that as little as six to ten times our RDAs of vitamin D can be toxic for small children. Twice as much as that can cause trouble for adults.

Although the U.S. RDA for vitamin D (400 units) applies to everyone, the RDA Committee notes that, "Since the requirement for the normal healthy adult seems to be satisfied by nondietary sources, no dietary recommendation is necessary. However, a dietary intake of 400 I.U. for normal individuals of all ages incurs no risk of toxicity."

---

*Vitamin D is also considered to be a hormone, because it is activated in one tissue to serve chemically in other tissues.

Vitamin K

The most striking function of this vitamin is suggested by the fact that it takes its initial from the German word for coagulation. By promoting clotting, vitamin K acts to help prevent hemorrhages in case of bodily injury.

While vitamin K is found in foods—especially green, leafy vegetables, cabbage, peas, and grains—there is not much in animal-source foods. On the other hand the vitamin is produced in quantity by the intestinal bacteria,* and deficiencies are virtually unknown under normal conditions. But prolonged use of antibiotics calls for some care because antibiotic therapy can knock out the K-producing bacteria.

The food form and the form produced by bacteria serve much the same function.

Vitamin E (Tocopherols)

From the beginning, realities have forced scientists to change and rechange their theories about this vitamin. It was first identified in 1922 as an unknown factor in the fertility of rats. By the time it was isolated, in 1936, it was closely identified with reproduction, so much so that it was named *tocopherol,* from the Greek meaning "to bear young." During the next decade numerous exciting deficiency signs were identified in animals—liver degeneration and muscular dystrophy in chicks and rabbits, heart damage in calves, and retarded growth in rabbits. The prospects for use in curing human ills looked important.

But none of these deficiency signs were found in humans; nor were any identifiable ailments. Indeed, over a period of eight years, starting in 1953, experiments were conducted (under the auspices of the National Research Council) in which volunteers were kept on low levels of the vitamin. For six years they were closely watched for physical or mental effects. Nothing seemed to happen.**

Vitamin E—really a group of eight different forms of an unusual

---

*Vitamin K is unusual in that it is one of the few nutrients which can be absorbed from the *large* intestine.

**When low levels of plasma vitamin E were induced in human volunteers for three years, however, red blood cell levels decreased slightly.

alcohol—appears mainly to be an antioxidant in humans, regulating the destructive oxidizing of cell membranes and vitamin A, and probably preventing some blood disorders. It is not known to have any enzymatic role. Its function is suggested by the fact that it can prevent oxidation (and thus rancidity) of oils; in fact, it is a common additive to oily foods. Some scientists have even questioned whether, technically, tocopherols ought really to be called vitamins at all.

If we look back at the deficiency effects in rats, we can see why some enthusiasts have assumed that all sorts of benefits derive from vitamin E—including greater sexual potency, the cure or prevention of heart disease, prevention of miscarriages, and the cure of ulcers and burns. The idea that the vitamin can slow the oxidation of cell membranes has led to the idea that it might somehow prevent some effects of aging, and this in turn has led to a wide sale of vitamin E in cosmetics. There is no evidence that it is useful. Scientifically, interest in a possible relationship between tocopherols and aging continues; but whatever else has been learned, we know that massive doses of E will not stop the clock.

An RDA for vitamin E was set in 1968, with 30 I.U. per day as the upper recommendation. (An I.U. of vitamin E is essentially equal to a milligram of the most active form, *alpha-tocopherol*. This provides a standard based on the true active amount of the vitamin, avoiding the confusion invited by the variances among the many natural forms.) Since typical Americans get only from 10 to 20 I.U., without evidence of any problems, in 1974, the RDA Committee cut the recommendation in half (although the U.S. RDA remains 30 I.U.).

Vitamin E needs rise with increased consumption of polyunsaturated fats. This is generally not a problem, however, because most foods high in polyunsaturated fat, such as vegetable oils, are also high in vitamin E. And, conversely, our needs fall when we eat less of such foods. It is hard to envision much of a problem; but our knowledge of vitamin E is far from complete. (For example, it appears that, for little-understood reasons, consumption of the trace mineral selenium lessens our need for E.)

Should one take vitamin E supplements, just to be safe? Remember, that as a fat-soluble vitamin, E can be stored in the body. And excess storage can be harmful. As for benefits from supplements, consider these two statements, made after careful review by respected authorities:

"Vitamin E has not been proved scientifically to have any of the 'miraculous' effects being claimed for it. And FDA sees no reason for persons in good health and eating a well-balanced diet to use a dietary supplement." (FDA in a report to consumers.)[8]

"Misleading claims that vitamin E supplementation of the ordinary diet will cure or prevent human ailments . . . are not backed by sound experimentation or clinical observations. Some of these claims are based upon deficiency symptoms observed in other species. Careful studies over a period of many years attempting to relate these symptoms to vitamin E deficiency in human beings have been unproductive. The wide distribution of vitamin E . . . makes a deficiency in humans very unlikely." (The National Research Council's Committee on Nutritional Misinformation.)[9]

Are There Any Other Vitamins?

Those which we have listed are the only ones which are generally recognized as vitamins for human beings. *Choline* is a vitamin for some animals, but it has not been established as a vitamin for humans, who can make it themselves. Other chemicals have sometimes been called *pseudo-vitamins.* These include PABA (*p-aminobenzoic acid*), really a part of folacin, *lipoic acid,* and *inositol;* choline is sometimes included in this grouping. These are mentioned mainly because health-food enthusiasts sometimes ascribe to these substances a need and value which has never found scientific support.

Some promoters have waxed eloquent over "vitamin B—15," *pangamic acid,* but it is not known to be a vitamin. Certainly "vitamin B—17" has been shown to be more myth than medicine; it is supposedly the active ingredient of *Laetrile,* an unaccepted cancer remedy sold at high prices to the desperate, despite Federal banning of the substance as valueless. This "vitamin" is derived from apricot pits, and some amateur attempts to make extracts at home have ended badly, for unless the extractor knows what he is doing, he can extract dangerous amounts of cyanide.

Lecithins are also commonly promoted as though they were vitamins, especially to lower blood cholesterol levels and prevent heart disease. These are useful fatty compounds which are known as *phospholipids,* and they are found in all cells. They are also useful as food additives, to emulsify lipids and give certain products smoothness. But they are not vitamins, and they do not prevent disease. Nor, despite claims made in popular magazines, do they move fatty deposits around on your body.

It would be smug to say that we have discovered the last true vitamin. As our ability to study the chemistry of the body at the level of the molecule improves, we may yet find more. But one thing is certain: the health-food maker or eccentric healer is not able to identify vitamin needs which the nation's major universities, clinics and laboratories cannot confirm. The scientific demand for hard evidence is not, as some claim, due to cronyism, a passion for form, or exclusivity; it is born of a responsibility that must insist on reality.

A BRIEF GUIDE TO MINERALS AND WATER

Underwood was sure he had solved the mystery in 1935, but he could not explain why. For some years, fat, well-fed sheep which had been moved onto certain Australian pastures and were given the best of care, had sickened and died. Underwood had found a difference in these pastures—a subtle lack of the metal cobalt in the soil. But not for a generation would the "outback" sheepmen know the significance of cobalt—that extremely tiny amounts are needed by sheep to make vitamin B—12.

How tiny? A decade before Underwood's discovery, Elvehjem of Wisconsin had found cobalt in living creatures and had estimated that a rat's body contained about one two-million-eight-hundred-thousandths of an ounce. We humans also need cobalt (which we must get in our vitamin B—12), but not in very large amounts. For example, B—12 deficiency in a vegetarian might be prevented by a glass or two of milk a day—and the amount of cobalt in this milk is on the order of a millionth of an ounce.

Not all our minerals are needed in such minute amounts, but even our largest mineral requirements are not really very big. For example, our calcium need is among the largest, being needed to build the skeleton. Nevertheless, in the same half glass of milk, an excellent calcium source, there is only about one 200th of an ounce of the mineral.

So while minerals in food were detected quite early—Menghini found iron in the blood in 1747—knowledge of their functions had to await a more sophisticated chemistry. And the truth is that even today, with microscopes which can look deep into the molecule, our knowledge of minerals is quite limited. We can begin to see why when we recall that the proper function of giant, complex molecules may depend on the inclusion and correct placement of a single atom.

It is not easy to define the term "mineral" in terms of human nutrition. It is a hangover from 19th century chemistry, when, on the burning of plant or animal materials, the residual ash was considered the mineral matter, at first looked upon as a kind of single food factor—as *the* protein and *the* vitamins were once seen. In every-day terms, a mineral is anything which is not vegetable or animal; but in nutritional terms, a mineral is surely part of both.

The broad definition of a nutritional mineral has to be something like—*An inorganic substance which is essential in small quantities for life processes. Inorganic,* in the chemical sense, refers to matter which is not constructed with a carbon skeleton. What we are really discussing here are the needs for some special atomic elements for making essential life structures and chemicals. Let us see what these are, confining our discussion largely to what we know about nutritional needs and how to meet them.

Calcium

Almost everyone knows that calcium is a basic material of the bones and teeth. The dairy people hardly let us forget. But most of us tend to think of the human skeleton much as if it were like the steel web of a skyscraper—solid, fixed, and constructed but once in the original building process of childhood, to be forgotten behind the more fragile exterior parts, until it begins to creak and crack with age.

Actually, our bones are dynamic and very much alive, constantly changing and interacting with the rest of the body. We may read that some ninety-nine percent of our calcium lies in teeth and bones, and that only one percent is at work in the blood and nerves, and general body chemistry. And thus we may easily be deceived. For we have the picture of a mass of immutable calcium locked in the skeleton on the one hand (some two to three pounds in all, really), and on the other of perhaps a dozen grams dispersed in a precarious balance throughout our body chemistry. So we might believe that at any moment, a tiny shortage could cause muscle spasms or let our nerves go awry.

As the late Adelle Davis explained: "Calcium is used by the nerves in the transportation of impulses. When calcium is undersupplied, nerves become tense and irritable . . . In children we see . . . temper tantrums, unpleasant dispositions, chewing of fingernails and restlessness in sleeping . . . The calcium-deficient adult is inclined to be quick-tempered, grouchy, and irritable, and to have a feeling of tenseness or uneasiness. He will often exhibit restless habits such as tapping the arm of a chair or swinging his feet."[10] What to do? Miss Davis urged milk, saying that ". . . the calcium soothes the nerves, and restful sleep usually follows." With our huge calcium reserves, these ideas are absurd.

Some of calcium-related chemistry is central to life. For example, the calcium in the fluid which bathes heart tissue plays an important role in the regulation of the heartbeat. To name just a few functions, calcium is essential to the clotting of blood, to the digestion and absorption of other nutrients, and to the transmission of nerve impulses. These functions have high priority, and the body is equipped to protect them and to guarantee that they continue. Bones and even teeth serve as storage centers (not just for calcium, but for other elements as well). Except in cases of extreme privation, the calcium for such processes is simply transported from the skeleton. (True, milk is soothing to many—but not for its calcium content. The effect is mainly like that of sucking one's thumb, which of course is reminiscent of our earliest milk drinking.)

One cannot wisely continue borrowing calcium from one's skeleton indefinitely, however. For there will be an over-all loss of calcium ions, and eventually the total body calcium can be compromised. The object of good nutrition is to replace the bodily losses in the adult, and of course to supply proportionately larger amounts to the child, who is enlarging his skeleton. For similar reasons, the pregnant or nursing mother also has greater calcium demands. Repeated pregnancies without adequate calcium intake can harm the mother—for her baby's needs take priority.

The losses in such body chemistry and the requirements of growth determine our calcium needs. Unfortunately, we cannot yet judge these amounts with anything like precision. For one thing, calcium absorption from the intestine can vary. It averages about 30 percent of our calcium intake. But if we get too little total calcium, our absorption efficiency increases, up to double the normal. If we get very high levels in our food, we may absorb as little as 10 percent. This suggests a protective mechanism. Calcium needs are also confused by inter-relationships of absorption and use that involve vitamin D intake, lack or excess of protein and vitamin C consumption, oxalic and phytic acids in foods we eat (oxalic acid is found in spinach and rhubarb, for example, and excess phytic acid may be obtained by overeating grains), the amount of fat we take in, and so on.

These differences are not small. When subjects consumed some 600 grams of protein a day (perhaps five times ordinary intake), their urine contained *eight* times as much calcium.

United Nations experts recommend 400-500 mg. of calcium a day for adults; Canada recommends 500 mg.; the U.S. RDA is 1,000 mg. Plainly there is disagreement here. Some experts have opined that only 200 to 260 mg. a day are really needed by adults. And Hegsted points out that low levels are apparently consumed by large populations with no seeming harm.[11] For example, he cites one study of high calcium consumption in northern Central America and low consumption in Panama, with no observable bone difference. He mentions that, when a low-calcium diet is fed, urinary and fecal losses become very low, suggesting the body's adjustment mechanism, altering use to serve the need.

These arguments are worth noting, in part because calcium is not easy to get in quantity, except from a few rich sources, such as milk, cheese, and sardines (because the small bones are eaten). A cup of milk supplies about a third of the U.S. RDA, a one-ounce slice of cheese about a fourth, a small can of sardines better than a third. Green leafy vegetables are also good sources, at a level of some 12 to 18 percent of the U.S. RDA per serving. A number of foods, such as eggs, cabbage, bread, and some vegetables and fruits, are often noted as calcium sources, but usually contain only around three percent of the U.S. RDA. When calcium requirements go still higher, as we shall see with pregnant women, or must be obtained from fewer calories, as among some children and senior citizens, the problem increases. Indeed, that is mainly why milk products are given a separate grouping in the Basic Four Food Groups.

The problem of meeting the existing U.S. RDA for calcium leads some experts to believe that the requirements will be studied more closely, with an eye toward reducing allowances.

We can probably conclude that the normal healthy adult (aside from pregnant and nursing women) need not fear minor failures to meet current RDAs. Hegsted has concluded that: "Due to the high levels of calcium recommended . . . which exceed the intakes of many people . . . dietary data are commonly interpreted as showing that a large percentage of the U.S. population is deficient in calcium and . . . that increased intakes of calcium would be beneficial. There is simply no evidence that this is true and . . . a great deal of evidence that it is not true.'' [11]

Phosphorus

While phosphorus is a widely used element in any number of body processes, indispensable in energy use, for example, its main function is as a kind of nutritional teammate of calcium. Deficiencies are virtually unknown, because phosphorus is so often found in so many foods; it is almost always present in quantity when one finds calcium.

Moreover, since phosphorus is often found where there is little or no calcium, as in meats, there is little practical need to worry about getting enough. The U.S. RDA is 1,000 mg., the same as calcium, and typical U.S. intake is estimated to be about 1,500 mg. And while ideally the biochemist would like to see phosphorus consumed in fairly close ration to calcium, most people seem to tolerate rather wide swings of this ratio.

There is one sure way to compromise bodily phosphorus—by using lots of antacids regularly. If these are of the common type, which are not absorbed, phosphorus can become chemically bound and kept from absorption. Prolonged use of antacids should be only on doctor's orders (and doctors usually take a dim view of such use).

Magnesium

This is another important element with wide involvement in body chemistry. We have seen that broad use generally goes with easy availability from a wide variety of food, and this is true for this mineral. Magnesium is needed in many enzyme systems, and in such basic matters as maintaining the electrical potential (hence the ability to function) of all our nerves and muscles. Moreover, there is ample capacity for storage, with calcium and phosphorus in the bone materials. (About 70 percent of our bodily magnesium is in the bone salts.) We can't afford to run out.

Magnesium is closely associated with the maintenance of the body's fluids. So if diarrhea or vomiting are prolonged, large amounts of magnesium may be lost with the fluid. Along with the replacement of such lost water, we also need to restore the salts, for it can take time to muster the body's reserves and circulate them sufficiently. Loss of these *electrolyte* salts helps to explain the abdominal cramps and spasms, weakness, and other symptoms which we sometimes associate with the immediate aftermath of food poisoning or intestinal diseases.

The U.S. RDA for magnesium is 400 mg. for adults; and contrary to the promotions of some supplement makers, the RDA Committee finds we have no general problem getting this much.* We tolerate reasonable excesses well, but they accomplish nothing, and we may also absorb less of this mineral when we swallow too much.

The average American diet is estimated to contain about 210 mg. of magnesium in each 1,000 calories. Milk is the best common animal source, but the main sources are vegetable. About 20 percent of our magnesium probably comes from grains. Beans, peas, nuts, and green leafy vegetables are good sources.

OF WATER AND SALT

(Sodium, Potassium, Chloride and the Inner Sea)

Whether one believes that human life evolved slowly out of the sea or that it sprang whole from the hand of God, it is equally true that life survives in an inner sea. All of the nutrients flow and act within that sea, and water makes up about two-thirds of the weight of our bodies.

Ours is a salty sea, and the saltiness is due to the minerals of life. Much of the function of the inner body of water depends upon its content of sodium, potassium, and chloride.

Even without these other micronutrients, water has basic essential functions. It accounts for all the fluidity of the blood and the lymph; it is the body's transportation system; it is the buffer and shock absorber between the cells; it is the principal coolant which guards

---

*Some individuals, however, who disdain milk, grains, legumes, and green vegetables may have marginal consumption.

the need of the inner body to stay within a narrow temperature range, whether on a winter mountain or a midsummer beach. (Much of our cooling is done by evaporating water from our skin, about half in perceivable perspiration and the other half evaporated so subtly that it is known as "insensible perspiration.") Water is the lubricant of our joints and the carrier of digestion. It is the indispensable chemical of hydrolysis. Finally, water is our waste remover, through urine and feces.

Our need for water is probably more acute than for any other nutrient. Vitamin deficiencies take weeks or months to cause symptoms. The absence of water will cause death within days. Our loss of water is steady and rather large. It must, for example, carry the heat of our chemical reactions out from our deepest cells to the skin. This job alone, in extreme heat, can require eight quarts of water in a day. An athlete commonly loses four or five quarts in a practice session.

We get much of our water in our "solid" food, in addition to such liquids as milk and fruit juices, which are usually over 90 percent water. Fruits and vegetables are generally at least 80 percent water. Meats are half water. Even bread is a third water by weight. Under ordinary conditions we can make do with the water in our "solid food"—about six to seven eight-ounce glasses (whether it be spring water, coffee, or root beer).

A hot climate or vigorous activity can boost this need dramatically. And what we eat or drink can raise it even more. For example, an ounce of pure alcohol (something more than two ounces of whiskey) can require eight ounces of water to be metabolized. The dry mouth after a few alcoholic drinks means that alcohol has caused dehydration no different than that of a couple of sets of tennis. In a somewhat dehydrated state, either because of exercise, high temperature, or perhaps the low humidity of a pressurized jetliner, the alcohol which is consumed becomes an unusually large percentage of the blood. The drinker can become a road menace much more quickly on a hot August day. A couple of glasses of water can help as a preventive.

The old idea that athletes should not drink water during a game or practice makes no physiologic sense. An hour-by-hour schedule of regular water intake will help performance and can prevent collapse. Notwithstanding popular opinion to the contrary, what is drunk, and the temperature of it, scarcely matters, with certain exceptions: An athlete obviously should not be drinking alcohol; he should not drink beverages with caffeine during exercise, since caffeine stimulates urination; and he should not consume beverages high in fat, such as milkshakes. Special "sports drinks" have no special value. (The art of managing body fluids in athletics has been carefully spelled out by Dr. Nathan Smith.)[12] The rapid loss of weight during vigorous sports activity is of course due mainly to lost fluid, and has little to do with fat.

Sodium, Potassium and Chloride

These are three of the major regulators of the body fluids. To suggest a little of how they work, consider that about 40 percent of the body's water is inside the cells *(intracellular water)*. Here the water contains a fair amount of potassium. Outside and surrounding each of the cells, is *extracellular water.* Its main mineral is sodium. Much of both the sodium and potassium are combined with chlorine, forming chlorides of the two metals. The two fluids are separated by the cell membrane.

The difference of electrical potential between the two fluids has a number of effects. There is a chemical "push-pull" force between the two minerals across the cell wall. Sodium, by attracting a flow of water, can help move nutrients to and into the cell through the membrane. Increases in the sodium concentration also serve to draw potassium out of the cell. The electrical changes produced by changes of sodium and potassium concentrations, inside and outside the cell, are intrinsic to the way in which the electrical impulses of the nervous system are transmitted from cell to cell, from nerves to muscles, to cause contraction and relaxation.

In a sense, we may see the cells as tiny batteries. When potassium is fairly high within a cell, it is primed to "fire"; in the case of a muscle cell, it is ready to contract. Sodium has the effect of relaxing the cell, helping some of the potassium to leave through the cell wall.

How much of these minerals do we need? There are no RDAs or U.S. RDAs, partly because the minerals are so plentifully available from foods. For example, table salt consists of some 40 percent sodium and 60 percent chlorine.

Bodily needs of sodium can be met by from 500 to 1,000 mg. a day. Estimated intake of sodium chloride (table salt) is from 6,000 to 18,000 mg. daily; that is, from 2,400 to 7,200 mg. of sodium and from 3,600 to 10,800 mg. of chloride. Since the need for chloride is roughly of the same magnitude as that for sodium, the problem for either is more apt to be excess rather than inadequacy. The need for salt is perhaps a tenth to a thirtieth of what we consume. In fact, because sodium and chloride are so common in foods, and because of the use of so many sodium-containing products in cooking (from soy sauce to baking soda or powder, to garlic salt, ketchup and the like) we would probably do very nicely with no added salt from the shaker.

Do we need extra salt when it is hot? The RDA Committee indicates that sweat losses of more than 4 liters call for extra salt. Such losses would be signaled by the loss of some eight pounds. For replacement, the Committee recommends two grams (roughly a teaspoon) of table salt for each extra liter (a little over a quart) of water (sweat) lost. The salt we put on our food usually supplies this much, and salt tablets are generally not needed.

Potassium, despite some commercial promotion to the contrary, is not a deficiency problem for normal Americans. The RDA Committee estimates a need of about 2,500 mg. a day. The usual intake is from 2,000 to 4,000 mg. Earlier we noted some good sources—such as bananas, potatoes, tomatoes, carrots, celery, citrus juice, meat, poultry, fish, and cereals. We will also see that a dietary shift toward better sources of some of the more marginal micronutrients will automatically increase potassium intake.

THE TRACE ELEMENTS

Some 17 other minerals are known to have biological functions, in quantities much smaller than those needed in the so-called *macrominerals* (those needed in relatively large quantity) discussed above. There is still considerable uncertainty about the need for some of these *microminerals* (needed in tiny amounts). Others are clearly essential to human chemistry, however.

Iron

We have seen the importance of iron and the fact that it is a troublesomely scarce mineral in our diets. It is a critical factor not only in the hemoglobin of the blood, but in other life chemicals, including some enzymes.

One of the problems with iron is that we seem to absorb and use only about 10 percent of what we consume, and we do not understand this absorption well. Our meat consumption gives us a good deal, especially in blood iron. And this is certainly one reason why adult males and most children over the age of six have enough. But infants and women of menstrual age consistently show shortages. The most conservative estimates are that perhaps two-thirds of young American women are short of iron.

One reason for this shortage may be the shift in our dietary habits, away from starchy sources of iron—wheat, beans, potatoes, etc.—and away from green vegetables.

The RDA for most children and adult males is 10 mg. But the RDA for women from adolescence into middle age is 18 mg. So the U.S. RDA has been set at the higher level, 18 mg. This can be hard to get, unless one consumes foods especially rich in iron, such as liver and egg yolk. For this reason the Food and Nutrition Board has recommended iron supplementation for most women. This supplementation should not be overdone, however. Remember that one probably has a start of eight to twelve mg. a day from a typical diet—and that excess iron intake can cause constipation.

The form in which the iron is found affects how well it is absorbed. Absorption is highest for such complexes as *ferrous sulfate, ascorbates, fumarates,* and *citrates.* These latter complexes are sometimes called *chelates,* and lately, there has been quite a lot of promotion for them. Keep in mind that "chelated iron" supplements sold at high prices in health-food stores are nothing new and are just the complexes described above, which can be bought more cheaply in the supermarket. Iron phosphates, carbonates, and EDTA complexes are not well absorbed and it is best not to count on them, especially in situations such as pregnancy, when adequate iron is most urgent.

(There is a current fad for amino-acid chelates of various minerals. Their only extra value is the one you pay at the checkout stand. And it should be emphasized that there is no valid reason why a normal person needs supplements of most minerals, chelated or otherwise, unless there is a condition worth a doctor's prescription.)

There is also a simple way to make your own iron supplements. That is, by cooking foods in old-fashioned utensils—iron pots and pans. If there is a somewhat acidified cooking medium—a little vinegar, red wine, citrus juice, tomato juice, or almost anything else that tastes rather sour—small amounts of iron will dissolve out of the pan and be eaten with the food. One cannot say very precisely how much iron you will get this way, but some rather casual testing indicates that it is substantial. And most young women are short of only a few milligrams.

Even though iron supplements are generally cheap and readily available, it is still a good idea for women to work on improving their consumption of iron-rich foods. For the resulting dietary pattern, as we shall see, tends to increase the consumption of other sometimes inadequate nutrients.

Copper

All mammals require this element. The U.S. RDA is 2 mg., an amount believed to be consumed by most of us who eat ordinary diets. But some newer evidence suggests that some people may be slipping below this intake, and that actually the RDAs may, in this unusual case, be close to the borderline of our needs.

Aside from liver and shellfish, most of the better sources of copper are in the vegetable world, and are rather consistently the good sources of iron, except that green, leafy vegetables are not as valuable for this mineral. Among the better sources are dried peas and beans, potatoes, raisins, nuts, and grains. Meats are not a bad source, but again, it is hard to depend on them for all the need.

Once again, the curative powers of copper, sometimes heralded in the literature of health-food stores, are limited to those who suffer from deficiencies. Except in some special circumstances, true copper deficiency symptoms are almost unknown in our society.* For aside from a few rich sources, there are small amounts throughout the world of food.

Iodine

One of the great popular misunderstandings is that mineral values of foods are dependent upon the mineral content of the soils in which they grow. In general, the mineral content of plants is governed by

*However, there has been discussion of the possible importance of a good balance between copper and zinc which might affect health, with concern about too little copper intake to balance the zinc.[13]

heredity, not by soil. But there are exceptions to the rule, and iodine is one of them. The iodine content of a plant, and sometimes of a food from an animal which eats the plant, can be increased by ample iodine in the soil. Even the iodine content of milk and eggs can vary, depending upon the content of the soil on which the dairy or poultry feed was grown.

Endemic goiter is the most striking result of an iodine shortage in a regional soil. This is evidenced by a swelling of the neck, due to enlargement of the thyroid gland, for iodine is an essential in the secretions of that gland and in its normal function.

How common is such an iodine deficiency? In 1960, the World Health Organization estimated that perhaps 200 million of the world's people suffered from iodine shortage. In the U.S., at the 1969 White House Conference, endemic goiter was said still to be a problem in a number of the Plains states, especially those toward the Canadian border. Such iodine shortages seem to be created by the leaching of iodine from the soils, as it is carried away in streams and rivers. The seas are rich in iodine. And usually the food of coastal areas, especially food taken from the sea, offers ample iodine.

The White House Conference decided that, since *iodized salt* could eliminate all question of iodine shortage, it was inexcusable not to make use of such salt universal. The taste is not changed, there is no reasonable problem with excess, and the shortage can thus be eliminated.

But for some reason many processors do not use iodized salt, and often the salt which is bought in bulk by food chains and schools is not iodized—a pathetic oversight, and one which could so easily be remedied.

Fluorine

Fluorine—or in nutritional terms, *fluoride*—is often thought to be merely an additive which can help to prevent tooth decay. If fluoride is incorporated in the diet in childhood, it certainly does reduce the incidence of dental caries, an extremely costly and destructive problem which is almost universal. The cost of adding fluoride to water is pennies per capita; the saving in dental work is many dollars per capita, even if we ignore the saving in discomfort.

But fluoride's importance goes beyond this important attribute.

The Food and Nutrition Board recognizes fluoride as an essential element. Fluoride functions as a decay-saver by taking part in the formation of calcium structures, as *fluor-apatite.* What this means is that these structures deposit and hold calcium better, in effect maturing earlier. Tooth decay takes time. A child's new teeth are relatively soft, developing their hardness slowly. Added fluoride speeds up that process, building a kind of shield.

Although the matter is not fully understood, it has been inferred by some scientists that the deposition and retention of calcium in the skeleton is also improved by fluoride. It is possible that adults may lose less calcium from bone if fluoride is adequately consumed, perhaps preventing *osteoporosis*—a decalcification of bone which increases risk of fracture—which is common in the elderly.

The natural contribution of fluorides in drinking water varies from some 0.3 mg. to 3.1 mg. on the average. The effects of such variation were clearly seen in an early test. In Quincy, Illinois, the fluoride content of the water was no more than 0.2 parts per million, and more than three times as many cavities as there were in Galesburg, not far away, where there were 1.9 parts of fluoride to a million parts of water.

Many American communities have now fluoridated their water— often to levels no greater than the natural fluoridation in other areas. The reduction in decay has been 50 percent or more. Most nutritionists, if they happen to live in areas where the anxious block fluoridation of the water, buy bottled water containing traces of fluorides.

No U.S. RDA has been set for fluoride.

Zinc

Zinc is the only other mineral for which a U.S. RDA has been set— 15 mg., though less seems to maintain an equilibrium. There is little indication of intakes below this amount among the majority of our populace. For zinc is closely linked to animal protein, and as we have seen, there are few Americans who do not get adequate animal protein.

For vegetarians, zinc must come from eggs, milk, and whole grains. If eggs and milk are not consumed, there is a problem. For zinc can be bound up by phytic acid (found in grains). Should a vegetarian depend chiefly on grains for his protein, he may end up short of zinc.

By and large, there is little indication of a zinc problem in U.S. nutrition. Little zinc is found in our water, and some shift away from galvanized (zinc-coated) pipes to copper may be reducing our water intake of this nutrient. But there is little concern here, at least for the meat eater.

Some Other Trace Minerals

In the future, there may be many interesting discoveries about the needs of other trace minerals in the diet of man. Indeed, we now know that some of these are essential, but we do not know of deficiencies, and we do not know enough to measure precise needs or set recommended allowances.

Chromium is essential in glucose metabolism. Manganese is essential in bone construction. Molybdenum is important in an essential enzyme. Selenium—another of the elements in which soil content influences food content—may or may not be essential for humans; it is present in most U.S. diets. Nickel, tin, vanadium, and silicon have been found essential in animals, but one cannot say what this means for man.

Yet again, returning to the realities of food choice, there would seem to be little question that certain strategies in planning our meals, in reading a menu or a supermarket ad, will deal nicely, not only with the problem nutrients of which we are now aware, but with those we may possibly find in the future. Let us now examine how our knowledge of nutrition can shape our strategies of food choice.

REFERENCES
1. Berkman, R. *Vitamins: Do they really cure everything from colds to menstrual cramps to schizophrenia?* Glamour, Mar. 1971.
2. Harper, A. E. Letter to Sen. William Proxmire.
3. Task Force on Vitamin Therapy in Psychiatry, *Megavitamin and orthomolecular therapy in psychiatry,* in Nutr. Rev., July, 1974, p. 44.
4. Adams, R. and Murray, F. *Megavitamin Therapy,* Larchmont Books, New York, 1973, 136—64.
5. Pauling, L. *Vitamin C and the Common Cold,* Bantam, New York, 1971.
6. Nittler, A. column in Let's Live, Jan., 1974.
7. National Nutrition Consortium and Deutsch, R., *Nutrition Labeling,* National Nutrition Consortium, Bethesda, 1975, p. 99.

8. FDA, *Vitamin E—Miracle or myth?* FDA Consumer, Jul./Aug., 1973.
9. Food and Nutrition Board, *Supplementation of Human Diets with Vitamin E,* A statement, Nat. Acad. Sci., Washington.
10. Davis, A. *Why You Need Calcium* (Part 9, Vitality Through Planned Nutrition), Bestways, May, 1976.
11. Hegsted, D. *Calcium and Phosphorus* in Modern Nutrition in Health and Disease, Lea and Febiger, Phila. 1973.
12. Smith, N. *Food for Sport,* Bull, Palo Alto, 1976.
13. Klevay, L. *Coronary heart disease: The zinc-copper hypothesis,* Amer. J. Clin. Nutr. 28:764—74, 1975.

General References

14. Sebrell, W. and Harris, R. eds. *The Vitamins,* Academic Press, New York, 1972.
15. Goodhart, R. and Shils, M. eds. Sections 5,6,7,8 of Part I, The Foundations of Nutrition, in *Modern Nutrition in Health and Disease,* Lea & Febiger, Phila., 1973.
16. Robinson, F. *The Vitamin Co-factors of Enzyme Systems,* Pergamon Press, 1966.
17. RDA Committee, *Essential Fatty Acids and Fat-Soluble Vitamins, Water-Soluble Vitamins* and *Mineral Elements,* chapters in Recommended Dietary Allowances, Nat. Acad. Sc., Washington, 1974. (*NOTE. References on micronutrients being extremely numerous, the reader is referred to the selected references relevant to specific nutrients, as shown in Ref. 17 above, and to the General References for this book. Some additional references, relevant to special applications of vitamins and minerals, are listed below.)
18. Joint Committee of Amer. Acad. Pediatrics Committees on Drugs and on Nutrition, *The use and abuse of vitamin A,* Pediatrics, 48:655, 1971.
19. Statement of the Amer. Acad. Pediatrics, *Vitamin C and the common cold,* Newsletter of the Amer. Acad. Pediatrics, November 1, 1971.
20. Stare, F. *Not quite cricket,* Nutr. Today, Jan./Feb., 1971.
21. Passmore, R. *New nostrom,* Nutr. Today, Jan./Feb., 1971.
22. Smith, R. *The vitamin healers,* The Reporter, Dec. 16, 1965.
23. Council on Foods and Nutrition, *Improvement of nutritive quality of foods,* JAMA, 205:160—1, 1968.
24. Davies, I. *The Clinical Significance of the Essential Biological Metals,* Thomas, Great Britain.
25. White, H. *Should food iron be increased,* Illinois Med. Jrnl., June, 1969.
26. Norman, C. *Iron enrichment,* Nutrition Today, Nov./Dec., 1973.
27. Hodges, R. *Vitamin E: Uses and misuses,* Nutrition & the M.D., May, 1975.
28. Hodges, R. *Megavitamin therapy with ascorbic acid,* Nutrition and the M.D., May, 1975.
29. Beal, V. *The iron controversy,* Food Prod. Devel., May, 1975.
30. Fox, M. *The essential trace elements,* FDA Papers 5, pp. 8—14.
31. Herbert, V. *Megavitamin therapy; Facts and fictions,* Food & Nutrition News, Mar./Apr., 1976.
32. La Chance, P. ed. *Nutrition for food executives,* Food Prod. Devel. (a series) 1973—74, passim.
33. Davis, T. et al. *Review of studies of vitamin and mineral nutrition in the United States, (1950—1968),* J. Nutr. Ed. 1:2 Fall, 1969.
34. Jukes, T. *When Friends and Patients Ask About Megavitamin Therapy,* lecture, unpub.
35. Hegsted, D. *Problems in the use and interpretation of the RDA,* Ecol. Food Nutr. 1:255, 1972.

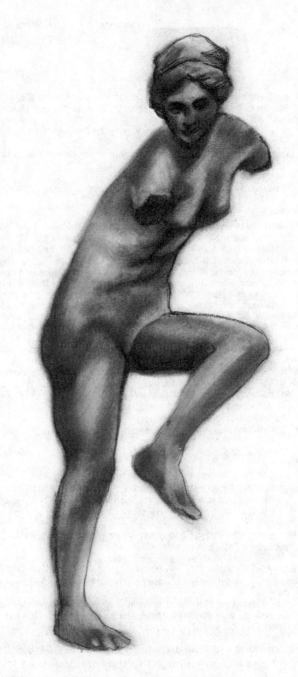

Balance, always understood to be the great art of life, is equally the art of the nutritionist. *Balancing Aphrodite, Goddess of Beauty and Fertility. Greek bronze, c. 200 B.C.*

chapter 12

BALANCE—THE SCIENTIFIC ART OF EATING

From the first, nutritionists have had the same purpose—to find a balance between the foods we eat and the chemical needs of life.

As late as the early 19th century, that balance was still obscure. For example, in London of that time, of every eight babies fed without mother's milk, seven died.[1]

By the early 20th century, science had coined the phrase "the balanced diet." But only three nutrients were known—protein, fat and carbohydrate—and when McCollum fed these to his rats in what was believed the perfect proportion, they began to sicken and die, and he predicted that we would find something more.

We have found more, both in nutrients and in foods to furnish them, but perhaps too much more, so that now when we look at our many foods and our many requirements, too often the result is utter confusion. Why should this information be confusing? Some simple mathematics will help to explain.

The Mathematics of Confusion.

If we recap our discussion of life and its nourishing chemicals, we see that we have examined, as essentials: fats and carbohydrates and 22 amino acids, water, some 22 vitamins and minerals, fiber and an unspecified number of trace elements.

In terms of requirements, we have reviewed 17 RDAs and 20 U.S. RDAs. The RDAs are different for 17 population groups—so we have been provided with recommendations, for 289 dietary necessities.

In meeting these recommendations, we have been using food-composition tables such as USDA Handbook No. 456. It lists 2,483 foods, with perhaps an average of three sublistings for each in terms of quantity, quality, and variations in processing. So we have 7,449 basic listings, with 15 different nutritive qualities for each, or 111,735 basic bits of information (to meet the 289 recommendations).

In reality, however, many supermarkets are said to offer not some 2,500, but some 11,000 different foods. So in theory, there could be 774,716 pieces of data appropriate to a proper choice of foods. Except, we may also want information on sodium, potassium, chloride, cholesterol, the three main types of fats and fiber—and the theoretical number of informational bits increases geometrically.

The point of all these numbers is to explain why the practical nutritionist must use some shortcuts in dietary analysis and planning. These shortcuts enable us to make some simple, safe estimates of what we need to eat. And they enable us to compensate intelligently for whatever are our personal tastes, food beliefs and physical conditions. One can construct a good diet for the blubber-eating Eskimo, the taro-eating Tahitian, the pasta-eating Italian, or the burger-eating American.

The endless bank of data about nutrition gives us check points that help us with some of the refinements of balance. For example, we need this welter of detail sometimes to check on foods which are within groups, to make certain that there are no important dissimilarities. For the grouping of foods is the nutritionist's principal technique for analyzing and planning.

UNDERSTANDING FOODS IN GROUPS

One simple way of using foods in groups is the *exchange system.* This has probably been used most in helping diabetics. For example, if the diabetic is selecting his meats, he looks at the meat *exchanges.*

He finds that similar amounts of pork and beef provide suitable exchanges for one another.

Since this system originated when carbohydrate limitation was still considered important for the diabetic, it was heavily oriented toward the carbohydrate content of foods. Secondly, it was concerned with calorie value, because, as we have seen, obesity has long been recognized as a factor in diabetes mellitus. In the group of cereal and grain products, five saltines were an exchange for a slice of bread. An avocado has much more fat than most fruits, so it is looked upon in the exchange system as a swap for a small pat of butter.

These exchange systems work, up to a point. But if we look closely, we will see that they have definite limitations.

Foods Are Not Sources of Single Nutrients

Each food is unique in its nutritional profile. If one exchanges beef for pork, one loses quite a bit of thiamin, of which pork happens to be an especially rich source. If one eats an avocado instead of a pat of butter, one gains a broad spectrum of nutrients, of the sort generally found in green vegetables, because butter has few nutrients other than fat.

Yet thinking about foods in terms of single nutrients is a popular way of looking at nutrition in our society, and one which has been carefully fostered by commercial interests. They sell the foods that are identified with certain glamorized nutrients. Almost everyone knows that citrus is a good source of vitamin C, so a powder which is colored orange and contains vitamin C may be substituted for the orange, without general realization of the fact that vitamin A, folacin, fiber and other nutrients are lost. On the other hand, an informed consumer knows that vitamin C-source foods are plentiful; he may derive his daily requirement from a number of lesser sources during the day—possibly a banana, some lettuce, a few cherries, some string beans. But each of these adjustments changes the dietary balance.

Food Exchanges Must Be Realistic

In these comparisons we can see a suggestion of the key flaw in the use of food groups as a guide. It is that one may put foods into the groups on too narrow a basis.

For example, if we look back at our examples of diabetic exchanges, the substitution of beef for pork gives us only one important dissimilarity, the sacrifice of thiamin. In realistic terms, there are probably very few of us who regularly depend on pork for thiamin. So the chance is not great that there will be a thiamin shortage for a day because we eat the beef.

On the other hand, if we were to substitute butter for our avocado, we might be unwise. A substitution of margarine or salad oil for the butter would be fine, because like butter, they are mainly sources of fats. (A small amount of vitamin A would be lost by using the salad oil—margarines are generally fortified with A—but the loss would be minor.) The avocado, however, is used differently in the diet. It might be compared more to string beans. Although the avocado has much more fat than string beans do, its place in the diet generally is much more like other vegetables than it is like the basic sources of fats.

In other words, the grouping of foods must be broadly based, and attention to a single dimension of its nutritive value may be a poor basis for selecting the grouping of a particular food. We can see that the grouping of foods in a realistic way can be tricky. Let us look at how it has been done.

THE BASIC FOOD GUIDES

As nutrition science began to take modern shape in the 1930s, various methods were tried for effective instruction about balanced nutrition. The greatest success was found with food groups in the "Basic Eleven." As the name indicates, this method placed foods in 11 groups, according to their similarities of nutritive value and role in diet, and also on the basis of what were seen as foundation nutrients. An obvious food group, for example, was the protein suppliers.

This system proved too cumbersome, however—who could really get a clear view of eleven food groups? Gradually it was felt that the individual food groups could be enlarged and the whole concept simplified—and the concept was modified, and modified again, first to the "Basic Nine," then to the "Basic Seven," and finally to today's "Basic Four."

The four foundation groups are:

Milk Group

Two or more glasses of milk, or servings of cheese, ice cream, etc., daily.

Meat Group

Two or more servings a day of meats, fish, poultry, eggs—with dry beans, peas, or nuts as alternates.

Vegetables and Fruits

Four or more servings daily of vegetables and fruits—from a group comprised of dark green or yellow vegetables, citrus, tomatoes, etc.

Breads and Cereals

Four or more servings daily—either enriched or whole-grain.

Depending on the character of the foods used to meet these group requirements, their caloric value is usually estimated at anywhere from 1,250 to perhaps 1,750 calories daily. (This presupposes that standard servings will be used, such as a 3.5-ounce portion of meat, that the foods are not served in sauces or gravies, and that the grains are not made into products with very high fat or sugar content, such as coconuts or pies. It is assumed that the extra allowable calories (to the levels needed by different individuals) will be consumed in additional foods, or in food ingredients used in the preparation of the basic foods.)

What Makes the Basic Four Work?

How can the whole panoply of foods and the variety of nutrient needs be reduced so simply to so few groups? In the answer to this question rests the key which permits those of us who are not computer-equipped scientists to plan a nutritionally sound diet, and to choose our food wisely every day without a great deal of research and mathematics.

For the fact is that generally, different patterns of nutrients appear in broad families of foods. In fact, except for the scarcity of calcium in the food world, we might envision only three food groups. (And indeed, if we ate liberally and knowledgeably from the grain and the vegetable and fruit groups, we could get sufficient calcium. Milk and its products provide a shortcut.)

Of course there are considerable variations among the foods within each group, and hence among their nutrients. One sort of fish or lettuce, nut or bean may differ nutritively from others. But it is assumed that from day to day and season to season, we will select differently from each of these groups, so that over a period of time, the nutritional values will be balanced to a desirable mean.

How the Basic Four Solves—And Causes—Problems.

Let us examine the milk group for a moment, as an example of how the food-group concept works. In recent decades American consumption per capita of fluid milk has gradually declined. This reduction may relate to tendencies toward certain nutrient shortages.

According to surveys, many of us seem to be getting too little riboflavin and calcium in our diets. These nutrients are well supplied by milk, which is also a contributor, though to a lesser extent, of some other nutrients which many people appear to consume inadequately—vitamin A, B—6, and folacin. Certainly the decline in milk drinking has been a factor in all of these shortages. And if we used more milk, some of the shortages would certainly be alleviated. In other words, the food-group concept would help nutritionally if it were regularly used.

On the other hand, there are flaws in the system. And these flaws suggest the need for nutrition knowledge and planning beyond the Basic Four. For one thing, the idea was originated when our food supply was simpler. The supermarket has wrought changes which have complicated matters. There are now thousands of convenience foods in which "basic foods" are combined. How do you place frozen pizza or chicken-pot pie in a food group? In many instances small amounts from various food groups may be present, but not enough nutritively to constitute a serving of any one group.

Consider a frozen pizza, with Italian sausage. It has something of the meat group, but a low-protein, high-fat meat in a small quantity. The crust may be suitable as a serving from the bread and cereals group, and the cheese may or may not scrape through as a milk-group serving. But what of the tomato sauce? Does it really make a vegetable serving? And after the crushing and double cooking of the tomatoes, are they really suitable as a vitamin C source? The answers tend to equivocate.

If we check TV dinners, we find that often the servings on the tray are much smaller than those envisioned for the Basic Four. Also, even though there is considerable variety in frozen-dinner meats, the vegetable slots change little; the only green vegetables one sees are peas and string beans. The small pile of dehydrated mashed potatoes has lost its vitamin C. And so on.

Even when products fit into the groups, they may not supply the assumed complement of nutrients. The intended nutritive values may be diluted. For example, biscuits substituted for bread may add a good deal of fat without much wheat; a pastry may represent a lot of sugar.

The Basic Four system has also been criticized because some nutrient requirements were unknown at the time it was created. It has been pointed out that the plan made no certain provision for vitamin E, folacin, magnesium, or zinc. And folacin, at least, seems to be short in many people's diets.

Finally, the Basic Four makes little allowance for changes in the life cycle. (The principal exception is in the milk group—with two glasses for adults, three for children, and four for teenagers.) We have generally similar cells throughout life, and the materials they need are essentially the same. But as their function changes—especially with changes of growth and activity—the needed quantities can change greatly.

As an example, consider the reference five-year-old child. He is so active and is growing so rapidly that he daily consumes only 200 calories less than his mother (1,800 and 2,000 calories respectively). His growth makes other demands for nutrients, too, such as extra calcium. His calcium need is as great as his mother's, even though he is little more than a third as heavy and does eat somewhat less food.

Three glasses of milk a day are recommended for him, providing for his calcium needs entirely. They also provide 27 grams of protein, only three grams less than his total need. Yet two servings of meat are suggested additionally, and we must remember that he also gets protein (and calcium) from bread and cereals, from vegetables, and even fruits.

Or consider the child's grandfather. His cells are, of course, far less active, and he is not growing. So he needs much less protein and calcium in proportion to his weight. He does not drink milk, but he has met his calcium needs by eating substantial amounts of cheese and green vegetables throughout his life. However, now his caloric needs are lower; he needs 600 calories less than he did at age 21. Instead of two or three ounces of cheese for a snack, he eats just one. His vegetable portions are smaller, too. And since he is now alone, he depends quite a lot on prepared convenience foods (in which greens are lacking).

Suppose grandfather makes a try at the Basic Four. He treats a slice of process cheese (cheaper, since he has budget problems, but containing less calcium than natural cheese) as a milk-group serving. Two servings give him only about a fourth of his needed calcium.

So while food guides such as the Basic Four are useful tools, they cannot be depended upon to do the whole job, since really effective nutrition planning should take into consideration more specific characteristics of an individual or a group. Later, we shall come back to them—with some ideas about how to make them serve each of us in a more personalized way.

TOWARD A MORE PERSONAL BALANCE

It is helpful to remember that, despite our individuality as people, our food habits, tastes, and needs tend to fall into groups. For example, baby, though certainly unique, shares characteristics with all babies—growing fast and living mainly on milk. Because of the milk they will probably have few calcium or protein problems. But milk has very little iron. So by the age of six months, most authorities agree, babies need some food which is a good iron source.

Adult food habits are much more complex, but they do tend to fall into cultural patterns. And one can usually find certain faults and advantages in each culture's ideas about food. In some cultures, the members follow certain patterns so closely that their nutrition problems tend to be quite predictable and consistent.

If we look at Americans, we see that they mostly build their meals around an animal-source main dish. If we look at Moslem Americans, we find that pork is eliminated from the meats. If we look at a college, we see that fish is not served often, and other foods may be limited because of price and the need to select foods with wide acceptance. If we look at a commune, we may find that the group is making all the food decisions for each member.

The public-health nutritionist makes use of such group patterns to identify the nutritional problems of the particular group. This can be particularly evident where resources are marginal and cultural patterns play a critical role, as in a developing country or an impoverished Indian tribe. And we can use the same technique to explore our own food patterns—in as broad a universe as our nation, or in as small a group as our family.

Having identified the patterns of our eating, we can then relate them to our own unique characteristics and lifestyles, to understand what modifications of diet we may need. Let us see how this works.

The Caloric Dimension.

The first measure of a diet is the total caloric value. This dimension represents a kind of budget, within which we must provide our nutrient needs. Clearly, the smaller our budget, the more carefully we must choose our expenditures.

For example, an athlete, burning perhaps 5,000 calories a day, can live in nutritional luxury. His needs for protein, and most other nutrients, is no greater than average. But eating at least twice as many calories, he can afford some carelessness. If he and our exemplary grandfather are the same size, and so both need 56 grams of protein a day, grandfather's diet must contain twice as high a percentage of protein.

Our athlete's caloric need is closer to that of the average man in 1900, when the reference adult male is estimated to have burned some 4,000 calories a day. Today a man of the same size, far more sedentary, uses only 2,700 calories. Although some nutrient needs (mainly for some water-soluble vitamins) change with the number of calories we consume, most do not. So the man of today must get much the same quantity of nutrients from much less food. In terms of a nutrition budget, each calorie we spend must bring a higher nutritive return. Foods which supply many calories, but rather few nutrients, defeat this purpose. They *dilute* our diets.

Some Patterns of Dilution.

We know that the major energy sources of our diets are fats and carbohydrates. So if surveys tell us that many of us are short of some other nutrients, we must be getting too many calories from foods which provide ample fats and/or carbohydrates, but too few of those other nutrients. Since fats provide more than twice as many calories as carbohydrates, they are the first place to look for diluents of the diet. Let us look again at our high-fat meal plan (p. 221). In one view, this dinner and its appetizers may seem contrived and unrealistic. It contains 162.8 grams of fat, representing some 1,465 calories from that one source. And in all it offers 2,624 calories, more than enough for a whole day for our reference man. Yet the meal is representative of a dominant pattern of food selection in our culture. Here is an analysis of it:

Table 12–1.

The Appetizer

Food	Calo-ries	Pro-tein (g.)	Fat g.	Carbo. g.	Calc. mg.	Phos. mg.	Iron mg.	Vit.A I.U.	Thia. mg.	Ribo. mg.	Niac. mg.	C mg.
Cashews 2 oz.	318	9.8	26	16.6	22	106	2.2	60	.24	.14	1.	—
Potato Chips, 20	228	2.2	16	20.	16	56	.8	—	.08	.02	2.	6
Whiskey, 1.5 oz.	110	—	—	tr	—	—	—	—	—	—	—	—
(Totals)	(656)	(12.0)	(42)	(36.6)	(38)	(162)	(3.0)	(60)	(.32)	(.16)	(3.)	(6.)

The Main Meal

Food	Calo-ries	Pro-tein (g.)	Fat g.	Carbo. g.	Calc. mg.	Phos. mg.	Iron mg.	Vit.A I.U.	Thia. mg.	Ribo. mg.	Niac. mg.	C mg.
Lettuce, ¼ head of Iceberg	18	1.2	.1	3.9	27	30	.7	450	.08	.08	.4	8
Blue-cheese dressing, 3 T.	228	2.2	23.4	3.3	36	33	tr	90	tr	.06	tr	tr
Chuck roast, cooked, 6 oz.	492	46.	32.6	—	20	228	5.8	60	.08	.36	7.2	—
Brown gravy, 2 T.	82	.6	7.	4.	—	4	.2	—	tr	.01	tr	—
Stuffing, top of stove	180	3.1	10.	18.	30.2	35	.9	—	.06	.08*	.9	—
Green peas, ½ cup	55	4.1	.5	9.5	15	69	1.5	480	.22	.07	1.4	10.5
Pecan pie, 1/6 of pie	577	7.	31.6	70.8	65	142	3.9	220	.22	.1	.4	—
Vanilla ice cream, 4 oz.	127	3.	7.	13.7	96	76	tr	290	.03	.14	1.	1
Cloverleaf roll	119	2.9	3.	19.6	16	36	.7	30	.09	.09	.8	—
Coffee, 6-oz. cup	2	tr	tr	tr	4	7	.2	—	—	—	.5	—
Cream, 1 T.	20	.5	1.8	.7	16	13	—	70	tr	.02	tr	tr
Butter, tsp.	34	tr	3.8	tr	1	1	—	160	—	—	—	—
(Totals)	(1968)	(70.5)	(120.8)	(143.5)	(326.2)	(674)	(13.9)	(1850)	(.78)	(1.01)	(11.7)	(19.5)
Total, Meal and Snack	2624	82.5	162.8	180.1	364.2	836	16.9	1910	1.1	1.17	14.7	25.5
Percent U.S. RDA	—	126.9%*	—	—	36.4%	83.6%	94%	38%	73.3%	68.8%	84.5%	42.5%

*Based on 65 grams as 100%—see text

Testing the Fat Meal by the Basic Four.

We might first test this meal for nutritive value, according to the Basic Four method. In these terms, it looks like this:

Table 12–2

Food	Milk	Meat	Veg. & Fruit	Cereal	Extra
Cashews		*(1)			
Potato chips			*(1)		
Whiskey					*
Lettuce			*		
Salad dressing					*
Beef roast		**(2)			
Gravy					*
Stuffing			*		
Green peas			*		
Pecan pie		*(1)			
Ice cream	*				
Roll				*	
Coffee					*
Cream					*
Butter					*

(1) Partial serving
(2) Two servings

So we have one serving from the milk group, the equivalent of three from the meat group (the cashews and pecan pie together furnish 16.7 grams of protein, enough to make a serving), two from the vegetable group, and two from the cereal group. The addition of a glass of milk or a cube of cheese, two slices of bread, a tomato, and some fruit juice during the day would have been all that was needed to fulfill Basic Four requirements. Keep this fact in mind, while we look at the meal more closely.

Is this Meal Realistic?

The general outline of our dinner would be quite typical throughout much of America, particularly for a meal for guests. In fact, there might have been a dip for the chips, and some people might easily have added a second cocktail, wine for dinner, and another cup of coffee.

The high caloric value of this menu is also realistic, in light of the fact that many of us skip breakfast—in a recent survey it was discovered that only 5 percent of those studied ate a "good" breakfast—and that others skimp on lunch. Many eat just one full meal and snack throughout the rest of the day. Experts suggest that much of our "meal-eating" is vanishing.[1]

If we concentrate our intake of so many calories in the one main-meal period, however, it will have to supply most of our nutritive needs. Alas, as our detailed menu analysis shows, often it doesn't. We can see shortages for vitamin A, water-soluble vitamins, and calcium, and a number of nutrients which are not shown on this chart are also insufficiently furnished. Only protein is provided adequately, in fact to excess.

Thus, although this meal might be said to be consistent with the Basic Four Plan, it is nutritionally lacking. It is overly diluted calorically. Let us examine why.

Fat-Density and Nutritive Dilution.

It is common for fats to make up a large part of our snacks. For example, our cashew nuts are certainly good food, but they contain 26 grams of fat, or 234 calories, almost 75 percent of the total calories of the nuts. Some of these fats are essential; of the 26 fat grams, 1.8 are in linoleic acid (the main essential fatty acid).

True, the nuts supply almost 10 grams of protein, over 2 mg. of iron, and a number of other micronutrients. But their caloric penalty is high, as it is for the chips, which represent an additional 16 grams of fat, and 144 fat-source calories. The chips supply some protein, iron, and even 10 percent of the U.S. RDA for vitamin C. But again the caloric price is high.

When added to the single cocktail, these appetizer foods use about a fourth of a reference man's daily caloric budget. In U.S. RDAs, it returns about a fifth of our protein, some four percent of calcium, an eighth of our iron, a little over one percent of our vitamin A, about a fifth of thiamin, less than a tenth of riboflavin, a seventh of niacin, and a tenth of vitamin C.

Does this mean that these are "bad" foods or "junk" foods? No.

But calorically, and nutritively, they must be thought of as *luxury* foods. We all like a little luxury in our lives. But how much can we afford?

In our sample meal, the butter, supplying little nutritively except calories and a thirtieth of our vitamin A, costs 34 calories, almost twice the energy of the lettuce, which gives us about a fifth of our A, a fourth of our vitamin C, and so on. Similarly, consider the 284 calories of fat in the pecan pie, the 210 calories of fat in the blue-cheese salad dressing, the 63 calories of fat in the gravy.

As a comparison of fat sources, weigh the calories and nutrients of the pie against those of the roast. The serving of roast furnished the whole U.S. RDA of protein, a third of a woman's iron (and more than half of a man's), and substantial quantities of other nutrients. It has about 80 calories less than the pie. Now compare the salad dressing with the small scoop of ice cream. With 100 fewer calories, the ice cream is a much better nutrient buy.

Let us total the calories for the most obvious sources of fat dilution, those with the poorest nutritive return:

Table 12–3

Food	Fat Content (grams)	Fat Calories
Cashews, 2 oz.	26	234
Potato Chips, 20	16	144
Cheese dressing, 3 T.	23.4	210
Brown gravy, 2 T.	7	63
Pecan pie, one sixth	31.6	284
Butter, 1 tsp.	3.8	34
Cream, 1 T.	1.8	16
Totals	109.6	985

Of the 1,487 total calories in the servings of these foods, almost 1,000 are from fat. From these total calories (55 percent of the reference man's daily energy supply) we get the following nutrients: protein (21.7 grams, generally of low quality), 156 mg. of calcium, 660 I.U. of vitamin A, 0.63 mg. of thiamin, 0.25 mg. of riboflavin, 3.4 mg. of niacin and 6 mg. of vitamin C—relatively modest percentages of the RDAs. The nuts make the picture somewhat brighter by adding substantially to protein and iron. And fats play a large part, even among the somewhat more nutritive foods in the meal—from the roast to the rolls, from the ice cream to the stuffing.

Alcohol and the Diet.

To include alcohol as a nutrient is to acknowledge a simple reality. Some 85 million Americans use alcohol in some form, some 8 million to the extent that they are considered "alcoholics." (The term is variously defined, but it generally describes a person who drinks to a self-destructive extent.)

A glance at our meal chart shows that alcohol provides scarcely any nutritive value except calories. Beer has more food value (for example, supplying such trace elements as chromium), but the 150 calories in a 12-ounce can provide little except niacin, which is amply furnished by almost any U.S. diet. Beer and wine are commonly thought of as mild alcoholic drinks. But they are drunk in so much greater volume than whiskeys that their diluent effect may be as great.

A "couple of drinks," or beers, or glasses of wine, give most Americans up to 10 percent or more of their daily calories, thus representing a luxury, and adding to the nutritive burden which must be borne by the rest of their diets. A "couple" for lunch, and again before dinner, then some wine and liqueur, can easily add up to a fourth of the food budget and more. A "few" can become a serious nutritional handicap.

Like any other source of energy, alcohol becomes either fuel or stored fat. It can be balanced into the diet, with the trade-offs and allowances we have seen necessary for such balancing. But when consumed in quantity, alcohol poses a difficult barrier to the inclusion of adequate nutrients in the day's food. By blurring our perceptions, it can also interfere with bodily controls over caloric consumption. And it can interefere with the processes of digestion and absorption.

(It may be helpful to compare the cocktail in our menu—noting that a drink using a sweetened mixer could add some 80 calories extra—with the green peas. The alcohol in our cocktail is the caloric equivalent of a whole cup of the peas—which could furnish some 8 grams of protein, almost a third of a man's iron, a fourth of a woman's vitamin A, almost half of her thiamin, a tenth of her riboflavin and niacin, and over 40 percent of her vitamin C.)

Carbohydrate-Density and Nutrient Need

As we have seen, carbohydrate is the primary energy source. Table sugar and similar sweeteners are very compact sources of carbohydrate, but are virtually without other nutritive value. Soft drinks made with sugar—colas and uncolas alike—supply only energy, as do the sweeteners we add to coffee or tea.

Some sweeteners are widely, but erroneously, supposed to be nutritively valuable. Honey is an example. In terms of the most significant nutrients—a teaspoon in a cup of tea will provide 1/3000th of a day's calcium and a little over 1/5000th of the day's protein, in exchange for some 21 calories. The tea itself, with scarcely any calories, contributes about five percent of adult magnesium RDAs and a meaningful amount of fluoride.

(There is an important principle of dietary analysis here. Tea and coffee are generally thought of, even by some nutritionists, as non-nutritive. But while their mineral content is unimpressive in terms of a single cup, a person who drinks six cups a day may get a third of his desired magnesium. When an individual's eating habits include heavy use of a food, that food should be given close attention, for its nutritive values are greatly magnified. For example, the use of shrimp, herring, sardines, or liver paté as frequent appetizers can provide an important source of protein, as well as other nutrients. The cookie-eater who nibbles ten chocolate chip cookies a day adds more than just 495 calories. He gets 5.7 grams of protein (10 percent of male RDA), almost 2 mg. of iron (20 percent of male and 11 percent of female RDA), a little vitamin A, and some B vitamins.)

Sweeteners are obvious in our evening menu. But as we have seen, they can make important caloric contributions. If one drinks six cups of coffee or tea a day and adds two teaspoons of sugar to each, one gets some 200 calories of extra energy. However, most of our sugar, like our fat, tends to be hidden in food, and taste is not necessarily a good guide to how much. A sour lemonade may conceal a lot. And our piece of pecan pie may contain perhaps nine teaspoons of sugar, making it far more sugar-dense than the ice cream.

While only the pie and ice cream represent obvious sugar in our meal plan, most of us get some sugar from a host of foods throughout the day, from the cereals at breakfast to the much larger amounts in canned fruits and pastries.* But sugar is also a very common additive to commercial food products, not just for sweetness, but also as a general flavor enhancer. Roughly a fourth of our added sugar comes

---

*In our food plan, examples are the donuts, chocolate drink, cookies, and soda pop.

from corn syrup (which many people think of as nutritively different from table sugar).

THE MAKING OF THE COMPACT DIET

Foods which are concentrated sources of energy can be the main barriers to balancing most American diets. For as we have seen repeatedly, some nutrients tend to be short in our diets. Clearly, if we have to add more foods to provide those nutrients, without removing something, we will add to our calories—and probably exceed our appetites.

It should be obvious that the simplest way to deal with calorically dense foods is to eat less of them. For example, a three-ounce serving of the roast, instead of six ounces, would save us some 16 grams of fat and almost 250 calories overall. We then would get only 23 grams of high-quality protein. But this is half the U.S. RDA. The rest of the main meal, exclusive of the appetizers, gives us about the same amount again, of mostly lower-quality protein. But remember that we do well to get even a third of our protein from high-quality sources, and that dinner is not our only meal. The same pattern of smaller servings can be applied to all the high-calorie foods on the menu—less salad dressing, gravy, pecan pie, etc.

Alternatively, we can make some substitutions of foods which incorporate less fat or sugar (though fat is the primary diluent in most of our diets) without losing needed nutrients or palatability. Six ounces of a fish such as halibut supplies more protein per ounce, and much less fat, than does the roast—12 grams of fat (including the butter) to the meat's 32. This can help to balance out the calories of a rich dessert. Alternatively, angel-food cake instead of the pecan pie can balance the fat of beef.

Water and fiber may also dilute foods; most fruits and vegetables are good examples. These foods vary as well in micronutrient density. The darker green of some leaves indicates greater biological activity, and more dense concentrations of micronutrients. Our wedge of head lettuce weighed about five ounces. It provided 450 I.U. of vitamin A. The same weight of the leafier, greener romaine lettuce would offer well over 2,500 units. Notice, too, that vitamin A was low, as it tends to be in U.S. diets. Eliminating one tenth of the blue-cheese dressing would make caloric room for the romaine. And of course, the lettuce provides not only vitamin A but a broad spectrum of water-soluble vitamins and minerals.

Of course, this much lettuce is a lot to eat, 2.5 cups. The same weight of leaves in cooked form (assuming foods such as spinach, which are usually served hot) provides only a cup or less. And these leaves, greener still, have even higher nutrient values, as we saw in our earlier look at mustard greens.

In seeking a more compact diet, however, with greater density of nutrients per calorie, we need to have some specific nutrient objectives. For example, crowding more protein into our food would be pointless for most of us. We need to know what our goals are—which nutrients are plentiful and which may be lacking. Let us look at some special problems and compare them to the general nutritional patterns of our culture.

For while all of us have changing nutritive needs with each passing year and with each important change in the style and circumstance of our lives, we all eat from essentially the same food supply, and we share many tastes and habits.

NUTRITIONAL BALANCE AND THE LIFE CYCLE

As we have suggested, the broad precepts of good nutrition and well chosen food apply to all humans. But the application of these precepts and choices varies, especially during three phases of the life cycle. These are the periods of growth to maturity, pregnancy and lactation, and the advanced years.

Many of the nutritional problems of these periods actually have economic, social, psychological and political origins. Others are essentially medical—such as dental difficulties, which are extremely widespread, or the particular digestive problems prevalent among the elderly. We will not attempt to deal with many of these, some which are beyond individual control. And the medical matters require individual advice from the health professional. But there are important areas of nutritional choice where information can help.

NUTRITION WITH ADVANCING YEARS

We have already set down the most basic nutrition problem of older people. It is the decline in the intake of calories. And it provides an exaggerated instance of the problems of most adults. The older person needs an especially nutrient-dense diet.

There are special social problems, however, which often accompany aging—loss of friends, close family, and money. They can inspire a general depression or indifference, in which the consumption of calories falls even below the reduced need. The most difficult nutritional problem for the older person may be that often he simply doesn't care.

The solution ot that problem is a sense that life is worth living, that there is something to do, and people who care whether or not it is done. There is, of course, no solution in biochemistry, no supplement to take. The seniors must first be motivated to care. And then, excepting their medical problems, they require mainly to seek nutrient density. Their cells may be less active. They may eat less. But their nutrient needs, like all their other human needs, are basically no different.

Indeed, one of the most important nutrition problems of our seniors is that promoters commonly single them out to be duped, convincing them that their nutritional needs are unique and cannot be met by ordinary foods. There are many pathetic reports of the results. Too commonly the elder person will spend much of the money he needs for ordinary food (not to mention housing and small diversions) on special foods which are sold to him with special promises.

There is no nutritional cure for aging. And in fact, because the aging person's diet must come from some 20 percent less food, there is a greater chance that a false reliance on health foods and special supplements, or experiments with eccentric and unbalanced diets, will do him harm.

DIET FOR A SMALL LIFE

So rapid is a baby's growth that if his mother grew as quickly, within a year she would be at least eight feet tall and weigh over 400 pounds. Such growth requires a lot of food; if the baby's father ate a commensurate amount, he would consume about 8,200 calories a day.

An infant's micronutrient needs are also extraordinary; he needs half the calcium, three-fourths of the vitamin C, and as much iron and vitamin D as his father. Clearly, inadequacies of nutrition in this high-speed growth period can quickly lead to trouble.

Most people believe that mother's milk is the perfect source of all the infant's required nutrients, but some nutrients are quite low. This is not troublesome at first. For by the time of birth the well-nurtured infant has stores of such minerals as iron and copper, and of such fat-soluble vitamins as A and D.

Mother's milk is a little richer than cow's milk in vitamin C,* but most pediatricians prescribe a supplement of this vitamin, along with vitamin D, either in drops or through small feedings of fruit juice. Except for these two vitamins, a well-fed mother can adequately furnish her baby's nutrient needs for some months.

But as the infant's reserves run down, other food must be added. Iron stores may be the key. By most estimates, iron stores are adequate for two to six months, when supplemental feeding is prescribed to head off any deficiency.

There is another factor which may contribute to the need for extra food. For mother's milk is not a constant thing. For example, the protein content of the milk has decreased by about a third at the end of the second month of nursing; zinc has fallen off by half. A number of other nutrient values continue to decline. This change may be harmless for a time, however, because the baby consumes larger and larger quantities of milk, compensating for its reduced nutrient density.

Breast or Bottle?

It is hard to find a nutritionist who does not emphasize breastfeeding (which is probably possible for more than 90 percent of mothers). There are both psychological and biochemical advantages. During the first weeks, the mother's immunities are conferred through her milk; there is no problem with contamination in breastfeeding; and the chemistry of the milk is unique. Cow's milk may be ideal for calves, but (to choose one example) the calf's digestive system is different from that of the baby; while the main protein of cow's milk is casein, that of human milk is *lactalbumin,* which is much better suited to the baby's digestion.

Modern infant formulas are designed to resemble human milk, with

---

*The mother who consumes more vitamin C provides more in her milk.

adjustments of proteins and carbohydrates, and even an increase in polyunsaturated fatty acids, to mimic the higher content of these lipids in breast milk. Moreover, the nutrients which decline in the changing milk, and which may become depleted in the baby's reserves can be kept constant in the formula—if this is desirable. If breastfeeding is not chosen, however, prepared formula rather than cow's milk is the better alternative. The differences between them are considerable.

Lamentably, the trend has been away from breastfeeding in the U.S. About two-thirds of babies were breastfed in the 1940s. By 1958 only a fourth of even 7-day-old babies were breastfed. By 1973, only 10 to 15 percent of 2-month-old babies were breastfed, and only five percent of six-month-olds. More than 70 percent of young infants are on formula, and a small percentage are on home made evaporated milk formulas. Interestingly, breastfeeding is most common among higher income and education groups, ironic in light of the economy of breastfeeding.

In one way the use of commercial formulas is similar to the problem with vitamin pills: not all the known nutrients can be added to the formula, only those for which there are established requirements.* Many nutritionists feel that there is no reason to assume, for example, that all the trace elements present in human milk are also present in cow's milk, and that precise chemical differences are all known.

The frequency of feeding discourages some mothers from nursing; for some who work it is impossible. But a combination of breast and bottle can work well, so long as the breast predominates.** Some pediatricians suggest that the father fill in at such times as middle-of-the-night feedings, with "relief" bottles, to encourage the mother (and perhaps to build a better psychological relationship between father and baby).

The Solid-Food Controversy

Medical tests usually agree that solids ought to be part of the diet by six months, but there is little agreement as to exactly when they are necessary. In the 1920s solids were seldom given before one

---

*Although no health problems of consequence have been documented for formula-fed infants in the U.S., some pediatricians do maintain that breast-fed babies have fewer problems, especially of digestion.

**If milk production is not amply stimulated, it falls off rapidly.

year. By 1963, 83 percent of infants between one and two months old were eating them. Studies indicate that infants can tolerate cereals by the second or third day of life. There are no problems with vegetables at 10 days, meats at 14 days, and fruits at 17 days. There is no need for them so early, however. In realistic terms, the amount of solids fed at first is very little, and the solid-food feeding of the first months amounts to little more than training to accept and swallow. Because this learning takes time, most physicians start babies on such foods well before the six-month point at which such foods contribute nutrients in important amounts.

Since we know that the baby can eat most basic foods well before he is a year old, how do the critical factors in infant nutrition compare to those we have seen with respect to adults? They are very like. The baby can survive on a great variety of foods; if this were not so, only infants in certain favored crop and climate areas would live. The American mother may feed cereal which has been finely ground and mixed with formula; the Samoan mother takes a bite of taro root, chews it to a wet pulp and then feeds it; the Eskimo baby may get the benefit of a little seal oil and chewed meat. And all can be well nourished.

The Infant's Milky Way

The balance point of the infant's diet is milk. While the protein varies in different milks (human milk about 7 percent, formulas 9 to 14 percent, and cow's milk 20 percent of calories), by six months, when solids are contributing substantial nutritive value, most babies are using cow's milk. At this age babies require 0.9 grams of protein for each pound of weight. What this means is that three eight-ounce bottles of milk a day furnish the entire protein need for the baby until he weighs 30 pounds. A fourth bottle, making a total of a quart a day, will provide needed protein up to almost 40 pounds, the median weight for a four-to-five-year-old boy. In this light, consumer-advocate complaints that baby foods are low in protein seem somewhat misplaced.

We find here an analog to the balancing considerations of the adult diet. Protein is provided by milk. And although early eating experiences are important to teach a catholicity of taste for a wide variety of foods, there is no pressing nutritional reason to urge meat in quantity on an often reluctant baby. True, meat supplies iron. But a baby's need for iron is so large relative to his weight, and the meat portion he will eat is so small, that meat is unlikely to be a major contributor of iron. An ounce of meat will probably supply less than 10 percent of this need.

Balancing Baby Foods and Baby Needs.

Cereals, vegetables, and fruits, as with adults, will supply more critical nutrients than meats, with fewer calories, especially nutrients complementary to the milk which still forms the basis of the diet. Of course, it would take huge quantities of cereal to meet infant RDAs for iron, for example, so baby cereals are very heavily fortified; infant rice cereal has about 16 times the iron of adult rice cereal. We have noted the problem of iron deficiency in American children. There is evidence that this iron deficiency appears at about the time many parents discontinue infant cereals.

Despite the vogue for home-made baby foods, and the fact than an informed mother can make them perfectly well, there are some good arguments for the application of technology to simplify the job. Almost all infant fruit juices, for example, are fortified with vitamin C, since some juices are not very good sources of C, and the infant may drink little. For example, it takes about 100 ounces of apple juice to supply the infant RDA for vitamin C, unless the supplemented infant type is used.

Should sugar be eliminated from baby food? As with adults, only when it becomes too much of a nutritional diluent. There is no reason to believe that infants learn "sugar addiction." In theory, one would want the infant to have a nutritively compact diet, especially since adipose storage cells seem to multiply in response to overfeeding at this age. But if a few grains of sugar will get him to accept an acid fruit or a green vegetable or any other valuable food, there seems little reason to withhold it. Watching a baby spit out food is both unpleasant and counter-productive nutritionally.

A most important psychological factor also enters here, as we noted in discussing obesity. Patterns of coaxing, rewarding, and emotional upset and relief that center on food add life-long emotional connotations to eating, which can cause trouble later on. A little sugar may be better than a little neurosis. A tiny amount of salt may also be a flavor enhancer, but free child access to the salt shaker should probably be limited, just as one sensibly limits access to the sugar bowl. One fact is certainly clear—a baby's "natural" appetite is a poor guide to good nutrition, regardless of many myths to the contrary.

In the nutritional education of a child, the central aim should be the future well-nourished adult. This is especially important as one begins to deal with the toddler, who is forming and expressing narrow preferences; we should not teach our culture's esteem for the rich man's diet, heavily diluted with fat. We won't if we take a little time to analyze the composition of the child's food and the realities of his physiological needs.

As the simplest kind of example, look at the food of a nine-month-old girl who weighs 22 pounds. A quart of milk gives her much more protein than she needs, so this is no problem. It provides 650 calories of the 1,100 she consumes. If the milk is whole, it provides over 300 calories of fat, almost 30 percent of the diet. If a diet of 35 percent fat is desirable, this means that only 85 more fat calories (a little over 9 grams) will bring her diet to this level. An ounce of beef offers about 5 of those grams. The yolk of a medium egg provides 4.6 grams more. A slice of processed cheese has a little over 3 grams. How many plain cookies or crackers, at about 0.05 grams of fat each, do you want her to have? How much butter on the cracker?

For an answer we need only look to the analogies with the adult diet. We can ask, are the four full bottles of milk a day necessary? Food tables and RDAs show us that three supply her needs for protein, as well as for calcium and riboflavin, both scarce nutrients. Technology may be of use. Low-fat milk (not skim, which may not be advisable for the very young) has only some 20 grams of fat, instead of the 34 that are in whole milk—and because nonfat milk solids are added, it has more protein and calcium.

FROM TODDLER TO TEEN

Our look at other special groups will be relatively brief, for we have now established some patterns and some rather simple variables. The patterns are those of basic nutrient need, and the impact upon that need of cultural habit and food availability. The variables are largely those of activity and growth—though more personal variables can always upset our tidy designs.

The Slowing of Growth.

The first mushroom growth tapers off after about a year. For example, there is about a 300 percent increase in weight the first year, but only a 22 percent increase in the second. The first year sees an increase of nine or ten inches in height; the second about half as much. By the fifth year, weight increase is down to 12 percent (a yearly increment which continues for the next ten years for boys, and about eight years for girls). Girls reach a growth peak at about puberty. Boys continue childlike growth for perhaps two years longer (accounting for much of the general size difference between the sexes).

Nothing, however, quite equals the dramatic slowdown of the second year. And with this, food intake also declines. The typical nine-month-old consumes close to 1,000 calories a day, perhaps half the calories of its mother. About a year later, and perhaps 10 pounds (50 percent) heavier, the same child needs only about 1,300 calories.

It is not only growth that changes matters, but the whole pace of life. The newborn has a heart rate of about 130 beats a minute; the rate is down to 100 at age two. Body temperature increases slightly through the first year, then begins to go down. Breathing rate declines from 30 breaths a minute in the first year to 25 in the second. Even the infant's flow of body water differs; he takes in and excretes some 20 percent of his total body fluid daily, compared to the adult's 5 percent. These factors all contribute to the baby's very high rate of metabolism, which then drops rapidly as he enters the toddler stage.

The toddler may still eat considerable food, but in amounts related more to his size than to his rate of growth. Many of his nutrient requirements are closer to those of his parents, in relation to caloric intake. Some nutrients may be needed in the same, or nearly the same, quantities as for his elders, and the diet must become compact in terms of those nutrients. The two-year-old needs as much calcium, phosphorus, and vitamin D as his parents do. As we have seen, some three glasses of milk a day can protect him here. His RDA for vitamin C is almost as great as an adult's, so a rich source of vitamin C becomes important.

As a guide, using average numbers, we see that our two-year-old's caloric need is about half that of his father. So when the child's nutrient requirements are no more than half those of the father, they can be managed with the same sort of food choices. (See the RDA tables, App. B and C.) Iron provides the only very significant departure from this pattern, other than vitamin C and the nutrients provided by milk. The two-year-old needs 50 percent *more* iron than his father does. In other words, his food must be *three times* as dense in iron. Often some iron supplementation is necessary, especially since the two-year-old's meat consumption is not great.

In general, we can see that nutrient density is as important for the child as for the parent. And conversely, excessive dietary dilution with fats and pure sugars can be harmful.

Since this pattern holds throughout childhood, it explains why so many nutritionists are concerned with the nutritive qualities of children's snacks. One recent study showed that some 21.8 percent of pre-schoolers' calories came from snacks, and 17.4 percent of the calories of elementary school children. Other studies show even higher percentages. One difficulty here is that so large a proportion of commercial snacks are so low in nutrient density (except for calories). For this reason, snacks must be thought of, not as extras but as small auxiliary meals.

One particularly important variable which can help to balance the child's diet is exercise. The child has more leisure time than most adults, and a greater availability of games and other physical activities. A television set can be a great nutritional handicap.

Exercise is also the principal remedy for obesity in childhood and adolescence. Even in the teen years, when girls may have reached virtually mature height and weight, profound developmental changes are occurring. Caloric restriction requires a still greater dietary compactness. A number of nutrient requirements reach their peak in the adolescence years, particularly those for B vitamins and some minerals. Greater physical activity is therefore the only healthful alternative to caloric restriction. Adolescent girls, particularly (because of the cessation of growth, preoccupation with weight control, and reduced activity) are among nutrition's most important nutritional problem groups.

THE CREATION OF A NEW LIFE

In no phase of life does the need for a compact diet become more pressing than of the pregnant woman. Simple mathematics illustrate the problem.

Let us begin with our reference woman, five feet five inches tall and 128 pounds. The RDA Committee averages her caloric intake at 2,000 calories after age 23. Caloric excess is allowed during pregnancy—to cover the building of the fetus and the placenta (the uterine organ which helps to maintain the new life), to support a higher metabolic rate, and to move extra physical weight around.

Overall, an ideal weight gain is about 24 to 28 pounds during pregnancy. (An inadequate weight gain may offer as many health problems for mother and baby as an excess gain.) The gain should be fairly steady, about half a pound to a pound each week. (A pound a week is, however, quite a lot, except for a large woman.) The RDA Committee averages all of these factors into an extra recommended allowance of 300 calories a day. The increase is the same regardless of the woman's size, so it is a smaller percentage increase for the larger woman.

In the case of some nutrients, eating a little more of the ordinary diet can cover the needs. This is true for iron or for niacin (with increased RDA of 2 mg. each, or about 15 percent). But in most cases, the increased need for nutrients is proportionately greater than the increase in calories which must supply them. Vitamin A is to be increased by 25 percent; so is vitamin E, riboflavin, B—6, and iodine. On an even larger scale, the 15 percent more calories must provide 33 percent more vitamin C, thiamin, B—12, and zinc, 50 percent more magnesium, calcium, and phosphorus, 65 percent more protein, and double the usual folacin.

Some help is provided by supplements prescribed for pregnancy. But no one knows just what nutritive increases are required for nutrients for which there are no RDAs. A number of such preparations surprisingly overlook some of the increased nutrient needs entirely, and have a balance of nutrients which is hard to account for on a logical basis. One such supplement offers a tablet with the following nutrients, stated with reference to the U.S. RDA for pregnant women:

Iron, 214%; ascorbic acid, 167%; thiamin, 270%; B—6₃, 99%; riboflavin, 100%; niacin, 50%; pantothenic acid, 9%; vitamin A, 50%; vitamin D, 100%; calcium, 5%; B—12, 25%.

Note that zinc, magnesium, iodine, phosphorus, vitamin E, and folacin are ignored. (Folacin need is especially urgent because of its role in forming nucleic acids, essential to the rapid cell division of the fetus.)

Calcium and phosphorus are virtually never included in sufficient quantities in such preparations, and so must come from food. And of course, protein must also be supplied by the diet. Although for many women the protein intake is already at the level recommended for pregnancy, the need for increased nutrient density will make it a little harder to meet protein needs. For protein generally comes with fat, and an increase in protein density is often accompanied by an increase in fat density. It is important for pregnant women to be aware of protein sources which are lower in fat.

THE NURSING MOTHER

We have seen some of the advantages of breastfeeding. While we shall not examine the psychological rewards to the nursing mother in detail, they are many. On the other hand, it is an ancient adage of child-rearing that one of the most difficult and important aspects is releasing the child from its dependency. For some nursing mothers, the great satisfaction of providing food for a small new life from one's own body, coupled with a strong sense of feminine identity and capacity which may be evoked, are powerful incentives to maintain the nursing role as long as possible. Unfortunately, the same psychological factors may lead to a wish to remain the sole source of the infant's food beyond the limits of nutritive reality. By prolonging breastfeeding overlong, well-intentioned mothers may unwittingly cheat the infant of needed nutrition.

The caloric allowance for the nursing mother is increased even over the allowance for pregnancy. In biologic terms, we can see that, in effect, she is indeed now eating for two humans. The RDA Committee estimates the need for additional food at 500 calories a day.

How should those calories be used? Along the lines we have described for pregnancy. The increases in calories are not sufficient to allow for carelessness; a look at the RDAs for lactation will explain why. The recommendations for the nursing mother are only extensions of those for the pregnant woman. The principles are the same. But a look at the baby's intense demands, due to its extraordinary growth, makes clear that the extra calories allowed for breastfeeding are not to be spent recklessly. In effect, the mother at the table becomes the surrogate for the baby. So well as she eats, so well will her child be fed.

SOME NUTRIENT TRENDS.

In both the special and general nutrient needs of Americans, and in the ways most of us eat, we have seen certain basic patterns. The table below indicates some of the nutritional results in a more specific way.

Table 12–4

Nutrient	Ample in Typical Diets	Marginal or Lacking in Many Diets
Protein (1)	*	
Fat (1)	*	
Carbohydrate	*	
Vitamin A		*
Vitamin C	*	
Thiamin		*
Riboflavin		*
Niacin	*	
Calcium (2)		*
Iron		*
Vitamin D	*	
Vitamin E	*	
Vitamin B_6		*
Folacin		*
Vitamin B_{12} (3)	*	
Phosphorus (1)	*	
Iodine		*
Magnesium		*
Zinc (2)	*	
Copper		*
Biotin	*	
Pantothenic Acid	*	
Sodium (1)	*	
Fluorine		*
Trace Elements		*
Fiber		*

Notes:
(1) May be excessive in some diets.
(2) Required amount (calcium), or intake (zinc) is somewhat controversial.
(3) May be marginal in some vegetarian diets.

What conclusions are implied here? First, our excesses tend toward those of the "rich man's diet," high in animal foods, and thus high in fat and protein. Our ability to afford oils, a food luxury in some regions of the world, contributes to this excess. (Salt, too, while now amply available in most of the world, has been an historical food luxury.)

This diet tends to yield much more phosphorus than calcium; for protein is often accompanied by phosphorus, but not calcium. This imbalance is considered undesirable, since the two minerals are used in a related way. In our sample fatty meal, the roast is ten times as high in phosphorus as in calcium, the nuts and peas five times as high. Here is an example of the fact that heavy emphasis on any group of foods is likely to have undesirable implications, some of them quite subtle.

Among the nutrients classified as generally ample are some that are not ample for everyone. The larger and more recent nutrition surveys,* especially the Ten State Survey, have shown rare indications of marginal protein, vitamin C, and even vitamin D. The Ten State Survey was largely of a low-income group. The families surveyed generally had annual incomes of less than $3,000, very few of over $5,000.

Five vitamins are listed as potentially deficient for many people—vitamin A, thiamin, riboflavin, vitamin B—6, and folacin. And we see that only one, vitamin A, is fat-soluble. The rest are water-soluble vitamins, appearing in small amounts in any one serving of food (though they are distributed quite widely). What do these vitamins have in common which could explain the shortages? Some of their richest sources are vegetable foods—grains, vegetables and fruits. And these are the foods which tend to be excluded from the "rich man's diet."

Why is the fat-soluble vitamin on the list? Largely because the main source of vitamin A is not its pure form (retinol), as it is found in animals, but its precursor form (the carotenes), as it is found in plants.

Grains, legumes, and green vegetables are especially good sources of these vitamins. Thiamin and riboflavin are not especially high in greens, whereas vitamin A, B-6, and folacin are. Many fruits are good sources of folacin and vitamin A.

*Providing some of the impetus and nutritional focus for federal food plans, especially Food Stamps and special helps such as the WIC (Women, infants and children) supplemental foods.

Aren't thiamin and riboflavin found in meats? Yes, but except for a couple of special sources—such as thiamin in pork and riboflavin in liver—their concentration isn't very high in any food. Here is where we feel the pinch of dietary dilution. The high caloric density of pure fats and carbohydrates displaces lower-calorie foods which would contribute small amounts of thiamin and riboflavin and provide adequate totals. The avoidance of starches particularly, in favor of "protein" foods rich in fats, has reduced our intake of all these vitamins.

Six minerals are also on our critical list. Shortages of two of these, iodine and fluorine, are related to lacks in the soil and water. Both are easily added, of course—iodine through iodized salt and fluorine through drinking water.

Of the other four, calcium is in some ways a special case. The decline in per capita milk consumption is often said to be to blame. But we must also consider that calcium is widely available in many foods in smaller amounts, especially those of plant origin, such as legumes. Some greens really have quite substantial amounts, and grains provide a little. In other words, were such foods consumed in greater quantity, the calcium shortage would certainly be lessened. (Of course, if calcium requirements are lowered, on the U.N. model, fewer diets will appear to be calcium-deficient.)

Of the three remaining problem minerals, iron is the only one with a broad and well documented pattern of deficiency. The same dietary strategem—less calorically dense food, more foods of plant origin—would alleviate the iron shortage (though probably not entirely for women, who need more iron and eat less food).

Any marginal magnesium or copper deficiencies—and it is not generally believed that either of these lacks is widespread—can be handled in the same way. In fact, this pattern of a reduction in nutritional diluents, and the replacement of these with more valuable grains, vegetables and fruits, is very likely to take care of whatever problems Americans may have with trace elements. In addition, the consumption of more of these same neglected foods will increase our fiber intake. And since we must consume greater volume of them to get many calories, the resulting bulkier diet should make weight maintenance easier.

Of course one further balancing factor for most of us is exercise. For apart from its other health benefits, exercise increases the total amount of food we can consume, and hence the quantity of nutrients.

While these general patterns of balance probably hold for most Americans, they do not hold for all. And the only way to know how they apply to the individual is by keeping track of the foods consumed for a period—three days is usually considered to be a minimum for accuracy—then examining the trends of intake. A nutrient-by-nutrient analysis is probably unnecessary, unless the individual departs from the trends.

Indeed, common sense and a little knowledge of how the food groups contribute to the diet quickly suggest which foods are neglected or overemphasized.

A Second Look at Basic Food Guides.

We have already seen that the Basic Four, while including most of the nutrients we need, may not include all, and can permit serious errors of nutritional dilution and distortion. On the other hand, if the principles of nutritive compactness which we have discussed are taken into account, basic food guides can become much more reliable. And they do have the merit of suggesting how the sources of nutrients are grouped in the world of foods.

It may well be that the chief value of these guides is for people who have very little other information about nutrition. On the other hand, there is evidence that, after forty years of persuasion, repetition and refinement, the food guides have not made much impact on the public's eating habits. Indeed, they seem to have a tendency to confirm our troublesome overemphasis on protein, through emphasis on two of the four groups which are good suppliers of protein.

In fact, because of the apparent ways in which people identify foods within the groups, selecting often those which are high in caloric dilution and low in nutrients, perhaps we ought to take one step backward toward the old Basic Seven. An update of this concept, developed by Dr. Philip White and the Council on Foods and Nutrition, suggests a food-group method of planning which, it should now be apparent, helps put in better focus the roles which plant-source foods play in our diets. It looks like this:

Table 12–5

Food		Child	Preteen & Teen	Adult	Aging Adult
	A Council on Foods and Nutrition Guide*				
Milk and its products		2–3	3–4 or more	2 or more	2 or more
Meat, fish, proteins		1–2	3 or more	2 or more	2 or more
Green and yellow vegetables		1–2	2	2	at least 1
Citrus and tomatoes		1	1–2	1	1–2
Potatoes, other fruits and vegetables		1	1	1	0–1
Bread, flour & cereal		3–4	4 or more	3–4	2–3
Fats		2	2–4	2–3	1–2

*Slightly adapted

One may note at once that no special provisions are made for the pregnant or lactating woman. Her diet should be presumed to look something like that of the typical adult, except for the addition of another milk-group serving, and a need for greater concentration on nutrient density in all her food selection.

Anyone who uses such a guide as this should keep some other ideas in mind. First, in choosing among foods, points ought to be given to those foods which meet the food-group suggestions without an excess contribution of fat or sucrose. Ice cream is not really a substitute for milk. The Council points out that it takes 2-3 large scoops to equal one glass of milk. There is a good reason why we can't have a donut as one cereal-group contributor—its fat content.

Beef is excellent food, but consistent choice of beef will result in the payment of a higher caloric price for protein than the choice of diets with chicken or fish.

The nutrient density of fruits and vegetables is important. The Council guide suggests this by dividing these into three groups. But even in these groups, we must remember that string beans are no nutritive match for the lamentably neglected green leafy vegetables.

Every nutrition author has his prejudices, and this one holds as a major (and documentable) prejudice the idea that a return to consumption of the darker greens—from kale to mustard, chard to turnip tops and even dandelion greens—would be both easy and meaningful. Season them with vinegar and herbs, put them in salads, where they add tangy spice of their own, use them to flavor stews (boiling them down slowly to join the juice of the dish), brew them open-handedly into soups (as the Italians do with spinach and escarole and endive, or in the Judaic tradition of *schav*), chop chives into omelets (in the Chinese foo yung manner), or fluff out sandwiches with cress, and nutritional gaps begin to close.

Much has been written in nutrition circles urging supplementation of the items of the Basic Four with nutritive snacks. The idea is commendable. But there are those of us who enjoy the pecan pie and the wine and the potato chips. When nutrition education challenges pleasure, education wears stark and sober robes, and pleasure tends to win. And yet there is no quarrel at all between pleasures and life. There is only the problem of our lessened need for energy versus our tendency to dilute our basic nutritive foods.

It is perhaps the central thesis of this book that we need not stifle pleasure to survive. We need only be realists when we look at our pleasure and at the essentials of our survival. For each gustatory joy, there is a balance of good sense. Chocolate cream pie and banana splits are not evils; they are only caloric hurdles. The knowledge of nutrition is, in the fullest sense, not an injunction to somber sacrifice. It is only a guide to balance, to the use of reason and hard-won knowledge as aids to better lives, not as restrictive penalties for living.

Let us match these goals against the realities of the food which the markets give us to eat.

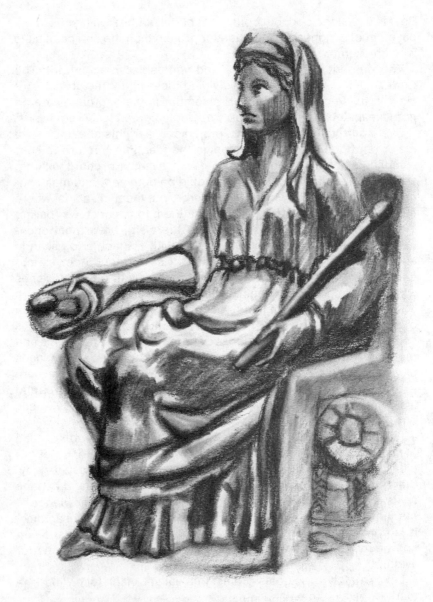

The making of food has been much the subject of religious and spiritual meaning and belief. *Vesta, Goddess of the Hearth, as Goddess of the Baker's Guild. Marble. Rome. C. 100 A.D.*

chapter 13

THE REALITIES OF FOOD

In the last generation, as Americans have become more interested in nutrition, they have also become more suspicious of the quality of their food supply. They are encouraged in their fears by such statements as this one, from the editors of *Prevention* (and of *Organic Gardening and Farming*):

"For all our endless variety of available food, it is close to impossible to be well nourished on what you can buy at our deceptively plentiful supermarkets. Nature is perfectly willing to provide us with a richness of nutrition . . . But alas, nature is no longer in command . . . As a result the food does not reach us as proper food anymore."[1]

Is our food really inadequate for our health needs? There are basically two charges: (1) That nutrients are lost through farming methods and processing, and (2) That poisonous chemicals are introduced into the food by agriculture and industry. Let us consider what science knows of the realities.

ARE OUR SOILS DEPLETED?

According to Carlton Fredericks, a broadcaster who writes a column for *Prevention,* our soils have been depleted of some essential nutrients, with the result that our crops are missing certain nutritive values: "Many of our foods spring from soils which have been over-cultivated or under-fertilized . . . yielding vegetables and fruits below standard in vitamin-mineral content."[2]

To test this statement, and many like it, we must know something of the chemistry and biology of agriculture.

The Nutrition of Plants

Much of what we have discussed of human nutrition may also be applied to the nutrient needs of plants. Like us, they are actually organized groups of cells. Like us their cells must also be supplied with the raw materials of life, and the materials which they require are determined by the chromosomes in the nuclei of each of their cells. Their chemical makeup is, like ours, ordained by heredity.

If we think about it for a moment, we realize that the life chemistry of plants must be somewhat similar to our own. For we get all our fuel and all our structural materials, either by consuming the plants directly, or by eating animals which have been fed on plants. Of course there are also striking differences, of which two are especially pertinent to our discussion. One is that plants usually do not consume other life forms as we do to get their nutrients. Instead, they take in nutrients in very simple form and use chlorophyll to trap solar energy.

The other difference is that, unlike us, plants cannot move around to seek food. So they depend on natural phenomena, or on us, to bring them food. From the beginning of mankind's dependence on agriculture, we have tended to provide plants with a kind of room service. This service was unnecessary while our use of plants was "natural." We simply foraged over the earth, seeking out those plants which had managed to survive. But once we began modern agriculture some 9,000 years ago, by growing plants in batches for a more dependable and convenient food source, "unnatural" growing methods became essential to their survival and to ours.

At first glance, it may seem that there is a striking difference between the ways in which we and the plants take in food—we by eating and they through their leaves and roots. But there is a basic similarity. Like us, the plants can absorb and take into their cells only the simpler structural units of their food. Of course, we have digestive systems; we chew up food into small particles and then use enzymes to break out the nutrients, all within our own bodies, before absorbing them into our bloodstreams. The roots of a plant, however, may be seen as similar to our intestinal walls. The difference is that, if soil nutrients are in more complex form, the bacteria in the soil, with their enzymes, do the work of breaking foods apart into forms of nutrients useful for plants.

What sort of nutrients must plants take in? We have seen that the bulk of our own nutrients is composed of carbon, hydrogen, and oxygen; our fourth greatest need is for nitrogen. Some three pounds of our bodies consist of nitrogen. (Like all life forms, we must make proteins, and that requires nitrogen.)

Plants need the same elements, taking the first three (carbon, hydrogen, and oxygen) from air and water. Nitrogen, though critical, is the smallest of the major needs.

Our nitrogen comes from the protein we eat. The plant takes up its nitrogen in a simpler form from the soil, combined with oxygen as a *nitrate* (NO_3). That nitrogen comes mainly, in nature, from the protein of decaying plant materials, such as leaves and stems. The plant cannot absorb amino acids. It must wait for the soil bacteria to make nitrates from life forms, and for rainwater to carry these chemicals to its roots for absorption. Then, unlike us, the plant makes its own amino acids.

The plant cells have no problem getting their carbon, hydrogen, and oxygen from water and the carbon dioxide in the air. But they must get their nitrogen from the soil.

Early in the history of agriculture, we learned that we must keep the soil supplied with nitrogen, or plants will not grow, since without nitrogen they cannot form the proteins for new cells. By trial and error early farmers found that manures and decomposing life materials would keep soils fertile. (The manures contain the wastes from decomposed amino acids, such as *urea* and *creatinine*.)

Once we understood some of this chemistry, beginning in the past century, we realized that simpler, more concentrated sources of nitrogen supplied these needs faster and more efficiently. The speed of replacement can be important. For plants often use nitrogen to build new cells and life chemicals much faster than we do; many double their own weight in one to two weeks.

Our modern "chemical" fertilizers supply nitrates rapidly in a simple, immediately usable form. "Organic" farming, with its compost piles of decaying manure and plants, does not directly supply the nitrate which plants can absorb. Its nitrogen is tied up in elaborate carbon-skeleton molecules, in low concentration. Manures, for example, tend to be only about one half of one percent to one percent nitrogen; our pure nitrates may offer ten to twenty times this concentration. The ironic reality of "organic" farming is that the plants cannot use nitrogen in organic form.

Of course, plants need more than nitrogen to grow. These other, smaller needs are also somewhat parallel to those of humans. Plants do not have to take in vitamins whole, as we do; they make their own (and ours, too). But they must have minerals. The minerals come from the rock and soil of the earth. The plants need as wide a variety as we do—where else would we get ours? Dominant among their needs are phosphorus, potassium, sulfur, and calcium. Phosphorus and potassium are needed especially, and during the last century we began to seek out deposits, grind them up, modify them so that they were most useful, and return them to our fields.

Phosphorus is usually incorporated in ammonium phosphates (combinations with ammonia and oxygen) or calcium phosphates. Potassium is acquired almost entirely from mined potassium chloride ores. Calcium sulfate (calcium, sulfur and oxygen) is another "chemical" fertilizer. And of course the other trace minerals, such as iron, which we seek for our own nutrition, are part of the hereditary plant chemistry. Else, for example, we could not depend on getting our iron from our potatoes and beans.

Does Agriculture Deplete Soil Minerals?

Certainly. That is why we use fertilizers to supply more than just nitrogen. "Organic" food enthusiasts fear that regular supermarket foods may be missing some of the needed minerals, because the soils may have lost them. "Won't foods grown by ordinary agricultural practices," ask the editors of *Prevention,* "fill the same need as organically grown foods? Unfortunately, most foods raised today are likely to be short in minerals . . ."

Is this true? Except for a few exceptional cases, no. The plants, responding to their hereditary necessities, need these minerals just as much as we do. These minerals are called for by the plant's chromosomes; if they are missing, the plants cannot grow.

What if the minerals are not entirely missing, but are merely in short supply? Then only as many plants as can be nourished by the available minerals will grow; or, like undernourished humans, they will be stunted and deformed. In other words, the farmer who works soil which is truly depleted of minerals gets no crop; or, if the minerals are in short supply, he may get a crop, but it will be a sparse one. As surely as human development is thwarted by inadequate nutrition, so is the development of plants. The farmer who exploited his soil would learn the hard way from a crop with very poor yield.

So any food which exists at all must be genetically complete food. It must contain a full complement of types of cells—otherwise, it could not exist.

May There Be Unobservable Deficiencies?

A few trace elements can be low. These elements (though essential for animal life) may play little role in the plant chemistry, and are taken into the plant by incidental absorption. There are only a few—chiefly iodine, selenium, cobalt, and zinc. Fluorine might be considered another. Of this group, there are easy safeguards against shortages for two, iodine and fluorine—iodine by the iodizing of salt and fluorine through water treatment. Most "organic" food enthusiasts oppose both.

The nutritional roles of selenium and cobalt were identified largely through inadequacies in the diets of pasture-raised livestock, mainly sheep and cattle. Nutritively, our main sources of these elements are animal foods. (Recall, for example, that the cobalt is a critical constituent of vitamin B—12) Where these elements may be lacking in the soil, the deficiency signs are quickly apparent in the animals, before the age at which they will be slaughtered, and in general they are easily supplemented, by adding either chemicals to the soil or to feeds.

(Note that shortages of such minerals as these are not due to farming practices, but to regional soil problems. Plants in certain areas will, for example, contain little iodine, and if used for compost will obviously not correct any problem in the soils in which they themselves grew.)

All of the elements which are known to be essential in the nutrition of humans are quite easily identified in soils by modern analytic methods. Our soils and foods are regularly tested, for at least three major reasons.

First, the farmer has an acute economic interest in his soil; it is his most costly and basic asset. A flawed soil, untreated, will produce a poor crop or none at all. The fertilizers which the farmer adds are expensive. He cannot afford to guess; so he has his soil analyzed.

Second, the soils are important economic assets to the society, especially in those states which produce most of our food. California, for example, if it were a separate nation, would be the world's seventh largest food producer, all by itself. Governments of agricultural states have an interest in keeping watch over their soils.

Third, under the newer Federal laws, to be able to make advertising and labeling claims about the nutritive values of food, one must make analyses of that food. The data from such tests are generally available to regulatory agencies and are plugged into a Federal data processing system. No evidence of general soil or food insufficiency (except as indicated above for iodine, etc.) has come to light. What is more, 10 years of research at the Michigan Experiment Station, 25 years of work at the U.S. Plant, Soil and Nutrition Laboratory at Ithaca, New York, and 34 years of testing on an experimental farm in England have discovered no nutritive differences between "natural" farming products and those on our general market.

Yet claims continue. Consider this statement from the *Organic Directory:* "Trace minerals—essential for enzyme action in performing your body's vital functions—are tailormade for your body only when you get them from organic foods. Don't wait for a mineral deficiency to strike. Get your minerals . . . from organic foods."[1]

Except for the home gardener, the use of plant and animal wastes for fertilizer can add greatly to price. A survey by U.S.D.A. provides rather graphic evidence of the costs of special foods.

Table 13-1

Food	Supermarket Price	Health Food Price
Canned apple juice	$0.29	$0.75
Dried pitted peaches	0.73	1.68
Cornmeal	0.14	0.44
Honey	0.55	1.05
Cucumber	0.19	0.69

The price of the fertilizer illusion is indeed high.

CAN WE LIVE ON PROCESSED FOOD?

Almost anyone who acquires any abundance of food—whether by planting a backyard fruit tree or a crop of lettuce or tomatoes, or by buying a whole tray of peaches—soon learns a stern reality. Unless one is informed and willing to take some trouble, one encounters a crisis of waste.

Since early in history, the perishability of food has been one of man's major technological problems. Killing a deer or finding a tree of ripe fruit, and being unable to make use of more than a small part of either, has always been unacceptably wasteful. The problem is especially acute with respect to plant foods, which have limited seasons of edibility. Without preservation, the end of those seasons would mark the beginning of hunger.

So our preserving techniques are aimed at maintaining a constant food supply. As society became more organized, and dependent on efficient agricultural production, the need to prevent waste became acute.

Roasting, drying and pounding food has long been known. The Egyptians of the First Dynasty, about 3,000 B.C., not only knew much about cooking and salting and drying, but had learned to preserve milk by making cheese. By 2,000 B.C. they were baking bread and brewing beer. Alcoholic beverages were as important for food preservation as for revelry in the ancient world. And indeed almost every primitive culture seems to have developed comparable use for fermentation. (American pioneers found that the land along the Ohio River was fine for growing corn. But how could they move the corn to a buyer? Their answer was to make it into a corn whiskey, which was shipped on rafts down the Ohio and Mississippi Rivers to New Orleans, and thence around the world. Kentucky still produces fine bourbon.)

Some Objectives of Food Processing

One of the first objectives of food processing, preservation, has two broad aspects. The preserver first seeks to combat *deterioration*. This is the result of changes occurring within the food itself; it may be entirely the result of the food's own chemistry, or it may result partly from such outside influences as light, heat, oxygen, and so on.

A second general aspect is really a part of our age-old competition with other life forms for food. For just as we must defend our berries from the crows, and our grain from the rat, so must we compete with the micro-organisms which would flourish on our food. *Spoilage* is the term used by food technologists to denote the damage (such as the molding of bread) wrought by micro-organisms.

Micro-organisms may also contaminate food, so that it becomes a carrier, either of disease organisms or of harmful toxins. For example, ingesting *salmonella* bacteria with egg or chicken results in our developing *salmonellosis* (with its digestive upheavals). On the other hand, *botulinum* organisms are not the direct cause of lethal *botulism;* it is the toxin they produce which can kill. *Staphylococcus* can do both—either cause an infection or make us ill with its toxin.

These organisms are all about us. Bread molds are everywhere. There is botulinum in virtually every American soil. So when we undertake the preservation of our food, we must process so as to defend our food and ourselves against a vast microbial world.

The idea has become widespread in recent years that processing for preservation is primarily for the convenience and profit of the seller. True, we could not have our well-stocked supermarket shelves without such processing. And many food-producing countries leave their food in a more "natural" state. But what is the result? A Brookings Institution study reports:

> "There is little question that large portions of food produced in low-income countries are lost . . . The Food and Agriculture Organization (FAO) estimates world food losses at between $24 and $48 billion a year. In Latin America, annual losses are believed to be about 40 percent of the total crop, in tropical Africa over 30 percent. It has been estimated that if *half* of the world's storage losses were prevented, enough calories would be saved *to satisfy the diets of half a billion people.*"[3]

(Italics are added.)

One important aspect of food utilization is transportion. More and more, the trend has been to center food production so as to take advantage of the best climate, soil, etc.

In this sense, warfare and empire-building have been important factors in the evolution of food preservation, the need being to supply armies on the march. Modern food preserving is often said to have begun with Napoleon's forays. (In 1810, the French brewer, Francois Appert, was awarded a prize of 12,000 francs for developing canning. He had sealed food in jars and then heated them in boiling water, a process which was believed to work because the food was shut away from air. It was not until much later that science understood that the process actually worked because the heat destroyed microbes in the food and the sealing prevented new infections.) The American Civil War and World War II both provided impetus for the preserving of food for shipment.

Today we grow most of our wheat in the Great Plains, freeze orange juice in Florida, and produce most of our fruits and vegetables in California. And almost all our important foods are available the year around: This would not be possible without processing.

Processing also serves another function, which we might characterize as the preparation of food for eating. In this sense, it is really an industrialized cookery.

Most of this work centers about two general concepts, just as our home cooking does: First we select the part of the food we want to eat and separate it from the part we don't want—as in taking the peas from a pod or a banana from its skin. And second, we modify the food for a specific eating purpose; the same wheat may go into a breakfast cereal, or a hamburger bun for lunch, or a cake for dinner. It may be boiled or baked, combined with other foods, seasoned, or perhaps nutritionally enriched or fortified. Of course most of this sort of processing has to do with sensory values.

Overall, this system provides us with perhaps eight to ten thousand foods in our markets, most of which are available to use continuously through the seasons, at a generally constant price scale. But what, many ask, does it do to our nutrition?

What Is "Natural" Food?

Of late considerable emphasis has been placed on distinctions between processed and "natural" foods. The terms are widely used without question—except by nutritionists. Recent marketing studies show that the word "natural" is a powerful stimulus for buyers, who seem to feel that "natural" food is much more healthful, that "processed" food may be the cause of anything less than optimal health.

As an example of such beliefs, consider the text developed by La Leche League, a national organization which laudably tries to encourage breastfeeding of infants and takes an active role (especially in regard to nutrition) in pre-natal and post-natal education of mothers: "In the presence of natural food," their official book advises pregnant women, "the appetite is virtually foolproof. In man, as in all other animals, if the opportunity for a natural selection is there, the appetite will always direct itself and demand the right foods at the right times."[4]

Alas, the evidence is that appetite is often a poor guide to nutritive food choice. But why should "natural" foods have this power? What are they? La Leche League includes among them pizza, pastrami on rye, and chop suey; and adds, "Modern transportation and mechanization make possible a varied and diverse selection of foods all through the year." Such confusion is typical.

Post's *Grape-Nuts* are billed as a "Natural Wheat and Barley Cereal." But in its long list of ingredients are malted barley—meaning that the grain has been broken down by hydrolysis into short-chain maltoses—and eight added vitamins. Kellogg's *All-Bran* is sold as "A Natural Food Fiber Cereal." It is so called, presumably, because its first ingredient is wheat bran. Wheat bran does have much fiber, and it is part of natural growth. But what sort of *unnatural* fiber could possibly be put into a cereal—polyester fiber? (Even this would have some claim to "naturalness"—it would have been made from petroleum, organic decayed material.) Other "natural" cereals have such ingredients as corn syrup or nonfat dried skim milk, which are certainly manufactured.

Clearly—although there is no precise definition of "natural" food—the intent of the consumer is to get food which is as close to its original state as possible. And equally clear is the belief that such food is more healthful. Let us see if we can test these ideas.

Does Processing Affect Nutritive Value?

There is little question that the preparation of food for consumption or storage usually has some effect on nutritive value. But we should keep in mind that, if our concern is about really substantial effects of such change: (1) There must be real (not simply cosmetic) changes in the food; (2) These changes must be substantial enough to make a difference in the nutrition of the individual; and (3) The changes must be meaningful in the context of the whole diet.

Perhaps the easiest way to understand these evaluations is to cite examples in the home preparation of food. Suppose we begin by having some freshly squeezed orange juice. The juicing of the orange is a form of processing.

First, which orange did we select? In 100 grams of whole orange, California navels have about 60 mg. of vitamin C, which is one of the most fragile and easily dissipated nutrients. Midseason Florida oranges have about 51 mg., and late Valencias have only about 37 mg. Even when we cut the orange, some vitamin C is lost to the oxygen in the air. If the juice sits out on the table, uncovered, for half an hour before being drunk, more vitamin C will be lost. As a result, the final product will contain from 20 mg. to 80 mg. of vitamin C in each 100 grams. Of course, we could use reconstituted frozen juice, made from a mixed batch of many oranges, professionally squeezed and packaged; it averages about 45 mg. of vitamin C per 100 grams.

How does all of this affect nutrition? Very little. For in terms of the whole diet, we are probably getting substantial amounts of vitamin C from other sources during the day—from tomatoes, potatoes, greens, other fruits, and so on. Adult male RDA for vitamin C is 45 mg. Does the "naturalness" matter? One must conclude that processing here makes no difference in terms of effect on health.

In the context of our orange juice, let us consider the pasteurization of milk. This process protects against many diseases. It also sacrifices a small amount of vitamin C. You as a consumer must decide whether a few milligrams of vitamin C matter in this context— considering the risk of diseases such as tuberculosis from "raw" milk. (Another factor is the deactivation of enzymes from pasteurized milk. Remember, these are cow enzymes, which will mostly be broken into their constituent amino acids after we swallow them, before they can enter our bloodstreams.)

There is often a nutrient loss when we select one part of a food and discard the rest. We eat "refined eggs." For most of us throw away the shell during "home processing." Yet the shell is very high in calcium. Shall we crush it into our scrambled eggs?

The outside leaves of our head of lettuce are rather dirty, torn, and unattractive. But they contain up to five times as much calcium as the inner leaves. Shall we throw away the outside leaves—and thus process the lettuce?

In making an apple pie, shall we peel the apple and lose over 30 percent of the vitamin C? The canning of tomato juice costs an average of one third of its vitamin C; should we squeeze fresh juice?

White flour has been milled until it loses some 60 percent of its calcium—but this may only represent about 3 milligrams of the 800-1,000 of our recommended daily allowance.

As for our use of fresh foods, we must be aware that food begins to change as soon as we take it from the plant. Freshly picked, a snap bean has about 18 mg. of vitamin C per 100 grams. After three days, only about 15 mg. are left—after six days, only about 8 mg. Then consider cooking time, the amount of water used, the temperature of the water, the pressure in the cooking vessel. In general, the commercial processor has tight controls over all these factors and takes pains to rush the crop from the field to his production line. The home cook may or may not be so scrupulous, and may actually squander far more nutrients.

With all this, how are we to make comparisons? Our tables of food composition show average differences between processed and fresh forms of foods; we have only to look them up. Labeling also tells us much. The values shown in either case are not exact, but they are perfectly good general guides.

Of course, not all the nutrients are shown either in ordinary food-composition tables or on labels. But if we use our knowledge of the chemical groupings of nutrients, we can make some deductions, using as guides a few nutrients which serve as fairly good indicators of processing losses. For example, vitamin C and thiamin are about the most easily lost of the water-soluble vitamins. As we have seen, vitamin C is especially vulnerable. Losses from heating, air exposure, or cooking with water should show up for these two. If these losses are minimal, chances are that they will be small for folacin and other water-soluble vitamins.

Vitamin A is a good indicator for losses of fat-soluble vitamins. And the retention of iron is a pretty good signal that the general mineral content has survived refinement, unless an ingredients label tells us that the iron has been added.

If, as in wheat flour, nutrients have been restored, only better-known nutrients may have been replaced, not the lesser known, such as trace elements. For example, iron may have been put back into a grain product, but magnesium omitted. To make realistic judgments, we must have a pretty good idea of the composition of the food *before* processing. And of course we must know something of human needs for the lost nutrients in order to say whether or not a loss is nutritionally significant.

The point is that when and if nutrient losses in processing are matters of concern, we ought to know specifically what has been lost and how much of it. Fantasies of loss have never been known to cause nutritional deficiencies.

WHAT DID THEY PUT IN YOUR DIET?

To turn again to the theses of *Prevention,* we see evidence of the concern that "processing" not only takes out the good, but adds substances that are dangerous to health: "We face the ineluctable fact that we are constantly being deluged with tiny bits of poison, coming to us from every conceivable purchase of food, some so stated on the label, most of them hidden and unmentioned . . . We can only counter this massive insult to our alimentary system and our health by trying to channel our food purchases through organic food shops or farms, and eating more vitamin supplements . . ."[1]

The public concern with food additives is often based in part on the idea that additives serve only the processors, and that they are not needed. As James Turner in the report of a Ralph Nader study group puts it: "The primary purpose of food additives to industry is to increase profits. Coloring, tenderizing or extending the shelf life of products to grind out more millions of dollars should not be tolerated if there is the slightest indication that a hazard to consumers might exist."[5]

Every banning of a food additive adds to the general suspicion and indignation (as in *cyclamate* or the food coloring *Red Number Two*). The public is outraged when industry tries to delay or appeal such banning. Many consumers are still more outraged when they see that nutrition science does not seem to be appropriately disturbed at a revelation that an additive which has been widely used is declared to be unsafe, especially if the additive is banned as cancer-causing.

The fact is that science and the public see food additives quite differently. And the core subject about which all the additive controversy swirls can be summed up in just one word—*safety.* Let us see what we can discern about the realities of additive safety and use.

Are Food Additives Safe to Eat?

A food additive may be defined simply as a substance which is added to a food to be consumed with that food. This definition takes in a lot of very different substances, from the *unintentional* additives, such as bacteria, rodent hairs, and pesticides, to the *intentional* additives—between 2 and 3,000 compounds which are mixed into our foodstuffs.

The public has a single question about all of these substances: Are they safe? In realistic scientific terms, the answer to that question can be extremely succinct. *No.* Then how can we dare to put additives in food? The scientist's answer, and a confusing one for the layman, is, "Because we don't think that they will hurt anyone."

The apparent conflict between these two answers is best understood by looking more closely at the meaning of safety. Webster defines safety as "freedom from danger, injury or damage." In these terms, stop to think of just one thing which you do or eat which is absolutely safe. Remember that, as a measurement, "freedom from—" must be considered as zero. Zero *what?* Zero *risk.*

Is it safe to cross the street at a quiet intersection with a traffic light and a policeman standing guard? One cannot really say that it is; there is a very low possibility that you will be hurt, but it is not zero. Is it safe to drink water or to eat a banana? One cannot really say that it is, scientifically. For anything we eat or drink can have a toxic effect, if we take enough of it, or take it under certain conditions.

It is hard for many people to understand that the only real measurement of "safety" is risk. In terms of crossing the street, for example, we may say that we feel secure, and mean that we think the risk is very low. At rush hour, the risk is somewhat higher, but not really threatening. And we have something to gain from crossing the street—getting to work, perhaps. So we derive a benefit from the crossing and undertake a very small risk. The balance in which the two are weighed is known as the *risk-benefit ratio.* It is in this same balance that a decision about whether to use an additive is made.

One problem with the term "risk-benefit ratio" is that it sounds menacing to most people. In crossing our quiet street, for example, we consider the risk seriously enough to look both ways for traffic; but we don't really fear the danger.

Measuring the Risk

These questions may seem quite semantic. But they have urgent practical implications. As an example, a primary aim in proving that a drug or additive can be used is to determine the *no-effect dose.* Suppose that a new drug is to be tested. We give animals 500 mg. of it and there is no harmful effect. Then we give 700 mg. and the animals' temperatures go up. We have found a "no-effect" dose and an "effect" dose. The measurements are important, for usually FDA requires that there be a 100-fold safety factor. In other words, usually the highest expected use of an additive should be less than one hundredth of the toxic amount (as determined by a well controlled, *long-term* study.)

For many people, even these huge safety factors are not enough. But consider. Would you try to consume vitamins A or D over a long period in quantities 100 times the RDA? At 10 to 25 times RDA they can be quite toxic. At only about 5 times some "normal" usage, ordinary table salt can cause harm. Imagine trying to get a no-effect test on water at 100 times the daily use. Remember, these margins are necessary because there is no way to prove absolute safety for anything.

As the National Academy of Science's Food Protection Committee puts the case: "No method is at hand—and none is in sight—for establishing, with absolute certainty, the safety of a food chemical under all conditions of use. Experience has shown, however, that properly conducted and interpreted animal experiments can provide that degree of assurance of safety reasonably expected in the evaluation of chemicals for use in human food."[6]

What is the result of such testing? We establish safety margins for the conditions and amounts in which an additive may be said to be "safe for intended use." This is all that we can hope for at the moment. But it is not enough for some.

Legislating Additive Safety

The safety programs of FDA began with Dr. Harvey Wiley; he used a volunteer "poison squad" of twelve men, who consumed quantities of food additives to see if they were harmful. For the first 52 years of FDA's existence (from 1906 to 1958) it was the Government's duty to prove danger, not the manufacturer's to prove "safety."

Then in 1958, Congress passed the Food Additives Amendment. As former FDA Commissioner Edwards explained it: "Prior to the enactment of this Amendment, the law did not prevent the addition to food of substances of unknown or uncertain toxicity . . . An item newly proposed for addition to food must now undergo strict testing designed to establish the safety of the intended use."[7]

Many people have difficulty understanding that the same substance can be both "toxic" and "safe," depending on how much is used and how it is used. Especially, they do not recognize the biological truth that there is no substance so toxic that the body cannot manage some tiny amount of it harmlessly; and there is none so safe that a great enough excess will not do injury. The result was the Amendment's "Delaney Clause," named for Congressman James J. Delaney of New York.

The Clause reads: "No additive shall be deemed to be safe if it is found to induce cancer when ingested by man or animal, or if it is found, after tests which are appropriate for the evaluation of the safety of food additives, to induce cancer in man or animals."

With this, an unrealistic demand for perfect safety became a part of our law. For no limit or condition was set upon the amounts of a substance or the terms of an experiment which might produce a tumor. All the much-publicized additive bannings of the last two decades stem from this legislation.

For example, massive doses of a compound called *trichlorethylene* (TCE), used as a cleaning agent and metal degreaser in industry, were fed to mice and rats over their entire lifetimes. Eventually, at these high doses, so large that they had to be forced into the animals through stomach tubes, some of the mice showed tumors. Tiny amounts of TCE were used in decaffeinating coffee. Ralph Nader's associates looked at the data and petitioned FDA to ban TCE. How high were the doses, however? Might they be consumed by real people? Compensating for the size differences between man and mouse, a person would have to drink at least *50 million cups of decaffeinated coffee every day,* for most of his life, to produce the same effects.

Cyclamates were banned because of tumors in mice, at intake levels equal to the sweetness of some 8 pounds of sugar a day over many years (ignoring the "no effect" results of lower levels of the material). Red Number Two dye was banned on the same basis. So it is easy to see that charges that there are known carcinogens (cancer causers) in our food are absurd. By law, if they are known, they *must* be removed from our food.

Recently, nitrates and nitrites, additives which are used in such meat products as sausages and bacon, mainly to prevent lethal *botulism,* have come under fire. Why? Because under certain conditions nitrites and amines can form *nitrosamines,* which have caused cancer in some animals, though not in humans. Because of the value of nitrites in protecting the healthfulness of meats, FDA checked 50 retail samples of sausage. Only three had formed even a *trace* of nitrosamine. Is this trace dangerous? Nitrites are formed during the digestion of nitrates, plentiful in many vegetables. Moreover there are nitrites normally present in our saliva, and we swallow enough in a day to equal the amount from several pounds of bacon. As for amines, we produce quite a lot every day during protein digestion. The nitrosamines in our abdomens far exceed those in our food.

Pressure grows to expand the Delaney Clause idea to other biologic effects of additives. In 1972, when one such bill went before the Senate Committee on Nutrition and Human Needs, the FDA Commissioner testified that, "The proposed new legislation would essentially ban all food ingredients and most foods."[7] As a matter of fact, this is probably the only route to "perfect safety."

Are There Reasons for Concern About Additives?

Most of the additives we use are in a group known as GRAS, or Generally Recognized as Safe. This is a list of substances which have been used for some time without any harm. The GRAS List began with the 1958 Additives Amendment, which emphasized safety testing for *new* additives, on the theory that the GRAS substances had all been tested by use. However, the 1969 White House Conference on nutrition recommended a gradual review of the GRAS List, and this is in progress.

In general, additives we use are not as "chemical" and "artificial" as most people think. Dr. Julius Coon helps to put additives in perspective with this overview of what they are:

"Most additives are flavoring agents. The majority are natural products such as . . . clove, dill, garlic, ginger, mustard, licorice . . . Some newer additives are the active chemicals isolated from plants that are responsible for the flavor of the natural . . . substances. Most of the remaining direct additives are also naturally occurring substances such as vitamins, minerals, inorganic and organic acids and salts, including amino acids . . . gums and colors, materials which enhance the quality or attractiveness of our food. It is surprising how few additives are synthetic materials unrelated to natural substances."[8]

Additives cannot be hidden; they must be listed as ingredients of foods. And there are Federal penalties for using additives to avoid sanitary processing or to conceal poor quality or bad handling. So we do know what additives have been put in our food intentionally. The older additives are being reviewed, and the new ones must pass a difficult and demanding muster before FDA will issue the order to admit them to our food supply.

At the moment, there is one main group of additives which are of questionable value in food and which have harmful aspects, which would probably bar them from FDA acceptance today. These are compounds which nature, not industry, has put into our foods. They include the deadly hydrogen cyanide, which kills criminals in the gas chamber (found in lima beans), arsenic (common in fish), the hallucinogen myristicin (in nutmeg), and many more. Clearly, we do not get enough of these substances in our food to do us in, a demonstration of the rule that toxicity is always a function of amount.

PESTICIDES AND UNINTENTIONAL ADDITIVES

One of the more unfortunate legal terms used in the world of foods is *filth*. A sure way to arouse reader alarm is with the news that more filth has been found in a food than the law allows. Invariably, some readers write outraged letters questioning why "filth" should be allowed in our food at all.

Filth is really incidental matter which usually gets into food while it is being grown, harvested, processed, or stored. It is not really as awful as it sounds. Consider "insect parts," one kind of filth. Generally these are not large juicy bug bits, but more often microscopic fractions of tiny aphids, mites, or weevils, members of the insect world which tend to live in and around the soil and food. Farms are in the country, often near woods and uncultivated lands, and city dwellers sometimes forget that there is an unpaved world of dirt and leaves, and that worms and beetles and bugs make their homes in the soils where our carrots grow (and even sometimes play valuable roles in agriculture). As neat and clean as farmers may be, some vestige of the country often remains with the food.

We must also keep in mind that wherever we assemble a great deal of food, whether harvested or still growing, we maintain a tempting buffet for some other creatures of the earth. Indeed, our unbalancing of nature, gathering food plants into concentrated growing grounds for convenience and economy, is one of the reasons why we must turn to pesticides.

Pesticides, a major public concern in food safety, are, like additives, regulated by Federal law. A special pesticides Amendment to the Food and Drug Act (passed in 1954) sets forth most of our current policies.

The pesticide question can be quite complex, with many ecological facets. The only problem of ecology we shall mention here is that of the human ecology.

Once again, we know quite a lot about how to identify pesticides in our food, and quite a lot about how pesticides affect our bodies. So we are able to make some measurements and do a fair job of determining how much we are endangered by these useful chemicals.

The Pesticides Amendment requires FDA to monitor pesticides in our food by sampling our market supplies. In 18 different market areas, FDA periodically buys a 2-week supply of varied foods, in the amounts suitable to a 19-year-old male's appetite. These are then prepared as for eating, and analyzed in the laboratory. In contrast to what is believed by many, the criteria for judging safe levels of pesticides in food are not set by business or agriculture, but are mainly determined by expert committees of the United Nations. By these standards, there is no known danger to health.

There is some limited evidence of pesticide contamination even in "organic" foods purchased during a New York investigation. In this study, 30 percent of the samples bought in "health-food" stores showed some small residues, as opposed to about 25 percent of food from supermarkets. In neither case was the amount of pesticide enough to hurt anyone. It is believed that the main source of such tiny residues of pesticides as do reach our food supply come less from the farm than from incidental contamination by such programs as weed or mosquito control.

Once again, remember that it is not possible to prove a negative. But neither government, nutrition science, nor medicine has seen significant evidence that pesticides are causing cancer, birth deformities, or genetic problems. Nor has there been any evidence of death or illness in North America from eating pesticides in food. (Accidental overdoses of pesticides inhaled or sprayed onto the skin of farm workers are unrelated.) Indeed, we now have very good evidence that small amounts of pesticides actually have the effect of stimulating the body's abilities to detoxify itself.

OF SCIENCE AND HUNGER

There is constant disagreement among nutrition experts and governmental authorities around the world about just how many hundred million people are malnourished, and how many tens of millions die each year of malnutrition. Whoever is right, the numbers are overwhelming. Certainly far more people than the total of the U.S. population are sick and often dying for lack of good food.

Major programs are going forward to give food gifts to the hungry. But probably the greater gift comes from the advances in food science and nutrition. The "Green Revolution" is teaching the science of agriculture in developing nations, to help these people produce their own food. Indonesian rice production has been boosted by a third. The Indian wheat crop doubled in six years. Latin America's corn output has risen by 50 percent. In ten years, West Pakistan has increased its wheat production by 76 percent.

New high-yielding seeds have been developed. Plants have been bred which produce less stalk to yield more rice. A breed of corn with tripled protein has been developed called Opaque 2. This astonishing grain has a protein value that approaches the quality of cow's milk. Even when it is the only protein source in the diet, it meets the hard test of curing kwashiorkor, the tragic protein-deficiency disease which has crippled so many of the world's children.

"The new seeds," says a Brookings Institution report,[3] "may affect the well-being of more people in a shorter period of time than any previous technical advance in history."

Meanwhile, in test programs, microorganisms are being grown as protein sources. As an indication of the potential of these new foods born of technology, the micro-organisms which yield single-cell protein (SCP) can double themselves in less than two hours in contrast to cattle which double their weight in one or two months. Some of these protein-making organisms can even live on waste from oil production, and it is estimated that the world's oil wastes could, if used this way, provide 700 percent of the planet's existing protein needs. There are many such rabbits coming out of food technology's hat: proteins taken from leaves, or from the crushed wastes of oilseeds of cotton and coconut.

But often there is a problem in persuading even the starving and the nutritionally deficient to accept and use what science has to offer them of life. Often, they cannot cross the barriers of old taboos, of unconscious fears and frightening myths, of suspicion of new food forms or tastes. Because they do not understand that science is not a new magic but merely a way to understand and use the physical realities of nature, they cling to the old folkways, often with closed eyes and ears and minds.

Are we really more advanced? Or are we as often victims of superstition, of an unwillingness to live according to the rational science which may well be the best product of our society and our time?

That decision belongs to you.

REFERENCES

1. *Organic Directory,* Rodale Press, Emmaus, Penna.
2. Fredericks, C., cited in Deutsch, R., *Where should you be shopping?,* Nutr. Rev., July, 1974.
3. Berg, A. *The Nutrition Factor,* The Brookings Institution.
4. La Leche League, *The Womanly Art of Breastfeeding,* La Leche League International, Franklin Park, Ill., 1973.
5. Turner, J. *The Chemical Feast,* Grossman, 1970.
6. Food Protection Committee, *The Use of Chemicals in Food Production, Processing, Storage and Distribution,* Nat. Acad. Sci., Washington, 1973.
7. Edwards, C. testimony before the U.S. Senate Select Committee on Nutrition and Human Needs, 1972.
8. Coon, J. *Protecting our internal environment,* Nutr. Today, Summer, 1970.
9. Symposium on *history of food science and technology,* Food Tech., Jan., 1975.
10. Wodicka, V. *FDA's view of food safety,* FDA Consumer, Oct., 1973.
11. IFT Expert Panel, *Organic Foods,* IFT Status Summary, Food Tech., Jan., 1974. (See also, other summaries by this panel.)
12. Duggan, R. and Dawson, K. *Pesticides: A report on residues in food,* FDA Papers, June, 1967.
13. *Some Questions and Answers about Food Additives,* FDA Fact Sheet, Oct., 1971.
14. Chem, L—F. and Lachance, P. *The nutritive profile of fast food meal combinations,* Food Prod. Devel., Oct. 1974.
15. Lachance, P. *Innovation versus nutrition as the criterion for product development,* Food Tech. 25 pp. 51—53.
16. Rasmussen, L. *Man and His Food 2,000 A.D.,* Food Tech. 23:56 1969.
17. Symposium, *Enrichment and fortification of food with nutrients,* J. Agr. Food Chem., 16:149, 1968.
18. Goodwin, R. *A Symposium on Chemical Additives in Food,* Little, Brown, Boston, 1967.
19. Stare, F. and Whelan, E. *Panic in the Pantry,* Atheneum, 1975.
20. Senate Committee on Nutrition, *Selected Papers on Technology, Agriculture Advances and Production,* June 1974, Washington.
21. Deutsch, R. ed. *Report of the California Conference on Food Advertising,* State of California Bureau of Marketing, 1975.
22. Council on Foods and Nutrition, Amer. Med. Assn., *Symposium on Vitamins and Minerals in Processed Foods,* Proceedings, 1971.
23. *The Buying Guide for Fresh Fruits, Vegetables and Nuts,* Blue Goose, Fullerton, Cal. 1971.

24. *Conserving Nutrients,* United Fresh Fruit and Vegetable Assn., Washington.
25. Joint FAO/WHO Expert Committee on Food Additives, *Evaluation of Food Additives,* Rome, FAO, 1971.
26. Joslyn, N. and Heid, J. *Food Processing Operations,* Avi, Conn., 1963.
27. Schroeder, H. *Losses of vitamins and trace minerals resulting from processing and preservation of foods,* Amer. J. Clin. Nutrition 24:562, 1971.
28. Ackroyd, W. *Food for Man,* MacMillan, New York, 1964.
29. *Protecting Our Food,* USDA, Washington, 1965.
30. Frazier, W. *Food Microbiology,* McGraw Hill, New York, 1967.
31. *Toxicants Occurring Naturally in Foods,* Nat. Acad. Sci. Wash., 1973.

GENERAL REFERENCES

NOTE ON USING THE REFERENCES.

The literature of nutrition is not only very large, it is also filled with overlapping, because the subject matter is so completely inter-related.

The *basic references* are listed below, which furnished the basic scientific information used in this book. These, of course, contain copious further bibliography of their own.

Specific references have been included for each chapter, indicating the sources of specific quotations or other information, for which the reader might wish a specific reference.

General references have also been supplied for each chapter. Usually, these are intended as guides to further information on subject matter which may not be found in the basic references. For effort has been made to avoid duplication of the listed works, though this has not always been possible. The intent is to provide avenues toward further reading in special subject areas, rather than to try to overwhelm the reader with an overlong and confusing reference list. References which are shown in the body of the text with double numbering (as, 2—13) indicate the repetition of a reference, later in the book in another context. In the example, the designation *2—13* means *reference number 13 in chapter two.* References are generally designated in the text by a single number, listed in the bibliography for that chapter.

BASIC REFERENCES

1. Goodhart, R. and Shils, M. (eds.) *Modern Nutrition in Health and Disease,* Lea & Febiger, Phila., 1973.
2. Pyke, R. and Brown, M. *Nutrition: An Integrated Approach,* Wiley, New York, 1967.
3. Food and Nutrition Board, *Recommended Dietary Allowances,* Nat. Acad. of Sciences, Washington, 1974.
4. Bogert, L., Briggs, G. and Calloway, D. *Nutrition and Physical Fitness,* Saunders, Phila. 1973.
5. *Report of the White House Conference on Food, Nutrition and Health, 1969,* U.S.G.P.O., Washington, 1970.
6. Fomon, S. et al. *Infant Nutrition,* Saunders, Phila. 1974.
7. Stare, F. and McWilliams, M. *Living Nutrition,* Wiley, N.Y. 1973.
8. Guthrie, H. *Introductory Nutrition,* Mosby, St. Louis, 1971.
9. Robinson, C. *Fundamentals of Normal Nutrition,* Macmillan, New York, 1973.
10. Williams, S. *Nutrition and Diet Therapy,* Mosby, 1973.
11. Watts, B. and Merrill, A. *Composition of Foods,* USDA Agriculture Handbook No. 8, USDA, Washington, 1963.
12. Mitchell, H. et al. *Cooper's Nutrition in Health and Disease,* Lippincott, Phila., 1968.
13. *Food for Us All,* 1969 Yearbook of Agriculture, USDA, Washington, 1969.
14. Beeson, P. and McDermott, W. *Cecil-Loeb Textbook of Medicine,* esp. section, Diseases of Nutrition, pp. 1187–1229, Saunders, Philadelphia, 1963.
15. Latham, M. et al. *Scope Manual on Nutrition,* Upjohn, Kalamazoo, 1970.
16. Adams, C. *Nutritive Value of American Foods: in Common Units,* Agriculture Handbook No. 456, USDA, Washington, 1975.
17. Deutsch, R. *Family Guide to Better Food and Better Health,* Meredith, Des Moines, 1971.

18. McWilliams, M. *Nutrition for the Growing Years,* Wiley, New York, 1971.
19. White, P. ed. *Let's Talk About Food: Answers to Your Questions about Foods and Nutrition,* AMA, Chicago, 1970.
20. Alfin-Slater, A. and Aftergood, L. *Nutrition for Today,* William C. Brown, Dubuque, Iowa, 1973.
21. Labuza, T. *Food for Thought,* Avi, Westport, Conn., 1974.
22. Leverton, R. *Food Becomes You,* Iowa State U., 1965.
23. National Nutrition Consortium and Deutsch, R. *Nutrition Labeling,* Bethesda, Md., 1975.

Foods and the History and Sociology of Nutrition
24. Galdston, I., *Human Nutrition: Historic and Scientific,* New York Acad. of Med. Monograph III, International Universities Press, New York, 1960.
25. Lowenberg, M. et. al. *Food and Man,* Wiley, New York, 1974.
26. Tannahill, R. *Food in History,* Stein and Day, New York, 1973.
27. Deutsch, R. *The New Nuts among the Berries,* in press.
28. McCollum, E. *A History of Nutrition,* Houghton-Mifflin, Boston, 1957.
29. Stewart, G. and Amerine, M. *Introduction to Food Science and Technology,* Academic, New York, 1973.
30. Goldblith, S. and Joslyn, M. *An Anthology of Food Science,* Avi, Westport, 1964.
31. Frazier, W. *Food Microbiology,* McGraw-Hill, New York, 1967.
32. Furia, T. *Handbook of Food Additives,* Chem. Rubber Pub. Co., Cleveland, 1968.
33. Lovelock, Yann, *The Vegetable Book,* St. Martin's, New York, 1973.
34. Montagne, P. *Larousse Gastronomique, The Encyclopedia of Food, Wine and Cookery,* Crown, New York, 1961.
35. Calhoun, A. *A Social History of the American Family,* Vol. I, 1607—1776, Vol. II, 1776—1865, Vol. III, 1865—1919, University, New York, 1960.
36. U.S. Senate, *National Nutrition Policy Study,* Vols. I—VII, Washington, 1974.
37. Economic Research Service, USDA, *The World Food Situation and Prospects to 1985,* Foreign Agricultural Economic Report No. 98, USDA Washington, 1974.

General References (Particularly applicable to Chapter 9.)
1. Lessing, L. *DNA: At the Core of Life Itself,* Macmillan, New York, 1967.
2. Watson, J. *The Double Helix,* Atheneum, 1968.
3. Barry, J. *Molecular Biology: Genes and the Chemical Control of Living Cells,* Prentice-Hall, Englewood Cliffs, N.J., 1965.
4. Mercer, E. *Cells: Their Structure and Function,* esp. "Cell, Plasma Membrane and Nucleus" and "The Cytoplasm" (chapters) Natural History Library—Doubleday, revised, 1967.
5. Lehninger, A. *Biochemistry,* Worth, New York, 1970.
6. *Report of an International Conference on Evaluation of Protein Quality,* Nat. Acad. Science, Pub. No. 1100, Wash., 1963.
7. Lachance, *Protein quality and PER,* Food Prod. Devel. 5:4, 1971.
8. Lachance, P. *Supplemental protein: Does the U.S. diet really need it?,* Food Prod. Devel. 6:5, 1972.
9. *Protein Supplement Health Hazards,* FTC staff report, Aug. 8, 1975.
10. *Lessons on Meat,* Nat. Livestock and Meat Board, Chicago, 1974.
11. Lappe, F. *Diet for a Small Planet,* Ballantine, New York, 1971.
12. Alfin-Slater, R. and Jelliffe, D. *Meat-centered diet high in calories, high in f,t and high in cost,* column, Los Angeles *Times* Home Magazine, Mar. 17, 1974.
13. Brown, L. *The world food prospect,* Science, Dec. 12, 1975.
14. *Protein,* chapter in *Recommended Dietary Allowances,* Nat. Acad. of Sci., Washington, 1974, pp. 37—48.
15. FAO/WHO Expert Group, *Protein Requirements,* WHO Tech. Report Series, No. 301, WHO, Geneva, 1965.
16. Brown, H. *Protein Nutrition,* Thomas, Springfield, Ill.

APPENDIX A—Nutrititive values for household measures and market units of foods

[Item numbers correspond to those in table 1 of Handbook No. 8, revised 1963. Values in parentheses denote imputed values usually from another form of the food or from a similar food. Zeros in parentheses indicate that amount of a constituent, if present, is probably too small to be measured. Dashes (—) denote lack of reliable data for a constituent believed to be present in a measurable amount. Calculated values, as those based on a recipe, are not in parentheses]

Food, approximate measures, units and weight (edible part unless footnotes indicate otherwise) (B)	Grams	Water (C) Percent	Food energy (D) Calories	Protein (E) Grams	Fat (F) Grams	Carbo-hydrate (G) Grams	Calcium (H) Milligrams	Phosphorus (I) Milligrams	Iron (J) Milligrams	Sodium (K) Milligrams	Potassium (L) Milligrams	Vitamin A value (M) International units	Thiamin (N) Milligrams	Riboflavin (O) Milligrams	Niacin (P) Milligrams	Ascorbic (Q) Milligrams
Almonds:																
1 oz	28	4.7	170	5.3	15.4	5.5	66	143	1.3	1	219	0	.07	.26	1.0	Trace
Anchovy:																
Flat—5 anchovies	20	58.6	35	3.8	2.1	.1	34	42	—	—	—	—	—	—	—	—
Apples:																
Raw, commercial varieties:																
2¾-in. diam—1 apple	150	84.4	80	.3	.8	20.0	10	14	.4	1	152	120	.04	.03	.1	6
Apple butter:																
1 tbsp	17.6	51.6	33	.1	.1	8.2	2	6	.1	Trace	44	0	Trace	Trace	Trace	Trace
Apple juice:																
1 fl. oz	31.0	87.8	15	Trace	Trace	3.7	2	3	.2	Trace	31	—	Trace	.01	Trace	Trace
Applesauce:																
Unsweetened—1 cup	244	88.5	100	.5	.5	26.4	10	12	1.2	5	190	100	.05	.02	.1	2
Apricots:																
Raw—1 cup	155	85.3	79	1.6	0.3	19.8	26	36	0.8	2	436	4,190	0.05	0.06	0.9	16
Canned, water pack, without artificial sweetener—1 cup	246	89.1	93	1.7	.2	23.6	30	39	.7	2	605	4,500	.05	.05	1.0	10
Sirup ack, heavy—1 cup	258	76.9	222	1.5	.3	56.8	28	39	.8	3	604	4,490	.05	.05	1.0	10
Cooked, fruit and liquid:																
Without added sugar—1 cup	250	75.6	213	4.0	.5	54.0	55	88	4.5	20	795	7,500	.01	.13	2.5	8
With added sugar—1 cup	270	66.2	329	3.8	.3	84.8	51	84	4.3	19	751	7,020	.01	.11	2.4	5
Frozen, sweetened—1 lb	454	73.3	445	3.2	.5	113.9	45	86	4.1	18	1,039	7,620	.09	.18	3.6	127
Apricot nectar:																
1 fl. oz	31.4	84.6	18	.1	Trace	4.6	3	4	.1	Trace	47	300	Trace	Trace	.1	1

APPENDIX A–Nutrititive values for household measures and market units of foods–Continued

[Item numbers correspond to those in table 1 of Handbook No. 8, revised 1963. Values in parentheses denote imputed values usually from another form of the food or from a similar food. Zeros in parentheses indicate that amount of a constituent, if present, is probably too small to be measured. Dashes (—) denote lack of reliable data for a constituent believed to be present in a measurable amount. Calculated values, as those based on a recipe, are not in parentheses]

Food, approximate measures, units and weight (edible part unless footnotes indicate otherwise) (B)	Grams	Water (C) Percent	Food energy (D) Calories	Pro-tein (E) Grams	Fat (F) Grams	Carbo-hydrate (G) Grams	Cal-cium (H) Milli-grams	Phos-phorus (I) Milli-grams	Iron (J) Milli-grams	Sodium (K) Milli-grams	Potas-sium (L) Milli-grams	Vitamin A value (M) Interna-tional units	Thia-min (N) Milli-grams	Ribo-flavin (O) Milli-grams	Niacin (P) Milli-grams	Ascor-bic (Q) Milli-grams
Artichokes:																
1 bud	300	86.5	50	3.4	.2	11.9	61	83	1.3	36	361	180	.08	.05	.8	10
Asparagus:																
Medium—4 spears	60	93.6	12	1.3	.1	2.2	13	30	.4	1	110	540	.10	.11	.8	16
Avocados, raw:																
All commercial varieties:																
Halved fruit served with																
skin—½ avocado	125	74.0	188	2.4	18.5	7.1	11	47	.7	5	680	330	.12	.23	1.8	16
Bacon:																
Slice, medium (approx. 20 slices per pound, raw)—2 slices	15	8.1	86	3.8	7.8	.5	2	34	.5	153	35	(0)	.08	.05	.8	—
Bananas:																
Medium—1 banana	175	75.7	101	1.3	.2	26.4	10	31	.8	1	440	230	.06	.07	.8	12
Barbecue sauce:																
1 cup	250	80.9	228	3.8	17.3	20.0	53	50	2.0	2,038	435	900	.03	.03	.8	13
Beans, common, mature seeds:																
Cooked, Great Northern or																
Navy—1 cup	180	69.0	212	14.0	1.1	38.2	90	266	4.9	13	749	0	.25	.13	1.3	0
With pork and tomato sauce—1 cup	255	70.7	311	15.6	6.6	48.5	138	235	4.6	1,181	536	330	.20	.08	1.5	5
Red, kidney, cooked—1 cup	185	69.0	218	14.4	.9	39.6	70	259	4.4	6	629	10	.20	.11	1.3	—
Beans, lima:																
Cooked—1 cup	170	71.1	189	12.9	.9	33.7	80	206	4.3	2	717	480	.31	.17	2.2	29
Beans, mung:																
1 cup	105	88.8	37	4.0	.2	6.9	20	67	1.4	5	234	20	.14	.14	.8	20

Food																
Beans, snap: 1 cup	125	92.4	31	2.0	.3	6.8	63	46	.8	5	189	680	.09	.11	.6	15
Yellow or wax: Cooked—1 cup	(125)	93.4	28	1.8	.3	5.8	63	46	.8	4	189	290	.09	.11	.6	16
Beef, trimmed to retail basis:																
Boneless chuck and chuck cuts:																
Cooked (braised or stewed), yield from 1 lb. raw beef—10.7 oz.	304	49.4	994	79.0	72.7	0	33	426	10.0	138	632	130	.15	.61	12.2	—
Chuck rib roasts or chuck rib steaks. Choice grade: yield from 1 lb. raw beef—10.7 oz.	304	40.3	1,298	68.1	111.6	0	30	334	8.8	119	545	210	.13	.52	10.6	—
Good grade: yield from 1 lb. raw beef—10.7 oz.	304	44.8	1,146	73.6	92.1	0	30	368	9.4	129	589	170	.14	.58	11.6	—
Flank steak: Yield from 1 lb. raw beef—10.7 oz.	304	61.4	596	92.7	22.2	0	43	456	11.6	162	742	40	.17	.70	14.0	—
Loin or short loin: Yield from 1 lb raw beef—10.6 oz.	301	37.2	1,400	59.3	127.0	0	27	506	7.8	145	664	220	.17	.48	12.6	—
T-bone steak. choice grade: Yield from 1 lb. raw beef—10.4 oz.	295	36.4	1,395	57.5	127.4	0	24	490	7.7	141	644	220	.17	.47	12.1	—
Loin end or sirloin: Yield from 1 lb. raw beef—11.7 oz.	331	43.9	1,281	76.1	105.9	0	33	632	9.6	186	852	180	.21	.60	15.6	—
Rib roast, choice grade: Yield from 1 lb. raw beef—11.7 oz.	331	40.0	1,456	65.9	130.4	0	30	616	8.6	161	738	250	.18	.50	11.9	—
Round steak: Yield from 1 lb. raw beef—10.7 oz.	304	54.7	793	86.9	46.8	0	36	760	10.6	213	973	80	.24	.67	17.0	—
Rump roast: Yield from 1 lb. raw beef—11.7 oz.	331	48.1	1,149	78.1	90.4	0	33	652	10.3	191	875	170	.21	.60	14.2	—
Ground beef: Lean with 10% fat: cooked (well done, oven-broiled, pan-broiled, or sauteed) Yield from 1 lb. raw ground beef—12 oz.	340	60.0	745	93.2	38.4	0	41	782	11.9	228	1,044	70	.32	.78	20.4	—
Beef and vegetable stew: 1 cup	245	82.4	218	15.7	10.5	15.2	29	184	2.9	91	613	2,400	.15	.17	4.7	17
Beef, corned, boneless: Cooked: yield from 1 lb. uncooked—10.7 oz.	304	43.9	1,131	69.6	92.4	0	27	283	8.8	2,867	182	—	.06	.55	4.6	0

APPENDIX A.–Nutrititive values for household measures and market units of foods—Continued

[Item numbers correspond to those in table 1 of Handbook No. 8, revised 1963. Values in parentheses denote imputed values usually from another form of the food or from a similar food. Zeros in parentheses indicate that amount of a constituent, if present, is probably too small to be measured. Dashes (—) denote lack of reliable data for a constituent believed to be present in a measurable amount. Calculated values, as those based on a recipe, are not in parentheses]

Food, approximate measures, units and weight (edible part unless footnotes indicate otherwise) (B)	Grams	Water (C) Percent	Food energy (D) Calories	Protein (E) Grams	Fat (F) Grams	Carbohydrate (G) Grams	Calcium (H) Milligrams	Phosphorus (I) Milligrams	Iron (I) Milligrams	Sodium (K) Milligrams	Potassium (L) Milligrams	Vitamin A value (M) International units	Thiamin (N) Milligrams	Riboflavin (O) Milligrams	Niacin (P) Milligrams	Ascorbic (Q) Milligrams
Canned corned-beef hash (with potato):																
Can, net wt. 15½ oz.—1 can	439	67.4	795	38.6	49.6	47.0	57	294	8.8	2,371	878	—	.04	.40	9.2	—
Beef, dried, chipped:																
Cooked, creamed—1 cup	245	72.0	377	20.1	25.2	17.4	257	343	2.0	1,754	375	880	.15	.47	1.5	1
Beef pot pie:																
Pie, whole (9-in. diam.)—1 pie	630	55.1	1,550	63.6	91.4	118.4	88	447	11.3	1,789	1,002	5,170	0.69	0.76	12.6	19
Beets, common, red:																
Cooked (boiled), drained, peeled:																
Diced or sliced—1 cup	170	90.9	54	1.9	.2	12.2	24	39	.9	73	354	30	.05	.07	.5	10
Beet greens, common, edible leaves and stems: Cooked (boiled), drained—1 cup	145	93.6	26	2.5	.3	4.8	144	36	2.8	110	481	7,400	.10	.22	.4	22
Beverages, alcoholic and carbonated nonalcoholic:																
Beer, can or bottle (12 fl. oz.)—1 container	360	92.1	151	1.1	0	13.7	18	108	Trace	25	90	—	.01	.11	2.2	—
Gin, rum, vodka, whisky: 80-proof Jigger [1½ fl. oz. or 44 ml.]—1 jigger	42	66.6	97	—	—	Trace	—	—	—	Trace	1	—	—	—	—	—
100-proof Jigger [1½ fl. oz. or 44 ml.]—1 jigger	42	57.5	124	—	—	Trace	—	—	—	Trace	1	—	—	—	—	—
Wines:																
Dessert: Wine glass (serving portion, 3½ fl. oz.]—1 glass	103	76.7	141	.1	0	7.9	8	—	—	4	77	—	.01	.02	.2	—
Table: Wine glass (serving portion 3½ fl. oz.]—1 glass	29	85.6	25	Trace	0	1.2	3	3	.1	1	27	—	Trace	Trace	Trace	—

Values for edible part of foods

Carbonated, nonalcoholic:																
Bottle (12 fl. oz.)—1 bottle	36.6	92	113	(0)	(0)	29.3	—	—	—	—	—	(0)	(0)	(0)	(0)	(0)
Cola type:																
Bottle or can (12 fl. oz.)—1 container	36.9	90	144	(0)	(0)	36.9	—	—	—	—	—	(0)	(0)	(0)	(0)	(0)
Cream sodas:																
Bottle or can (12 fl. oz.)—1 container	371	89	160	(0)	(0)	40.8	—	—	—	—	—	(0)	(0)	(0)	(0)	(0)
Fruit-flavored sodas:																
Bottle or can (12 fl. oz.)—1 container	372	88	171	(0)	(0)	44.6	—	—	—	—	—	(0)	(0)	(0)	(0)	(0)
ginger ale, pale dry and golden:																
Bottle or can (12 fl. oz.)—1 container	366	92	113	(0)	(0)	29.3	—	—	—	—	—	(0)	(0)	(0)	(0)	(0)
Root beer:																
Bottle or can (12 fl. oz.)—1 container	370	89.5	152	(0)	(0)	38.9	—	—	—	—	—	(0)	(0)	(0)	(0)	(0)
Special dietary drinks with artificial sweetener (less than 1 Cal. per ounce):																
Bottle or can (12 fl. oz.)—1 container	355	100	—	(0)	(0)	—	—	—	—	—	—	(0)	(0)	(0)	(0)	(0)
Biscuits, baking powder, baked from home recipe. Enriched flour:																
Biscuit, 2-in. diam. 1¼ in. high—1 biscuit	28	27.4	103	2.1	4.8	12.8	34	49	0.4	175	33	Trace	.06	.06	.5	Trace
Unenriched flour: Biscuit, 2-in. diam. 1¼ in. high—1 biscuit	28	27.4	102	2.1	4.8	12.8	34	49	.1	175	33	Trace	.01	.03	.1	Trace
Biscuit mix with enriched flour and biscuits baked from mix:																
Biscuits made with milk: Biscuit, 2-in. diam. 1¼ in. high—1 biscuit	28	28.5	91	2.0	2.6	14.6	19	65	.6	272	32	Trace	.08	.07	.6	Trace
Blackberries:																
1 cup	144	84.5	84	1.7	1.3	18.6	46	27	1.3	1	245	290	.04	.06	.6	30
Blueberries:																
Raw: 1 cup—1 cup	145	83.2	90	1.0	.7	22.2	22	19	1.5	1	117	150	(.04)	(.09)	(.7)	20
Frozen, not thawed: Unsweetened: 1 cup	165	85.0	91	1.2	.8	22.4	17	21	1.3	2	134	120	.05	.10	.8	12
Frozen, not thawed: Sweetened: Cup—1 cup	230	72.3	242	1.4	.7	61.0	14	25	.9	2	152	70	.09	.12	.9	18
Boston brown bread: canned: Piece, 3¼-in. diam. ½ in. thick—1 piece.	45	45.0	95	2.5	.6	20.5	41	72	.9	113	131	0	.05	.03	.5	0
Bouillon cubes: 1 cube.	4	4	5	.8	.1	.2	—	—	—	960	4	—	—	—	—	—

APPENDIX A—Nutritive values for household measures and market units of foods—Continued

[Item numbers correspond to those in table 1 of Handbook No. 8, revised 1963. Values in parentheses denote imputed values usually from another form of the food or from a similar food. Zeros in parentheses indicate that amount of a constituent, if present, is probably too small to be measured. Dashes (—) denote lack of reliable data for a constituent believed to be present in a measurable amount. Calculated values, as those based on a recipe, are not in parentheses]

(B) Food, approximate measures, units and weight (edible part unless footnotes indicate otherwise)	Grams	(C) Water Percent	(D) Food energy Calories	(E) Protein Grams	(F) Fat Grams	(G) Carbohydrate Grams	(H) Calcium Milligrams	(I) Phosphorus Milligrams	(J) Iron Milligrams	(K) Sodium Milligrams	(L) Potassium Milligrams	(M) Vitamin A value International units	(N) Thiamin Milligrams	(O) Riboflavin Milligrams	(P) Niacin Milligrams	(Q) Ascorbic Milligrams
Boysenberries:																
Canned, water pack, solids and liquid, without artificial sweetener—1 cup	244	89.8	88	1.7	.2	22.2	(46)	(46)	[2.9]	2	207	320	[.02]	[.24]	[1.7]	17
Frozen, not thawed: Unsweetened—1 cup	126	86.8	60	1.5	.4	14.4	32	30	2.0	1	193	(210)	.03	.16	1.3	16
Sweetened—1 cup	143	74.3	137	1.1	.4	34.9	24	24	.9	1	150	(200)	.03	.14	.9	11
Bran:																
Added sugar, salt, malt extract, vitamins—1 cup	60	3.6	144	7.6	1.8	44.6	50	598	5.8	493	466	2,820	( )	( )	( )	( )
Bran flakes:																
40% bran—1 cup	35	3.0	106	3.6	.6	28.2	19	125	12.4	207	137	1,650	.41	.49	4.1	12
Bran flakes with raisins:																
1 cup	50	7.3	144	4.2	.7	39.7	28	146	17.7	212	154	2,350	.58	.71	5.8	18
Brazil nuts:																
Shelled—1 oz. or 6–8 kernels	28	4.6	185	4.1	19.0	3.1	53	196	1.0	Trace	203	Trace	.27	.03	.5	—
Breads:																
Cracked-wheat bread—1 slice	25	34.9	66	2.2	.6	13.0	22	32	.3	132	34	Trace	.03	.02	.3	Trace
French or vienna bread: French—1 slice	35	30.6	102	3.2	1.1	19.4	15	30	.8	203	32	Trace	.10	.08	.9	Trace
Vienna: Piece, 4¾ in. wide, 4 in. high, ½ in. thick—1 slice	25	30.6	73	0.3	.8	13.9	11	21	.6	145	23	Trace	.07	.06	.6	Trace
Italian bread: enriched, 4½ in. wide, 3¼ in. high, ¾ in. thick—1 slice	30	31.8	83	2.7	.2	16.9	5	23	.7	176	22	(0)	.09	.06	.8	(0)
Raisin bread: 3¾ in. wide, 3⅜ in. high, ½ in. thick—1 slice	25	35.3	66	1.7	.7	13.4	18	22	.3	91	58	Trace	.01	.02	.2	Trace

Rye bread: American,																
slice, 4¾ in. wide,																
3¾ in. high, 7/16 in. thick—1 slice	25	35.5	61	2.3	.3	13.0	19	37	.4	139	36	(0)	.05	.02	.4	(0)
Pumpernickel: 5 in. wide, 4 in.																
high, ⅜ in. thick—1 slice	32	34.0	79	2.9	.4	17.0	27	73	.8	182	145	(0)	.07	.04	.4	(0)
Salt-rising bread, unenriched:																
4⅛ in. wide, 4½ in. high,																
7/16 in. thick—1 slice	24	36.5	64	1.9	.6	12.5	6	17	.1	64	16	Trace	.01	.01	.1	Trace
White bread, enriched: 4⅜ in.																
wide, 4 in. high, 9/16 in. thick—1 slice	28	35.6	76	2.4	.9	14.1	24	27	.7	142	29	Trace	.07	.06	.7	Trace
White bread, unenriched:																
4⅜ in. wide, 4 in. high,																
9/16 in. thick—1 slice	28	35.6	76	2.4	.9	14.1	24	27	.2	142	29	Trace	.02	.03	.3	Trace
Whole-wheat bread: 4 in. wide, 4 in.																
high, 7/16 7/16 in. thick—1 slice	25	36.4	61	2.6	.8	11.9	25	57	.8	132	68	Trace	.06	.03	.7	Trace
Breadcrumbs:																
Dry, grated (enriched)—1 cup	100	6.5	392	12.6	4.6	73.4	122	141	3.6	736	152	Trace	.22	.30	3.5	Trace
Bread pudding with raisins																
(made with enriched bread)—1 cup	265	58.6	496	14.8	16.2	75.3	289	302	2.9	533	570	800	.16	.50	1.3	3
Bread stuffing mix and stuffings:																
1 cup	200	61.4	416	8.8	25.6	39.4	80	132	2.0	1,008	116	840	.10	.18	1.6	Trace
Broccoli:																
Medium—1 stalk	180	91.3	47	5.6	.5	8.1	158	112	1.4	18	481	4,500	.16	.36	1.4	162
Brussels sprouts:																
1 cup	155	88.2	56	6.5	.6	9.9	50	112	1.7	16	423	810	.12	.22	1.2	135
Buckwheat flour:																
Light, sifted—1 cup	98	12	340	6.3	1.2	77.9	11	86	1.0	—	314	(0)	.08	(.04)	(.4)	(0)
Bulgur (parboiled wheat):																
Unseasoned—1 cup	135	56.0	227	8.4	.9	47.3	27	270	1.8	809	117	(0)	.07	.04	3.2	(0)
Butter:																
Regular (approx. ⅛ of stick—1 tbsp	14.2	15.5	102	.1	11.5	.1	3	2	0	140	3	470	—	—	—	0
Whipped type (approx. ⅛ of stick—1 tbsp	9.4	15.5	67	0.1	7.6	Trace	2	2	0	93	2	310	—	—	—	0
Buttermilk:																
1 cup	245	90.5	88	8.8	.2	12.5	296	233	.1	319	343	10	.10	.44	.2	2
Cabbage:																
Common varieties (Danish, domestic,																
pointed types): Raw—1 cup	90	92.4	22	1.2	.2	4.9	44	26	.4	18	210	120	.05	.05	.3	42

APPENDIX A–Nutrititive values for household measures and market units of foods—Continued

[Item numbers correspond to those in table 1 of Handbook No. 8, revised 1963. Values in parentheses denote imputed values usually from another form of the food or from a similar food. Zeros in parentheses indicate that amount of a constituent, if present, is probably too small to be measured. Dashes (—) denote lack of reliable data for a constituent believed to be present in a measurable amount. Calculated values, as those based on a recipe, are not in parentheses]

Food, approximate measures, units and weight (edible part unless footnotes indicate otherwise) (B)	Grams	Water (C) Percent	Food energy (D) Calories	Pro-tein (E) Grams	Fat (F) Grams	Carbo-hydrate (G) Grams	Values for edible part of foods									
							Cal-cium (H) Milli-grams	Phos-phorus (I) Milli-grams	Iron (J) Milli-grams	Sodium (K) Milli-grams	Potas-sium (L) Milli-grams	Vitamin A value (M) Interna-tional units	Thia-min (N) Milli-grams	Ribo-flavin (O) Milli-grams	Niacin (P) Milli-grams	Ascor-bic (Q) Milli-grams
Cooked—1 cup	145	93.9	29	1.6	.3	6.2	64	29	.4	20	236	190	.06	.06	.4	48
Red, raw—1 cup	90	90.2	28	1.8	.2	6.2	38	32	.7	23	241	40	.08	.05	.4	55
Cabbage, Chinese:																
1 cup	75	95.0	11	.9	.1	2.3	32	30	.5	17	190	110	.04	.03	.5	19
Cakes:																
Angelfood, tube cake (2½ in. arc: vol.. 20.6 cu. in.: 1/12 of cake)—1 piece	60	31.5	161	4.3	.1	36.1	5	13	.1	170	53	0	.01	.08	.1	0
Boston cream pie (3¼-in. arc: vol. 20.8 cu. in.: ⅛ of cake)—1 piece	103	34.5	311	5.2	9.7	51.4	69	104	.5	192	92	220	.03	.11	.2	Trace
Chocolate (devil's food): Without icing:																
2-layer, 9-in. diam.—1 cake	890	24.6	3,257	42.7	153.1	462.8	659	1,219	8.0	2,617	1,246	1,340	.18	.89	1.8	1
(2 × 2 × 2 in.: vol.. 8.0 cu. in.)—1 piece	39	24.6	143	1.9	6.7	20.3	29	53	.4	115	55	60	.01	.04	.1	Trace
With chocolate icing: 2-layer, 9-in. diam.—1 cake	1,193	22.0	4,402	53.7	195.7	665.7	835	1,563	11.9	2,804	1,837	1,910	.24	1.19	2.4	2
12.2 cu. in.—1 piece	75	22.0	277	3.4	12.3	41.9	53	98	.8	176	116	120	.02	.08	.2	Trace
Cupcake, 2¾-in. diam.—1 cupcake	44	22.0	162	2.0	7.2	24.6	31	58	.4	103	68	70	.01	.04	.1	Trace
Cottage pudding, made with enriched flour—1 cake	436	26.6	1,500	27.9	49.3	236.7	392	501	6.1	1,304	384	610	.65	.74	5.2	1
(2 × 4 × 1½ in.: vol.. 12.0 cu. in.)—1 piece	54	26.6	186	3.5	6.1	29.3	49	62	.8	161	48	80	.08	.89	.6	Trace
With chocolate sauce—1 piece	74	27.9	235	3.9	6.5	42.0	53	81	1.0	172	104	70	.09	.10	.7	Trace
Fruitcake: Made with enriched flour:																
Dark (¼ × 2 × 1½ in.: vol. 0.8 cu. in.)—1 slice	15	18.1	57	.7	2.3	9.0	11	17	.4	24	74	20	.02	.02	.1	Trace

Food																
Light: [¼ × 2 × 1½ in.: vol., 0.8 cu. in.]—1 slice	15	18.7	58	.9	2.5	8.6	10	17	.2	29	35	10	.02	.02	.1	Trace
Gingerbread: made with enriched flour [3 × 3 × 2 in.: vol. 18.0 cu. in.]—1 piece	117	30.8	371	4.4	12.5	60.8	80	76	2.7	277	531	110	.14	.13	1.1	0
Plain cake: Without icing [3 × 3 × 2 in.: vol. 18.0 cu. in.]—1 piece	86	24.5	313	3.9	12.0	48.1	55	88	.3	258	68	150	.02	.08	.2	Trace
With chocolate icing: [3 × 3 × 2 in.: vol. 19.9 cu. in.]—1 piece	123	21.4	453	5.2	17.1	73.1	77	128	.7	282	140	220	.02	.11	.2	Trace
Cupcake. 2¾-in.-diam—1 cupcake	47	21.4	173	2.0	6.5	27.9	30	49	.3	108	54	80	.01	.04	.1	Trace
Pound: Old fashioned [3½ × 3 × ½ in.]—1 slice	30	17.2	142	1.7	8.9	14.1	6	24	.2	33	18	80	.01	.03	.1	0
Sponge: Tube cake [1¾-in. arc: vol. 15.4 cu. in.]—1 piece	49	31	146	3.7	2.8	26.5	15	55	.6	82	43	220	.02	.07	.1	Trace
White: without icing (1 cu. in.)—1 cube	4.7	24.2	18	.2	.8	2.53	4	—	Trace	15	4	Trace	Trace	Trace	Trace	Trace
With coconut icing [1¾-in arc: vol. 13.4 cu. in.]—1 piece	78	21.3	289	2.9	10.4	47.3	35	56	.2	200	83	20	.01	.05	.2	Trace
With uncooked white icing [1¾-in. arc: vol. 12.4 cu. in.]—1 piece	78	20.0	293	2.6	10.1	49.1	37	51	.1	183	45	90	.01	.05	.1	Trace
Carob flour [St. Johnsbread]: 1 cup	140	11.2	252	6.3	2.0	113.0	493	113	—	—	—	—	—	—	—	—
Carrots: Raw—1 carrot	81	88.2	30	.8	.1	7.0	27	26	.5	34	246	7,930	.04	.04	.4	6
Cooked (boiled), drained: Sliced—1 cup	155	91.2	48	1.4	.3	11.0	51	48	.9	51	344	16,280	.08	.08	.8	9
Cashew nuts: 1 cup	140	5.2	785	24.1	64.0	41.0	53	522	5.3	21	650	140	.60	.35	2.5	—
Cauliflower: Raw—1 cup	100	91.0	27	2.7	.2	5.2	25	56	1.1	13	295	60	.11	.10	.7	78
Cooked (boiled), drained—1 cup	125	92.8	28	2.9	.3	5.1	26	53	.9	11	258	80	.11	.10	.8	69
Caviar, sturgeon: Granular—1 tbsp	16	46.0	42	4.3	2.4	.5	44	57	1.9	352	29	—	—	—	—	—
Celery, green [Pascal type]: Raw—1 stalk	40	94.1	7	.4	Trace	1.6	16	11	.1	50	136	110	.01	.01	.1	4
Chard, Swiss: Cooked (boiled), drained: Leaves and stalks—1 cup	145	93.7	26	2.6	.3	4.8	106	35	2.6	125	465	7,830	.06	.16	.6	23

APPENDIX A–Nutritive values for household measures and market units of foods—Continued

[Item numbers correspond to those in table 1 of Handbook No. 8, revised 1963. Values in parentheses denote imputed values usually from another form of the food or from a similar food. Zeros in parentheses indicate that amount of a constituent, if present, is probably too small to be measured. Dashes (—) denote lack of reliable data for a constituent believed to be present in a measurable amount. Calculated values, as those based on a recipe, are not in parentheses]

Food, approximate measures, units and weight (edible part unless footnotes indicate otherwise) (B)	Grams	Water (C) Percent	Food energy (D) Calories	Pro-tein (E) Grams	Fat (F) Grams	Carbo-hydrate (G) Grams	Cal-cium (H) Milli-grams	Phos-phorus Milli-grams	Iron (J) Milli-grams	Sodium (K) Milli-grams	Potas-sium (L) Milli-grams	Vitamin A value (M) Interna-tional units	Thia-min (N) Milli-grams	Ribo-flavin (O) Milli-grams	Niacin (P) Milli-grams	Ascor-bic (Q) Milli-grams
Cheeses, natural and processed; cheese foods; cheese spreads:																
Blue or Roquefort type—1 oz	28	40	104	6.1	8.6	.6	89	96	[.1]	—	—	[350]	.01	.17	.3	[0]
Brick—1 oz	28	41.0	105	6.3	8.6	.5	207	129	[.3]	—	—	[350]	—	.13	Trace	[0]
Camembert (domestic)—1 oz	28	52.2	85	5.0	7.0	.5	30	52	.1	—	31	[290]	.01	.21	.2	[0]
Cheddar (domestic type)—1 oz	28	37	113	7.1	9.1	.6	213	136	.3	198	23	[370]	.01	.13	Trace	[0]
Cottage cheese [cottage cheese dry curd with creaming mixture: 4.2% milk fat].																
Packed (large or small curd)—1 cup	245	78.3	260	33.3	10.3	7.1	230	372	.7	561	208	[420]	.07	.61	.2	[0]
Cottage cheese dry curd (without creaming mixture)—1 cup	200	79.0	172	34.0	.6	5.4	180	350	.8	580	144	[20]	.06	.56	[.2]	[0]
Cream: 3 oz—1 pkg	85	51	318	6.8	32.0	1.8	53	81	.2	213	63	[1,310]	[.02]	.20	.1	[0]
Whipped—1 cup	155	51	580	12.4	58.4	3.3	96	147	.3	388	115	[2,390]	[.03]	.37	.2	[0]
Limburger—1 oz	28	45	98	6.0	7.9	.6	167	111	.2	—	—	[320]	.02	.14	.1	[0]
Parmesan: prepackaged forms—1 oz	28	30	111	10.2	7.4	.8	323	221	.1	208	42	[300]	.01	.21	.1	[0]
Shredded—1 oz	28	25	120	10.9	7.9	.9	346	237	.1	223	45	[320]	.01	.22	.1	[0]
Swiss (domestic)—1 oz	28	39	105	7.8	7.9	.5	262	160	.3	201	29	[320]	Trace	[.11]	[Trace]	[0]
Pasteurized processed cheese:																
American, approx. 3½ × 3½ × ⅛ in.—1 slice or 1 oz	28	40	105	6.6	8.5	.5	198	219	.3	322	23	[350]	.01	.12	Trace	[0]
Pimiento (American)—1 slice or 1 oz	28	40	105	6.5	8.6	.5	53	—	—	—	—	[350]	—	—	Trace	—
Swiss—1 slice or 1 oz	28	40	101	7.5	7.6	.5	251	246	[.3]	331	28	[310]	[Trace]	.11	Trace	[0]
Pasteurized process cheese spread, American:																
Jar, net wt. 5 oz.—1 jar	142	48.6	409	22.7	30.4	11.6	802	1,243	[.9]	2,308	341	[1,240]	.01	.77	.1	[0]

Food																
Cheese souffle: Whole (yield from recipe), 7½×7½×1¾ in.—1 souffle	440	65.0	959	43.6	75.2	27.3	884	858	4.4	1,602	532	3,520	.22	1.06	.9	Trace
Cherries: Raw. Sour, red, without pits and stems—1 cup	155	83.7	90	1.9	.5	22.2	34	29	.6	3	296	1,550	.08	.09	.6	16
Sweet: without pits and stems—1 cup	145	80.4	102	1.9	.4	25.2	32	28	.6	3	277	160	.07	.09	.6	15
Candied, whole—10 cherries	35	12.0	119	.2	.1	30.3	—	—	—	—	—	—	—	—	—	—
Canned, solids and liquid: Sour (tart), red, water pack, pitted style—1 cup	244	88.0	105	2.0	.5	26.1	37	32	.7	5	317	1,660	.07	.05	.5	12
Sweet—1 cup	270	86.6	119	2.2	.5	29.6	37	32	.7	2	323	150	.05	.05	.5	7
Chestnuts: Shelled—1 cup	160	52.5	310	4.6	2.4	67.4	43	141	2.7	10	726	—	.35	.35	1.0	—
Chewing gum: 1 piece	1.7	3.5	5	—	—	1.6	—	—	—	—	—	—	(0)	(0)	(0)	(0)
Chicken, cooked: All classes, roasted: Light meat, without skin—1 cup	140	63.8	232	44.2	4.8	0	15	371	1.8	90	575	80	.06	.14	16.2	—
Dark meat, without skin—1 cup	140	64.4	246	39.2	8.8	0	18	321	2.4	120	449	210	.10	.32	7.8	—
Broilers, ready-to-cook, broiled flesh only: Yield from 1 lb. ready-to-cook broilers—7.1 oz.	201	71.0	273	47.8	7.6	0	18	404	3.4	133	551	180	.10	.38	17.7	—
Fryers, ready-to-cook, fried: Breast—½ breast	94	58.4	160	25.7	5.1	1.2	9	218	1.3	—	—	70	.04	.17	11.6	—
Drumstick—1 drumstick	56	55.0	88	12.2	3.8	.4	6	89	.9	—	—	50	.03	.15	2.7	—
Thigh—1 thigh	65	55.8	122	15.0	5.9	1.3	7	121	1.2	—	—	100	.03	.25	3.5	—
Wing—1 wing	50	52.6	82	8.8	4.5	.8	3	72	.6	—	—	80	.02	.08	2.1	—
Chicken, canned, meat only, boned—1 cup	205	65.2	406	44.5	24.0	0	43	506	3.1	—	283	470	.08	.25	9.0	8
Chicken a la king, cooked—1 cup	245	68.2	468	27.4	34.3	12.3	127	358	2.5	760	404	1,130	.10	.42	5.4	12
Chicken fricassee, cooked—1 cup	240	71.3	386	36.7	22.3	7.7	14	271	2.2	370	336	170	.05	.17	5.8	—
Chicken potpie: Pie, whole (9-in. diam.) ⅓ of pie—1 piece	232	56.6	545	23.4	31.3	42.5	70	232	3.0	594	343	3,090	0.26	0.26	4.2	5
Chili con carne, with beans, canned: 1 cup	255	72.4	339	19.1	15.6	31.1	82	321	4.3	1,354	594	150	.08	.18	3.3	—
Chives, raw (chopped) 1 tbsp	3	91.3	1	.1	Trace	.2	2	1	.1	—	8	170	Trace	Trace	Trace	2

APPENDIX A–Nutrititive values for household measures and market units of foods—Continued

[Item numbers correspond to those in table 1 of Handbook No. 8, revised 1963. Values in parentheses denote imputed values usually from another form of the food or from a similar food. Zeros in parentheses indicate that amount of a constituent, if present, is probably too small to be measured. Dashes (—) denote lack of reliable data for a constituent believed to be present in a measurable amount. Calculated values, as those based on a recipe, are not in parentheses]

(B) Food, approximate measures, units and weight (edible part unless footnotes indicate otherwise)	Grams	(C) Water Percent	(D) Food energy Calories	(E) Pro-tein Grams	(F) Fat Grams	(G) Carbo-hydrate Grams	(H) Cal-cium Milli-grams	(I) Phos-phorus Milli-grams	(J) Iron Milli-grams	(K) Sodium Milli-grams	(L) Potas-sium Milli-grams	(M) Vitamin A value Interna-tional units	(N) Thia-min Milli-grams	(O) Ribo-flavin Milli-grams	(P) Niacin Milli-grams	(Q) Ascor-bic Milli-grams
Chocolate:																
1 oz.	28	2.3	143	3.0	15.0	8.2	22	109	1.9	1	235	20	.01	.07	.4	0
Chocolate sirup:																
(or topping)—1 fl. oz. or 2 tbsp.	37.5	31.6	92	.9	.8	23.5	6	35	.6	20	106	Trace	.01	.03	.2	0
Chop suey with meat																
(without noodles)—1 cup	250	75.4	300	26.0	17.0	12.8	60	248	4.8	1,053	425	600	.28	.38	5.0	33
Chow mein, chicken (without noodles):																
1 cup	250	78.0	255	31.0	10.0	10.0	58	293	2.5	718	473	280	.08	.23	4.3	10
Citron, candied:																
1 oz.	28	18.0	89	.1	.1	22.7	24	7	.2	82	34	—	—	—	—	—
Clams, raw, meat only:																
Hard, soft, unspecified: Pint—1 pt. or 1 lb.	454	81.7	345	57.2	7.3	9.1	313	735	27.7	544	821	450	.45	.82	5.9	45
Cocoa and chocolate-flavored beverage powders:																
Cocoa powder with nonfat dry milk—1 oz. or approx. 4 heaping tsp.	28	1.9	102	5.3	.8	20.1	167	155	.5	149	227	10	.04	.21	.2	1
Cocoa powder without milk—1 oz. or approx. 4 heaping tsp.	28	1.3	98	1.1	.6	25.3	9	48	.6	76	142	—	.01	.03	.1	0
Coconut meat:																
1 cup	130	50.9	450	4.6	45.9	12.2	17	124	2.2	30	333	0	.07	.03	.7	4
Coconut milk:																
1 cup	240	65.7	605	7.7	59.8	12.5	38	240	3.8	—	—	0	.07	Trace	1.9	5
Cod:																
Cooked (broiled), with butter or margarine: 5 in. long, 2½ in. wide, ½ in. thick—1 fillet	65	64.6	111	18.5	3.4	0	20	178	.7	72	265	120	.05	.07	2.0	—

Coffee, instant, water-soluble solids:																
Dry powder: Ounce (yields approx.																
14 cups of beverage)—1 oz	28	2.6	37	Trace	Trace	(9.9)	51	109	1.6	20	923	0	0	.06	8.7	0
Coleslaw																
made with mayonnaise—1 cup	120	79.0	173	1.6	16.8	5.8	53	35	.5	144	239	190	.06	.06	.4	35
Collards: Cooked (boiled), drained: Leaves including																
stems, cooked in																
small amount of water—1 cup	145	90.8	42	3.9	.9	7.1	220	57	.9	36	339	7,830	.20	.29	1.7	67
Cookies:																
Assorted (sandwich type, shortbread, sugar wafers, butter flavored, chocolate chip, coconut bars, etc.):																
Brownies with nuts—1 brownie	20	9.8	97	1.3	6.3	10.2	8	30	.4	50	38	40	.04	.02	.1	Trace
Butter, thin, rich (butter-																
flavored cookies)—10 cookies	50	4.5	229	3.1	8.5	35.5	63	47	.3	209	30	330	.02	.03	.2	0
Chocolate chip: 2⅓-in. diam.—4 cookies	40	3.0	206	2.2	12.0	24.0	14	40	.8	139	47	40	.04	.04	.4	Trace
Commercial type:—10 cookies	105	2.7	495	5.7	22.1	73.2	41	120	1.9	421	141	130	.04	.07	.4	Trace
Fig bars (1⅝ × 1⅝ × ⅜ in.)																
4 cookies	56	13.6	200	2.2	3.1	42.2	44	34	.6	141	111	60	.02	.04	.2	Trace
Gingersnaps, 2-in. diam.,																
¼ in. thick:—10 cookies	70	3.1	294	3.9	6.2	55.9	51	33	1.6	400	323	50	.03	.04	.3	Trace
Ladyfingers, 3¼ × 1⅜ × 1⅛ in.																
4 ladyfingers	44	19.2	158	3.4	3.4	28.4	18	72	.7	31	31	290	.03	.06	.1	0
Macaroons, 2¾-in. diam.,																
¼ in. thick—2 cookies	38	4.4	181	2.0	8.8	25.1	10	32	.3	13	176	0	.02	.06	.2	0
Marshamallow (plain cooky with marshmallow topping, coconut- or chocolate- coated):																
Coconut-coated, 2⅛-in. diam.,																
1⅛-in. thick—4 cookies	72	9.8	294	2.9	9.5	52.1	15	41	.4	150	66	190	.01	.04	.1	Trace
Chocolate-coated, 1¾-in. diam.,																
¾ in. thick—4 cookies	52	9.8	213	2.1	6.9	37.6	11	30	.3	109	47	140	.01	.03	.1	Trace
Oatmeal with raisins, 2⅝-in. diam.,																
¼-in. thick—4 cookies	52	2.8	235	3.2	8.0	38.2	11	53	1.5	84	192	30	.06	.04	.3	Trace
Sugar wafer type																
1¾×⅛⅜×⅜ in.—10 cookies	70	2.3	331	7.0	13.4	46.9	29	81	.6	121	123	140	.05	.06	2.0	Trace

APPENDIX A–*Nutritive values for household measures and market units of foods*–Continued

[Item numbers correspond to those in table 1 of Handbook No. 8, revised 1963. Values in parentheses denote imputed values usually from another form of the food or from a similar food. Zeros in parentheses indicate that amount of a constituent, if present, is probably too small to be measured. Dashes (—) denote lack of reliable data for a constituent believed to be present in a measurable amount. Calculated values, as those based on a recipe, are not in parentheses]

Food, approximate measures, units and weight (edible part unless footnotes indicate otherwise)		Water	Food energy	Protein	Fat	Carbohydrate	Calcium	Phosphorus	Iron	Sodium	Potassium	Vitamin A value	Thiamin	Riboflavin	Niacin	Ascorbic
							Values for edible part of foods									
(B)	Grams	(C) Percent	(D) Calories	(E) Grams	(F) Grams	(G) Grams	(H) Milligrams	(I) Milligrams	(J) Milligrams	(K) Milligrams	(L) Milligrams	(M) International units	(N) Milligrams	(O) Milligrams	(P) Milligrams	(Q) Milligrams
Sandwich type (chocolate or vanilla):																
1¾-in. diam., ⅜-in. thick—4 cookies	40	2.2	198	1.9	9.0	27.7	10	96	.3	193	15	0	.02	.02	.2	0
Shortbread, 1⅝ × 1⅝ × ¼ in.:																
10 cookies	75	3.0	374	5.4	17.3	48.8	53	117	.4	45	50	60	.03	.04	.4	0
Sugar, soft, thick, with enriched flour, home recipe: cooked, 2⅛-in. diam.,																
¼-thick—10 cookies	95	1.4	461	4.7	18.4	69.7	34	76	.3	180	57	130	.01	.04	.5	0
Vanilla wafers: 1¾-in. diam.																
¼ in thick—10 cookies	40	2.8	185	2.2	6.4	29.8	16	25	.2	101	29	50	.01	.03	.1	0
Corn, sweet:																
Kernels, cooked on cob—1 ear	140	74.1	70	2.5	.8	16.2	2	69	.5	Trace	151	310	.09	.08	1.1	7
Corn fritters:																
(2-in. diam., 1½-in. thick)—1 fritter	35	29.1	132	2.7	7.5	13.9	22	54	.6	167	47	140	.06	.07	.6	1
Corn grits, degermed:																
1 cup	245	87.1	125	2.9	0.2	27.0	2	25	0.2	502	27	150	0.05	0.02	0.5	(0)
Corn flakes:																
Sugar coated, added salt, iron,																
vitamins—1 cup	40	2.2	154	1.8	.1	36.5	1	10	1.0	267	27	1,880	.46	.56	4.6	14
Corn pudding:																
1 cup	245	76.7	255	9.8	11.5	31.9	162	206	1.2	1,068	414	640	.07	.32	1.0	5
Cornbread, baked from home recipe:																
(2½ × 2½ × 1½ in.—1 piece	78	53.9	161	5.8	5.6	22.7	94	165	.9	490	122	120	.10	.15	.5	1
Spoonbread, made with white																
whole-ground cornmeal—1 cup	240	63.0	468	16.1	27.4	40.6	230	394	2.4	1,157	317	700	.22	.43	1.0	1

Food																
Cornmeal, white or yellow: Degermed, enriched: cooked—1 cup	240	87.7	120	2.6	.5	25.7	2	34	1.0	264	38	140	.14	.10	1.2	(0)
Cornstarch, stirred: 1 tbsp.	8	12	29	Trace	Trace	7.0	(0)	(0)	(0)	Trace	Trace	(0)	(0)	(0)	(0)	(0)
Cowpeas, including blackeye peas: Cooked (boiled), drained—1 cup.	165	71.8	178	13.4	1.3	29.9	40	241	3.5	2	625	580	.50	.18	2.3	28
Crab, including blue. Dungeness, rock king: Cooked (steamed)—1 cup	155	78.5	144	26.8	2.9	.8	67	271	1.2	—	—	3,360	.25	.12	4.3	3
Crab, canned, drained solids: 6½ oz—1 can	125	77.2	126	21.8	3.1	1.4	56	228	1.0	1,250	138	—	.10	.10	2.4	—
Drained contents from can: 6½ oz—1 can	180	77.2	182	31.3	4.5	2.0	81	328	1.4	1,800	198	—	.14	.14	3.4	—
Crab, deviled: 1 cup	240	63.3	451	27.4	22.6	31.9	113	329	2.9	2,081	398	—	.19	.26	3.6	14
Crackers: Animal—10 crackers	26	3.0	112	1.7	2.4	20.8	14	30	.1	79	25	30	.01	.03	.1	Trace
Cheese—10 crackers	31.3	3.9	150	3.5	6.7	18.9	105	97	.3	325	34	110	Trace	.03	.3	(0)
Graham: Cracker, 1 large rectangular piece, 1 or 2 or 4 pieces.	14.2	6.4	55	1.1	1.3	10.4	6	21	.2	95	55	(0)	.01	.03	.2	(0)
Saltines, 1⅞-in. square, ⅛-in. thick—10 crackers	28.4	4.3	123	2.6	3.4	20.3	6	26	.3	[312]	[34]	(0)	Trace	.01	.3	(0)
Soda—10 biscuits.	50.4	4.0	221	4.6	6.6	35.6	11	45	.8	554	60	(0)	.01	.03	.5	(0)
Cranberries: 1 cup	95	87.9	44	.4	.7	10.3	13	10	.5	2	78	40	.03	.02	.1	10
Cranberry juice cocktail: Bottled—1 cup	253	83.2	164	.3	.3	41.7	13	8	.8	3	25	Trace	.02	.02	.1	30
Cranberry sauce: Sweetened—1 cup	277	62.1	404	.3	.6	103.9	17	11	.6	3	83	60	.03	.03	.1	6
Cream, fluid: Half-and-half (cream and milk: 11.7% fat)—1 tbsp.	15	79.7	20	.5	1.8	.7	16	13	Trace	7	19	70	.02	.02	Trace	Trace
light, coffee, or table (20.6% fat)—1 tbsp.	15	71.5	32	.5	3.1	.6	15	12	Trace	6	18	130	.02	.02	Trace	Trace
Light Whipping or whipping (31.3% fat)	15	62.1	45	.4	4.7	.5	13	10	Trace	5	15	190	Trace	.02	Trace	Trace
Heavy or heavy whipping (37.6% fat)-1 tbsp.	15	56.6	53	.3	5.6	.5	11	9	Trace	5	13	230	Trace	.02	Trace	Trace

APPENDIX A—Nutrititive values for household measures and market units of foods—Continued

[Item numbers correspond to those in table 1 of Handbook No. 8, revised 1963. Values in parentheses denote imputed values usually from another form of the food or from a similar food. Zeros in parentheses indicate that amount of a constituent, if present, is probably too small to be measured. Dashes (—) denote lack of reliable data for a constituent believed to be present in a measurable amount. Calculated values, as those based on a recipe, are not in parentheses]

Food, approximate measures, units and weight (edible part unless footnotes indicate otherwise) (B)	Grams	Water (C) Percent	Food energy (D) Calories	Pro-tein (E) Grams	Fat (F) Grams	Carbo-hydrate (G) Grams	Cal-cium (H) Milli-grams	Phos-phorus (I) Milli-grams	Iron (J) Milli-grams	Sodium (K) Milli-grams	Potas-sium (L) Milli-grams	Vitamin A value (M) Interna-tional units	Thia-min (N) Milli-grams	Ribo-flavin (O) Milli-grams	Niacin (P) Milli-grams	Ascor-bic (Q) Milli-grams
Cream puffs with custard filling (approx. 3½-in. diam.. 2 in. high)—1 cream puff	130	58.3	303	8.5	18.1	26.7	105	148	.9	108	157	460	.05	.22	.1	Trace
Cress, garden: Raw—1 cup	135	92.5	31	2.6	.8	5.1	82	65	1.1	11	477	10,400	.08	.22	1.1	46
Cucumbers, raw: Slices [6 from large cucumber or 8 from small cucumber]—6 large or 8 small slices	28	95.1	4	.3	Trace	1.0	7	8	.3	2	45	70	.01	.01	.1	3
Custard, baked: 1 cup	265	77.2	305	14.3	14.6	29.4	297	310	1.1	209	387	930	.11	.50	.3	1
Dandelion greens: Cooked (boiled), drained—1 cup	105	89.8	35	2.1	.6	6.7	147	44	1.9	46	244	12,290	.14	.17	—	19
Dates, moisturized or hydrated—10 dates	80	22.5	219	1.8	.4	58.3	47	50	2.4	1	518	40	.07	.08	1.8	0
Doughnuts: Cake type, plain; 3½-in. diam.—1 doughnut	25	23.7	98	1.2	4.7	12.9	10	48	.4	125	23	20	.04	.04	.3	Trace
Eclairs with custard filling and chocolate icing—1 eclair	100	56.2	239	6.2	13.6	23.2	80	112	.7	82	122	340	.04	.16	.1	Trace
Eggs: Chicken: Raw, whole, fresh—1 egg	57	73.7	82	6.5	5.8	.5	27	103	1.2	61	65	590	.05	.15	Trace	0
Egg white of, large egg—1 white	33	87.6	17	3.6	Trace	.3	3	5	Trace	48	46	0	Trace	.09	Trace	0
Egg yolk of large egg—1 yolk	17	51.1	59	2.7	5.2	.1	24	97	.9	9	17	580	.04	.07	Trace	0
Cooked: fried—1 egg	46	67.7	99	6.3	7.9	.1	28	102	1.1	155	64	650	.05	.14	Trace	0

Food, approximate measure, and weight															
Hard cooked—1 egg	57	73.7	82	6.5	5.8	.5	27	103	1.2	61	65	590	.04	.14	Trace	0
Poached—1 egg	50	73.3	82	6.5	5.8	.5	27	103	1.2	136	65	590	.04	.13	Trace	0
Scrambled—1 egg	64	72.1	111	7.2	8.3	1.5	51	121	1.1	164	93	690	.05	.18	Trace	0
Eggplant, cooked (boiled), drained: 1 cup	200	94.3	38	2.0	.4	8.2	22	42	1.2	2	300	20	.10	.08	1.0	6
Endive (curly endive and escarole), raw—1 cup	50	93.1	10	.9	.1	2.1	41	27	.9	7	147	1,650	.04	.07	.3	5
Farina: Enriched: Cooked—1 cup	245	89.5	103	3.2	.2	21.3	10	29	(1)	353	22	(0)	.10	.07	1.0	(0)
Fats, cooking (vegetable fat, mixed fat shortenings)—1 cup	200	0	1,768	0	200.0	0	0	0	0	0	0	—	0	0	0	0
Figs: Raw: Medium, 2¼-in. diam. (approx. 9 per pound)—1 fig	50	77.5	40	.6	.2	10.2	18	11	.3	1	97	40	.03	.03	.2	1
Canned, solids and liquid: whole style: water pack—3 figs; 1¾ tbsp. liquid	80	86.6	38	.4	.2	9.9	11	11	.3	2	124	20	.02	.02	.2	1
Sirup pack, heavy—3 figs; 1¾ tbsp. liquid	85	77.2	71	.4	.2	18.5	11	11	.3	2	127	30	.03	.03	.2	1
Filberts (hazelnuts): Shelled (approx. 20 nuts)—1 oz	28	5.8	180	3.6	17.7	4.7	59	96	1.0	1	200	—	.13	—	0.3	Trace
Fishcakes, cooked: Fried—1 regular-size cake	60	66.0	103	8.8	4.8	5.6	—	—	—	—	—	—	—	—	—	—
Fish flakes, canned, solids and liquid—1 cup	165	72.1	183	40.8	1.0	0	81	383	1.3	—	—	—	—	—	—	—
Fish sticks, breaded, cooked frozen—1 fish stick or 1 oz	28	65.8	50	4.7	2.5	1.8	3	47	.1	—	—	0	.01	.02	.5	—
Flounder, baked with butter or margarine: Fillet, 6 in. long, 2½ in. wide, ¼ in. thick—1 fillet	57	58.1	115	17.1	4.7	0	13	196	.8	135	335	—	.04	.05	1.4	1
Fruit cocktail, canned, solids and liquid: Water pack, without artificial sweetener—1 cup	245	89.6	91	1.0	.2	23.8	22	32	1.0	12	412	370	.05	.02	1.2	5
Sirup pack, heavy—1 cup	255	79.6	194	1.0	.3	50.2	23	31	1.0	13	411	360	.05	.03	1.0	5
Fruit salad, canned solids and liquid: water pack, without artificial sweetener—1 cup	245	90.1	86	1.0	.2	22.3	20	27	.7	3	341	1,150	.02	.07	1.5	7
Sirup pack heavy—1 cup	255	80.0	191	.8	.3	49.5	20	28	.8	3	342	1,150	.03	.08	1.5	5

APPENDIX A—Nutritive values for household measures and market units of foods—Continued

[Item numbers correspond to those in table 1 of Handbook No. 8, revised 1963. Values in parentheses denote imputed values usually from another form of the food or from a similar food. Zeros in parentheses indicate that amount of a constituent, if present, is probably too small to be measured. Dashes (—) denote lack of reliable data for a constituent believed to be present in a measurable amount. Calculated values, as those based on a recipe, are not in parentheses]

Food, approximate measures, units and weight (edible part unless footnotes indicate otherwise) (B)		Water (C) Percent	Food energy (D) Calories	Protein (E) Grams	Fat (F) Grams	Carbohydrate (G) Grams	Calcium (H) Milligrams	Phosphorus (I) Milligrams	Iron (J) Milligrams	Sodium (K) Milligrams	Potassium (L) Milligrams	Vitamin A value (M) International units	Thiamin (N) Milligrams	Riboflavin (O) Milligrams	Niacin (P) Milligrams	Ascorbic (Q) Milligrams
	Grams															
Garlic:																
1 clove	3	61.3	4	.2	Trace	.9	1	6	Trace	1	16	Trace	.01	Trace	Trace	Trace
Gelatin, dry:																
1 envelope	7	13.0	23	6.0	Trace	0	—	—	—	—	—	—	—	—	—	—
Gelatin dessert powder and desserts made from dessert powder:																
Desserts made with water—1 cup	240	84.2	142	3.6	0	33.8	—	—	—	122	—	—	—	—	—	—
With fruit added—1 cup	240	81.8	161	3.1	.2	39.4	—	—	—	82	—	—	—	—	—	7
Ginger root, crystallized:																
(Candied)—1 oz.	28	12.0	96	0.1	0.1	24.7	—	—	—	—	—	—	—	—	—	—
Goose, domesticated, cooked [roasted]; total edible (flesh, skin, giblets); Yield from 1-lb. ready-to-cook goose—8½ oz.	240	39.1	1,022	56.9	86.4	0	(26)	[576]	[5.0]	—	—	—	[.19]	[.58]	[19.4]	—
Gooseberries:																
Raw—1 cup	150	88.9	59	1.2	.3	14.6	27	23	.8	2	233	440	—	.02	—	50
Granadilla, purple																
Passion fruit, raw—1 fruit.	35	75.1	16	.4	.1	3.9	2	12	.3	5	63	130	Trace	.02	.3	5
Grapefruit and grapefruit juice:																
pink, red, white-½ grapefruit	184	88.4	40	.5	.1	10.3	16	16	.4	1	132	80	.04	.02	.2	37
Grapefruit juice and grapefruit used for juice—1 cup	246	90.0	96	1.2	.2	22.6	22	37	.5	2	399	200	.10	.05	.5	93
Frozen concentrated juice:																
Unsweetened [6 fl. oz.]-1 glass.	185	89.3	76	.9	.2	18.1	19	31	.2	2	315	20	.07	.03	.4	72
Sweetened with nutritive sweetener—1 glass	186	87.8	87	.7	.2	21.2	15	26	.2	2	268	10	.06	.02	.3	61

Food																
Grapes:																
American type (slip skin) as Concord, Delaware, Niagara, Catawba—1 cup	153	81.6	70	1.3	1.0	15.9	16	12	.4	3	160	100	(.05)	(.03)	(.3)	4
European type (adherent skin) as Thompson Seedless, Emperor, Flame Tokay, Ribier, Malaga, Muscat—1 cup	160	81.4	107	1.0	.5	27.7	19	32	.6	5	277	(160)	.08	.05	.5	6
Seeded types—1 cup	160	81.4	102	.9	.5	26.3	18	30	.6	5	263	(150)	.08	.05	.5	6
Grapejuice:																
Canned or bottled—1 cup	253	82.9	167	.5	Trace	42.0	28	30	.8	5	293	—	.10	.05	.5	Trace
Frozen concentrate, sweetened with nutritive sweetener—1 glass	187	86.4	99	.4	Trace	24.9	6	7	.2	2	64	10	.04	.06	.4	7
Grape drink, canned (approx. 30% grapejuice)—1 glass	187	86.0	101	.2	Trace	25.8	6	7	.2	2	65	—	.02	.02	.2	30
Haddock, fried: (panfried or ovenfried)—1 fillet	110	66.3	182	21.6	7.0	6.4	44	272	1.3	195	383	—	.04	.08	3.5	2
Halibut, Atlantic and Pacific broiled with butter or margarine (quadrangular piece, 6½ in. long, 2–2¾ in. wide)—1 fillet	125	66.6	214	31.5	8.8	0	20	310	1.0	168	656	850	.06	.09	10.4	—
Heart: Beef, lean, cooked (braised)—1 cup	145	61.3	273	45.4	8.3	1.0	9	262	8.6	151	336	40	.36	1.77	11.0	1
Herring: Canned, solids and liquid: Plain, 15 oz—1 can	425	62.9	884	84.6	57.8	0	625	1,262	7.7	—	—	—	—	.77	—	—
Pickled: Bismarck herring, 7 in. long, 1½ in. wide, ½ in. thick—1 herring	50	59.4	112	10.2	7.6	0	—	—	—	—	—	—	—	—	—	—
Smoked, kippered, canned, drained solids: Drained contents from can can of net wt. 3¾ oz.—1 can	80	61.0	169	17.8	10.3	0	—	—	—	—	—	—	—	—	—	—
Honey, strained or extracted—1 tbsp.	21	17.2	64	.1	0	17.3	1	1	.1	1	11	20	Trace	0.22	2.6	Trace
Horseradish: Prepared—1 tbsp.	15	87.1	6	.2	Trace	1.4	9	5	.1	14	44	0	Trace	.01	.1	—

APPENDIX A—Nutrititive values for household measures and market units of foods—Continued

[Item numbers correspond to those in table 1 of Handbook No. 8, revised 1963. Values in parentheses denote imputed values usually from another form of the food or from a similar food. Zeros in parentheses indicate that amount of a constituent, if present, is probably too small to be measured. Dashes (—) denote lack of reliable data for a constituent believed to be present in a measurable amount. Calculated values, as those based on a recipe, are not in parentheses]

Food, approximate measures, units and weight (edible part unless footnotes indicate otherwise) (B)	Grams	Water (C) Percent	Food energy (D) Calories	Protein (E) Grams	Fat (F) Grams	Carbohydrate (G) Grams	Calcium (H) Milligrams	Phosphorus (I) Milligrams	Iron (J) Milligrams	Sodium (K) Milligrams	Potassium (L) Milligrams	Vitamin A value (M) International units	Thiamin (N) Milligrams	Riboflavin (O) Milligrams	Niacin (P) Milligrams	Ascorbic (Q) Milligrams
Ice cream and frozen custard, plain—1 cup	133	63.2	257	6.0	14.1	27.7	194	153	.1	84	241	590	.05	.28	.1	1
Ice milk: [5.1% fat]—1 cup	131	66.7	199	6.3	6.7	29.3	204	162	.1	89	255	280	.07	.29	.1	1
Ices: water, lime—1 cup	193	66.9	247	.8	Trace	62.9	Trace	Trace	Trace	Trace	6	Trace	Trace	Trace	Trace	2
Jams and preserves, sweetened with regular amount of nutritive sweetener—1 tbsp	20	29	54	.1	Trace	14.0	4	2	.2	2	18	Trace	Trace	.01	Trace	Trace
Jellies: 1 tbsp	18	29	49	Trace	Trace	12.7	4	1	.3	3	14	Trace	Trace	.01	Trace	1
Kale, leaves without stems, midribs: Cooked (boiled), drained—1 cup	110	87.8	43	(5.0)	(.8)	6.7	206	64	1.8	(47)	[243]	9,130	.11	.20	1.8	102
Kidney, beef, cooked (braised)—1 cup	140	53.0	353	46.2	16.8	1.1	25	342	18.3	354	454	1,610	.71	6.75	15.0	—
Kohlrabi, thickened bulb-like stems: Raw, diced—1 cup	140	90.3	41	2.8	.1	9.2	57	71	.1	11	521	30	.08	.06	.4	92
Cooked (boiled), drained—1 cup	165	92.2	40	2.8	.2	8.7	54	68	.5	10	429	30	.10	.05	.3	71
Kumquats, raw, medium size—1 kumquat	20	81.3	12	.2	Trace	3.2	12	4	.1	1	44	110	.01	.02	—	7
Lamb, retail cuts: Leg: cooked (roasted): Lean with fat (83% lean, 17% fat)—9.4 oz	267	54.0	745	67.6	50.5	0	29	555	4.5	166	757	—	.40	.72	14.7	—
Lean, trimmed of separable fat—9.3 oz	264	62.2	491	75.8	18.5	0	34	628	5.8	186	849	—	.42	.79	16.4	—

Food	Weight (g)	Water (%)	Calories	Protein (g)	Fat (g)	Carbohydrate (g)	Calcium (mg)	Phosphorus (mg)	Iron (mg)	Sodium (mg)	Potassium (mg)	Vitamin A (I.U.)	Thiamin (mg)	Riboflavin (mg)	Niacin (mg)	Ascorbic acid (mg)
Loin chops:																
Lean with fat (66% lean, 34% fat): raw																
Yield from 1 lb. raw chops with bone—10.1 oz	285	47.0	1,023	62.7	83.8	0	26	490	3.7	154	702	—	.34	.66	14.3	—
Rib chops:																
Lean with fat (62% lean, 38% fat):																
Yield from 1 lb. raw chops with bone—9.5 oz	268	42.9	1,091	53.9	95.4	0	24	418	2.9	132	604	—	.32	.56	12.3	—
Shoulder:																
Lean with fat (74% lean, 26% fat):																
Yield from 1 lb. raw lamb with bone—9½ oz	270	49.6	913	58.6	73.4	0	27	464	3.2	144	656	—	.35	.62	12.7	—
Lard:																
Tablespoon—1 tbsp.	13	0	117	0	13.0	0	0	0	0	0	0	0	0	0	0	0
Lemons, raw:																
Medium—1 lemon	110	90.1	20	.8	.2	6.0	19	12	.4	1	102	10	.03	.01	.1	39
Lemon juice:																
1 tbsp.	15.2	91.0	4	.1	Trace	1.2	1	2	Trace	Trace	21	Trace	Trace	Trace	Trace	7
Lemonade concentrate:																
Frozen—1 can	219	48.5	427	.4	.2	111.9	9	13	.4	4	153	40	.05	.06	.7	66
Lentils:																
Cooked—1 cup.	200	72.0	212	15.6	Trace	38.6	50	238	4.2	—	498	40	0.14	0.12	1.2	0
Lettuce, raw:																
Butterhead—1 cup	55	95.1	8	.7	.1	1.4	19	14	1.1	5	145	530	.03	.03	.2	4
Cos. or romaine—1 cup.	55	94.0	10	.7	.2	1.9	37	14	.8	5	145	1,050	.03	.04	.2	10
Crisphead varieties such as iceberg—1 cup.	55	95.5	7	.5	.1	1.6	11	12	.3	5	96	180	.03	.03	.2	3
Looseleaf or bunching varieties—1 cup.	55	94.0	10	.7	.2	1.9	37	14	.8	5	145	1,050	.03	.04	.2	10
Limes:																
1 lime	80	89.3	19	.5	.1	6.4	22	12	.4	1	69	10	.02	.01	.1	25
Limeade concentrate, frozen:																
6 fl. oz. (yields 1 qt. diluted juice)—1 can	218	50.0	408	.4	.2	107.9	11	13	.2	Trace	129	Trace	.02	.02	.2	26
Liver:																
Beef, cooked (fried): Slice, approx. 6½ in. long, 2⅜ in. wide, ⅜ in. thick—1 slice.	85	56.0	195	22.4	9.0	4.5	9	405	7.5	156	323	45,390	.22	3.56	14.0	23
Calf, cooked (fried)—1 slice.	85	51.4	222	25.1	11.2	3.4	11	456	12.1	100	385	27,800	.20	3.54	14.0	31
Chicken, whole, approx. 2 in. long, 2 in. wide, ⅝ in. thick—1 liver	25	65.0	41	6.6	1.1	.8	3	40	2.1	15	38	3,080	.04	.67	2.9	4

APPENDIX A.–Nutritive values for household measures and market units of foods—Continued

[Item numbers correspond to those in table 1 of Handbook No. 8. revised 1963. Values in parentheses denote imputed values usually from another form of the food or from a similar food. Zeros in parentheses indicate that amount of a constituent, if present, is probably too small to be measured. Dashes (—) denote lack of reliable data for a constituent believed to be present in a measurable amount. Calculated values, as those based on a recipe, are not in parentheses]

(B) Food, approximate measures, units and weight (edible part unless footnotes indicate otherwise)	Grams	(C) Water Percent	(D) Food energy Calories	(E) Protein Grams	(F) Fat Grams	(G) Carbohydrate Grams	(H) Calcium Milligrams	(I) Phosphorus Milligrams	(J) Iron Milligrams	(K) Sodium Milligrams	(L) Potassium Milligrams	(M) Vitamin A value International units	(N) Thiamin Milligrams	(O) Riboflavin Milligrams	(P) Niacin Milligrams	(Q) Ascorbic Milligrams
Lobster, northern:																
Cooked—1 cup	145	76.8	138	27.1	2.2	.4	94	278	1.2	305	261	—	.15	.10	—	—
Lobster Newburg:																
1 cup	250	64.0	485	46.3	26.5	12.8	218	480	2.3	573	428	—	.18	.28	—	—
Loganberries:																
1 cup	144	83.0	89	1.4	.9	21.5	50	24	1.7	[1]	245	[290]	[.04]	[.06]	[.6]	35
Lychees:																
10 fruits	150	81.9	58	.8	.3	14.8	7	38	.4	3	153	—	—	.05	—	38
Macaroni:																
Enriched: cooked—1 cup	140	73.0	155	4.8	.6	32.2	11	70	1.3	1	85	(0)	.20	.11	1.5	(0)
Unenriched—1 cup	140	73.0	155	4.8	.6	32.2	11	70	.6	1	85	(0)	.01	.01	.4	(0)
Macaroni (enriched) and cheese:																
1 cup	200	58.2	430	16.8	22.2	40.2	362	322	1.8	1,086	240	860	.20	.40	1.8	Trace
Mackerel, Atlantic:																
Broiled with butter or margarine:																
Fillet, 8½ in. long, 2½ in. wide, ½ in. thick—1 fillet	105	61.6	248	22.9	16.6	0	6	294	1.3	—	—	[560]	.16	.28	8.0	—
Mackerel, canned, solids and liquid:																
(No. 300); net wt. 15 oz.—1 can	425	66.4	765	89.7	42.5	0	1,105	1,224	9.4	—	—	130	.13	1.40	37.4	—
Mackerel, salted:																
Fillet, 7¾ in. long, 2½ in. wide, ½ in. thick—1 fillet	112	43.0	342	20.7	28.1	0	—	—	—	—	—	—	—	—	—	—
Malt:																
Dry—1 oz	28	5.2	104	.37	.5	21.9	—	—	1.1	—	—	—	.14	.09	2.6	—

Food															
Malt extract:															
Dried—1 oz.	28	3.2	104	1.7	Trace	25.3	14	83	2.5	23	65	—	.10	.13	2.8	—
Mangoes:															
Raw—1 fruit.	300	81.7	152	1.6	.9	38.8	23	30	.9	16	437	11,090	.12	.12	2.5	81
Margarine:															
Regular type and soft—1 tbsp.	14.2	15.5	102	.1	11.5	.1	3	2	0	140	3	470	—	—	—	0
Whipped type—1 tbsp.	9.4	15.5	68	.1	7.6	Trace	2	2	0	93	2	310	—	—	—	0
Marmalade:															
Citrus, sweetened—1 tbsp.	20	29.0	51	.1	Trace	14.0	7	2	.1	3	7	—	Trace	Trace	Trace	1
Milk, cow:															
Fluid (pasteurized and raw):															
Whole, 3.5% fat—1 cup.	244	87.4	159	8.5	8.5	12.0	288	227	.1	122	351	350	.07	.41	.2	2
Skim—1 cup.	245	90.5	88	8.8	.2	12.5	296	233	.1	127	355	10	.09	.44	.2	2
Low fat with 2% nonfat milk solids added—1 cup.	246	87.0	145	10.3	4.9	14.8	352	276	.1	150	431	200	.10	.52	.2	2
Canned: evaporated (unsweetened)—1 cup.	252	73.8	345	17.6	19.9	24.4	635	517	.3	297	764	810	.10	.86	.5	3
Condensed (sweetened)—1 cup.	306	27.1	982	24.8	26.6	166.2	802	630	.3	343	961	1,110	.24	1.16	.6	3
Dry: Whole, regular—1 cup.	128	2.0	643	33.8	35.2	48.9	1,164	906	.6	518	1,702	1,450	.37	1.87	.9	8
Nonfat, regular—1 cup.	120	3.0	436	43.1	1.0	62.8	1,570	1,219	.7	638	2,094	40	.42	(2.16)	1.1	8
Nonfat, instant—1 cup or envelope.	68	4.0	244	24.3	.5	35.1	879	683	.4	358	1,173	20	.24	1.21	.6	5
Malted:															
Dry powder—1 oz. or approx. 3 heaping tsp.	28	2.6	116	4.2	2.4	20.1	82	108	.6	125	204	290	.09	.15	.1	(0)
Chocolate drink, fluid, commercial:															
Made with skim milk—1 cup.	250	82.8	190	8.3	5.8	27.3	270	228	.5	115	355	210	.10	.40	.3	3
Made with whole 3.5% fat milk—1 cup.	250	81.5	213	8.5	8.5	27.5	278	235	.5	118	365	330	.10	.40	.3	3
Hot chocolate—1 cup.	250	80.5	238	8.3	12.5	26.0	260	235	0.5	120	370	360	0.08	0.40	0.3	3
Hot cocoa—1 cup.	250	79.0	243	9.5	11.5	27.3	295	283	1.0	128	363	400	.10	.45	.5	3
Milk, goat:															
Fluid—1 cup.	244	87.5	163	7.8	9.8	11.2	315	259	.2	83	439	[390]	.10	.27	.7	2
Milk, human:															
1 fl. oz.	30.8	85.2	24	.3	1.2	2.9	10	4	Trace	5	16	70	Trace	.01	.1	2
Molasses, cane:															
First extraction or light—1 tbsp.	20	24	50	—	—	13.0	33	9	.9	3	183	—	.01	.01	Trace	—
Second extraction or medium—1 tbsp.	20	24	46	—	—	12.0	58	14	1.2	7	213	—	.02	.02	.2	—
Third extraction or blackstrap—1 tbsp.	20	24	43	—	—	11.0	137	17	3.2	19	585	—	.02	.04	.4	—

APPENDIX A—Nutrititive values for household measures and market units of foods—Continued

[Item numbers correspond to those in table 1 of Handbook No. 8, revised 1963. Values in parentheses denote imputed values usually from another form of the food or from a similar food. Zeros in parentheses indicate that amount of a constituent, if present, is probably too small to be measured. Dashes (—) denote lack of reliable data for a constituent believed to be present in a measurable amount. Calculated values, as those based on a recipe, are not in parentheses]

(B) Food, approximate measures, units and weight (edible part unless footnotes indicate otherwise)	Grams	(C) Water Percent	(D) Food energy Calories	(E) Protein Grams	(F) Fat Grams	(G) Carbohydrate Grams	(H) Calcium Milligrams	(I) Phosphorus Milligrams	(J) Iron Milligrams	(K) Sodium Milligrams	(L) Potassium Milligrams	(M) Vitamin A value International units	(N) Thiamin Milligrams	(O) Riboflavin Milligrams	(P) Niacin Milligrams	(Q) Ascorbic Milligrams
Muffins, baked from home recipes:																
Plain, made with enriched flour																
Yield from approx.																
3 tbsp. of batter—1 muffin	40	38.0	118	3.1	4.0	16.9	42	60	.6	176	50	40	.07	.09	.6	Trace
Unenriched flour—1 muffin	40	38.0	118	3.1	4.0	16.9	42	60	.2	176	50	40	.02	.06	.2	Trace
Blueberry—1 muffin	40	39.0	112	2.9	3.7	16.8	34	53	.6	253	46	90	.06	.08	.5	Trace
Bran—1 muffin	40	35.1	104	3.1	3.9	17.2	57	162	1.5	179	172	90	.06	.10	1.6	Trace
Corn, made with enriched degermed cornmeal—1 muffin	40	32.7	126	2.8	4.0	19.2	42	68	.7	192	54	120	.08	.09	.6	Trace
Muffin mix, corn, and muffins and cornbread baked from mix:																
Muffins and cornbread; made with egg and milk—1 muffin	40	30.4	130	2.8	4.2	20.0	96*	152	.6	192	44	100	.07	.08	.6	Trace
Mushrooms:																
Agaricus campestris, cultivated commercially, raw—1 cup	70	90.4	20	1.9	.2	3.1	4	81	.6	11	290	Trace	.07	.32	2.9	2
Muskmelons:																
Casaba (Golden Beauty). Wedge. 7¾ in. long, 2 in. wide ½ melon	477	91.2	82	1.9	.3	20.4	38	44	1.1	33	682	9,240	.11	.08	1.6	90
at center—1 wedge	245	91.5	38	1.7	Trace	9.1	[20]	[22]	[.6]	[17]	[351]	40	[.06]	[.04]	[.8]	18
Honeydew; 7 in. long, 2 in. wide at center—1 wedge	226	90.6	49	1.2	0.4	11.5	21	24	0.6	18	374	60	0.06	0.04	0.9	34
Mustard greens:																
Cooked (boiled), drained—1 cup	140	92.6	32	3.1	.6	5.6	193	45	2.5	25	308	8,120	.11	.20	.8	67

Food, approximate measure	Grams	Water (%)	Food energy (cal.)	Protein (g)	Fat (g)	Carbohydrate (g)	Calcium (mg)	Phosphorus (mg)	Iron (mg)	Sodium (mg)	Potassium (mg)	Vitamin A (IU)	Thiamin (mg)	Riboflavin (mg)	Niacin (mg)	Ascorbic acid (mg)
Mustard:																
Prepared, yellow—1 tsp., pouch. or cup	5	80.2	4	.2	.2	.3	4	4	.1	63	7	—	—	—	—	—
Nectarines:																
Raw—1 nectarine	150	81.8	88	.8	Trace	23.6	6	33	.7	8	406	2,280	—	—	—	18
Noodles, egg noodles:																
Enriched—1 cup	160	70.8	200	6.6	2.4	37.3	16	94	1.4	3	70	110	.22	.13	1.9	(0)
Unenriched—1 cup	160	70.8	200	6.6	2.4	37.3	16	94	1.0	3	70	110	.05	.03	.6	(0)
Noodles, chow mein:																
Canned—1 cup	45	1.1	220	5.9	10.6	26.1	—	—	—	—	—	—	—	—	—	—
Oat products used mainly as hot breakfast cereals:																
Oat flakes, maple-flavored instant-cooking—1 cup	240	83.0	166	6.2	1.9	31.2	24	156	1.4	257	—	(0)	.14	.05	1.4	(0)
Oat and wheat cereal—1 cup	245	83.6	159	6.4	2.2	29.6	27	184	1.7	412	—	(0)	.22	.05	1.2	(0)
Oatmeal or rolled oats, regular—1 cup	240	86.5	132	4.8	2.4	23.3	22	137	1.4	523	146	(0)	.19	.05	.2	(0)
Oats, puffed, added sugar, salt, minerals, vitamins—1 cup	25	3.4	99	3.0	1.4	18.8	44	102	2.9	317	—	1,180	.29	.35	2.9	9
Ocean perch, Atlantic:																
Cooked, fried—1 oz.	28	59.0	64	5.4	3.8	1.9	9	64	.4	43	81	—	.03	.03	.5	—
Oils, salad or cooking:																
Corn, safflower, soybean oils, soybean-cotton-seed oil blend—1 tbsp.	13.6	0	120	0	13.6	0	0	0	0	0	0	—	0	0	0	0
Olive or peanut oil—1 tbsp.	13.5	0	119	0	13.5	0	0	0	0	0	0	—	0	0	0	0
Okra:																
Cooked (boiled), drained—1 cup	160	91.1	46	3.2	.5	9.6	147	66	.8	3	278	780	(.21)	(.29)	(1.4)	32
Olives, pickled; canned or bottled:																
Green: large—10 olives	46	78.2	45	.5	4.9	.5	24	7	.6	926	21	120	—	—	—	—
Ripe: Ascolano: large—10 olives	55	80.0	61	.5	6.5	1.2	40	8	.8	385	16	30	Trace	Trace	Trace	—
Mission—10 olives	46	73.0	73	.5	8.0	1.3	42	7	.7	297	11	30	Trace	Trace	Trace	—
Onions, mature (dry):																
Raw—1 cup	115	89.1	44	1.7	.1	10.0	31	41	.6	12	181	50	.03	.05	.2	12
Cooked (boiled), drained—1 cup	210	91.8	61	2.5	.2	13.7	50	61	.8	15	231	80	.06	.06	.4	15
Onions, young green:																
Chopped—1 tbsp.	6	89.4	2	.1	Trace	.5	3	2	.1	Trace	14	(120)	Trace	Trace	Trace	2
Bulb and white portion of top—2 medium or 6 small onions	30	87.6	14	0.3	0.1	3.2	12	12	0.2	2	69	Trace	0.02	0.01	0.1	8

APPENDIX A–Nutrititive values for household measures and market units of foods—Continued

[Item numbers correspond to those in table 1 of Handbook No. 8, revised 1963. Values in parentheses denote imputed values usually from another form of the food or from a similar food. Zeros in parentheses indicate that amount of a constituent, if present, is probably too small to be measured. Dashes (—) denote lack of reliable data for a constituent believed to be present in a measurable amount. Calculated values, as those based on a recipe, are not in parentheses]

Food, approximate measures, units and weight (edible part unless footnotes indicate otherwise) (B)	Grams	Water (C) Percent	Food energy (D) Calories	Protein (E) Grams	Fat (F) Grams	Carbohydrate (G) Grams	Calcium (H) Milligrams	Phosphorus (I) Milligrams	Iron (J) Milligrams	Sodium (K) Milligrams	Potassium (L) Milligrams	Vitamin A value (M) International units	Thiamin (N) Milligrams	Riboflavin (O) Milligrams	Niacin (P) Milligrams	Ascorbic (Q) Milligrams
Oranges, raw, used for peeled fruit: All commercial varieties: Whole fruit,																
2⅝-in. diam.—1 orange.	180	86.0	64	1.3	.3	16.0	54	26	.5	1	263	260	.13	.05	.5	(66)
California: Navels (winter oranges): medium, 2⅞-in. diam., size 88—1 orange.	206	85.4	71	1.8	.1	17.8	56	31	.6	1	272	(280)	.14	.06	.6	(85)
Valencias (summer oranges): medium 2⅝ in. diam. size 113—1 orange	161	86.5	62	1.4	.4	15.0	48	27	1.0	1	230	(240)	.12	.05	.5	(59)
Florida: Medium, 2 11/16-in. diam. size 100—1 orange.	204	86.4	71	1.1	(.3)	18.1	65	26	.3	2	(311)	(300)	.15	.06	.6	(68)
Orange juice, raw, and oranges used for juice:																
1 cup.	248	88.3	112	1.7	.5	25.8	27	42	.5	2	496	500	.22	.07	1.0	124
California: Navels (winter oranges)—1 cup.	249	87.2	120	2.5	.2	28.1	27	45	.5	2	483	500	.22	.07	1.0	152
Valencias (summer oranges)—1 cup.	248	87.8	117	2.5	0.7	26.0	27	47	0.7	2	471	500	0.22	0.07	1.0	122
Florida: All commercial varieties—1 cup.	247	88.8	106	1.5	.5	24.7	25	40	.5	2	509	490	.22	.07	1.0	111
Early and midseason (Hamlin, Parson Brown, Pineapple)—1 cup.	246	89.6	98	1.2	.5	22.9	25	37	.5	2	512	490	.22	.07	1.0	125
late season (Valencias)—1 cup.	248	88.3	112	1.5	.5	26.0	25	45	.5	2	503	500	ff+.22	.07	1.02	1.0
Temple—1 cup.	248	88.0	134	1.2	(.5)	32.0	(25)	42	.5	2	—	(500)	.22	.07	1.0	124
Orange juice, canned: Unsweetened—1 cup.	249	87.4	120	2.0	.5	27.9	25	45	1.0	2	496	500	.17	.05	.7	100
sweetened with nutritive sweetener—1 cup.	250	86.5	130	1.8	.5	30.5	(25)	45	1.0	2	(496)	500	.17	.05	.7	100

Values for edible part of foods

Food	Weight (g)	Water (%)	Cal.	Protein	Fat	Carb.						Vit. A				
Orange juice concentrate, frozen Unsweetened. Diluted with 3 parts water by volume—1 glass	187	87.2	92	1.3	.2	21.7	19	32	.2	2	378	410	.17	.03	.7	90
Orange juice, dehydrated: (Crystals)—1 oz	28	1.0	108	1.4	.5	25.2	24	38	.5	2	490	480	.19	.06	.8	102
Oysters: raw (chilled), meat only: Eastern Approx. 13–19 Selects (medium)—1 cup	240	84.6	158	20.2	4.3	8.2	226	343	13.2	175	290	740	.34	.43	6.0	—
Pacific and Western (Olympia)—1 cup	240	79.1	218	25.4	5.3	15.4	204	367	17.3	—	—	—	.29	—	3.1	72
Cooked (fried)—4 Select oysters	45	54.7	108	3.9	6.3	8.4	68	108	3.6	93	91	200	.08	.13	1.4	—
Oyster stew, home prepared: 1 part oysters to 2 parts milk by volume (approx. 6 medium oysters per cup)—1 cup	240	82.0	233	12.5	15.4	10.8	274	266	4.6	814	319	820	.14	.43	2.2	—
Pancakes, baked from home recipe. made with—Enriched flour: 4-in. diam.—1 cake	27	50.1	62	1.9	1.9	9.2	27	38	.4	115	33	30	.05	.06	.4	Trace
Unenriched flour: 4-in. diam.—1 cake	27	50.1	62	1.9	1.9	9.2	27	38	.2	115	33	30	.01	.04	.1	Trace
Pancake and waffle mixes and pancakes baked from mixes: Plain and buttermilk: with enriched flour, 4-in. diam.—1 cake	27	50.6	61	1.9	2.0	8.7	58	70	.3	152	42	70	.04	.06	.2	Trace
Pancakes, made with egg. milk: 4-in. diam.—1 cake	27	50.6	61	1.9	2.0	8.7	58	70	.2	152	42	70	.02	.05	.1	Trace
Buckwheat and other cereal flours: Pancakes, made with egg. milk: 4-in. diam.—1 cake	27	57.9	54	1.8	2.5	6.4	59	91	.4	125	66	60	.03	.04	.2	Trace
Papaws, common. North American type, raw:—1 papaw	130	76.6	83	5.1	.9	16.4	—	—	—	—	—	—	—	—	—	—
Papayas, raw: 1 papaya or 1 lb.	454	88.7	119	1.8	.3	30.4	61	49	.9	9	711	5,320	.12	.12	.9	170
Parsley, common garden: 1 tbsp.	3.5	85.1	2	.1	Trace	.3	7	2	.2	2	25	300	Trace	.01	Trace	6
Parsnips: Cooked (boiled), drained—1 cup	155	82.2	102	2.3	.8	23.1	70	96	.9	12	587	50	.11	.12	.2	16
Pâté de foie gras, canned: 1 tbsp.	13	37.0	60	1.5	5.7	.6	—	—	—	—	—	—	.01	.04	.3	—

372

REALITIES OF NUTRITION

APPENDIX A—Nutritive values for household measures and market units of foods—Continued

[Item numbers correspond to those in table 1 of Handbook No. 8, revised 1963. Values in parentheses denote imputed values usually from another form of the food or from a similar food. Zeros in parentheses indicate that amount of a constituent, if present, is probably too small to be measured. Dashes (—) denote lack of reliable data for a constituent believed to be present in a measurable amount. Calculated values, as those based on a recipe, are not in parentheses]

Food, approximate measures, units and weight (edible part unless footnotes indicate otherwise) (B)	Grams	Water (C) Percent	Food energy (D) Calories	Protein (E) Grams	Fat (F) Grams	Carbohydrate (G) Grams	Calcium (H) Milligrams	Phosphorus (I) Milligrams	Iron (J) Milligrams	Sodium (K) Milligrams	Potassium (L) Milligrams	Vitamin A value (M) International units	Thiamin (N) Milligrams	Riboflavin (O) Milligrams	Niacin (P) Milligrams	Ascorbic (Q) Milligrams
Peaches:																
Raw: whole: fruit, 2¼-in. diam.—1 peach	175	89.1	58	.9	.2	14.8	14	29	.8	2	308	2,030	.03	.08	1.5	11
Canned, solids and liquid:																
water packed—1 cup	244	91.1	76	1.0	.2	19.8	10	32	.7	5	334	1,100	.02	.07	1.5	7
Sirup pack, heavy—1 cup	256	79.1	200	1.0	.3	51.5	10	31	.8	5	333	1,100	.03	.05	1.5	8
Dried, sulfured (halves)—1 cup	160	25.0	419	5.0	1.1	109.3	77	187	9.6	26	1,520	6,240	.02	.30	8.5	29
Frozen, sliced, sweetened with nutritive sweetener—1 cup	250	76.5	220	1.0	.3	56.5	10	33	1.3	5	310	1,630	.03	.10	1.8	100
Peach nectar:																
Canned—1 cup	249	87.2	120	.5	Trace	30.9	10	27	.5	2	194	1,070	.02	.05	1.0	Trace
Peanuts:																
Roasted in shell (with skins)—10 nuts	27	1.8	105	4.7	8.8	3.7	13	74	.4	1	127	—	.06	.02	3.1	0
Roasted, salted (Spanish and Virginia types) 10 or 20 whole nuts or 1 tbsp., chopped	9	1.6	53	2.3	4.5	1.7	7	36	.2	38	61	—	.03	.01	1.5	0
Peanut butter made with moderate amounts of added fat, nutritive sweetener, salt—1 tbsp	16	1.7	94	4.0	8.1	3.0	9	61	.3	97	100	—	.02	.02	2.4	0
Pears:																
raw, including skin:																
Bartletts, 2½-in.—1 pear	180	83.2	100	1.1	.7	25.1	13	18	.5	3	213	30	.03	.07	.2	7
Boses, 2½-in. diam.—1 pear	155	83.2	86	1.0	.6	21.6	11	16	.4	3	183	30	.03	.06	.1	6
D'Anjous, 3-in. diam.—1 pear	220	83.2	122	1.4	.8	30.6	16	22	.6	4	260	40	.04	.08	.2	8

Food and measure															
Canned, solids and liquid: Water pack, without artificial sweetener—1 cup	244	91.1	78	.5	.5	20.3	12	17	.5	2	215	10	.02	.05	.2	2
Sirup pack. heavy—1 cup	255	79.8	194	.5	.5	50.0	13	18	.5	3	214	10	.03	.05	.3	3
Dried, sulfured (halves)—10 halves	175	26.0	469	5.4	3.2	117.8	61	84	2.3	12	1,003	120	.02	.32	1.1	12
Pear nectar:																
Canned—1 cup	250	86.2	130	.8	.5	33.0	8	13	.3	3	98	Trace	Trace	.05	Trace	Trace
Peas, green, immature:																
Canned—1 cup																
Cooked (boiled), drained—1 cup	160	81.5	114	8.6	.6	19.4	37	158	2.9	2	314	860	.45	.18	3.7	32
Peas, mature seeds, dry:																
Split, cooked—1 cup	200	70.0	230	16.0	0.6	41.6	22	178	3.4	26	592	80	0.30	0.18	1.8	—
Peas and carrots, frozen:																
Yield from 10 oz., frozen peas and carrots—1¾ cups	278	85.8	147	8.9	.8	28.1	70	158	3.1	234	436	25,850	.53	.19	3.6	22
Pecans:																
large (64–77 per pound)—10 nuts	65	3.4	236	3.2	24.5	5.0	25	99	.8	Trace	207	40	.30	.04	.3	1
Peppers, hot, chili:																
Immature, green—1 cup	245	93.9	49	1.7	.2	12.3	12	34	1.0	—	—	1,490	.07	.07	1.7	167
Canned, chili sauce—1 cup	245	94.1	51	2.2	1.5	9.6	22	39	1.2	—	—	23,500	.02	.22	1.5	74
Dried, chili powder with added seasonings—1 tsp.	2	8.5	7	.3	.2	1.1	5	4	.3	31	20	1,300	Trace	.02	.2	Trace
Peppers, sweet, garden varieties:																
Immature, green: Raw: No. 1 grade, 2¾-in. long, 2½-in. diam.—1 pepper	90	93.4	16	.9	.1	3.5	7	16	.5	10	157	310	.06	.06	.4	94
cooked: Boiled, drained: No. 1 grade—1 pepper	73	94.7	13	.7	.1	2.8	7	12	.4	7	109	310	.05	.05	(.4)	70
Stuffed with beef and crumbs—1 stuffed pepper	185	63.1	315	24.1	10.2	31.1	78	224	3.9	581	477	520	.17	0.81	4.6	74
Mature, red, raw: No. 1 grade—1 pepper	90	90.7	23	1.0	.2	5.2	10	22	.4	—	—	3,280	(.06)	(.06)	(.4)	151
Persimmons, raw:																
Native—1 persimmon	30	64.4	31	.2	.1	8.2	7	6	.6	Trace	76	—	—	—	.2	16
Pickles:																
Cucumber: Dill: Medium, approx. 3¾-in. long, 1¼-in. diam.—1 pickle	65	93.3	7	.5	.1	1.4	17	14	.7	928	130	70	Trace	.01	Trace	8
Bread-and-butter—2 slices	15	78.7	11	.1	Trace	2.7	5	4	.3	101	—	20	Trace	Trace	Trace	1
Sour: Medium—1 pickle	65	94.8	7	.3	.1	1.3	11	10	2.1	879	—	70	Trace	.01	Trace	5

APPENDIX A—Nutrititive values for household measures and market units of foods—Continued

[Item numbers correspond to those in table 1 of Handbook No. 8, revised 1963. Values in parentheses denote imputed values usually from another form of the food or from a similar food. Zeros in parentheses indicate that amount of a constituent, if present, is probably too small to be measured. Dashes (—) denote lack of reliable data for a constituent believed to be present in a measurable amount. Calculated values, as those based on a recipe, are not in parentheses.]

(B) Food, approximate measures, units and weight (edible part unless footnotes indicate otherwise)	Grams	(C) Water Percent	(D) Food energy Calories	(E) Protein Grams	(F) Fat Grams	(G) Carbohydrate Grams	(H) Calcium Milligrams	(I) Phosphorus Milligrams	(J) Iron Milligrams	(K) Sodium Milligrams	(L) Potassium Milligrams	(M) Vitamin A value International units	(N) Thiamin Milligrams	(O) Riboflavin Milligrams	(P) Niacin Milligrams	(Q) Ascorbic bic Milligrams
sweet: Whole, gherkins—1 pickle.	35	60.7	51	.2	.1	12.8	4	6	.4	—	—	30	Trace	.01	Trace	2
Chowchow or mustard pickles:																
Sour—1 cup.	240	87.6	70	3.4	3.1	9.8	77	127	6.2	3,211	—	—	—	—	—	—
Sweet—1 cup.	245	68.9	284	3.7	2.2	66.2	56	54	3.7	1,291	—	—	—	—	—	—
Relish, finely cut or chopped, sweet—1 tbsp.	15	63.0	21	.1	.1	5.1	3	2	.1	107	—	—	—	—	—	—
Pies:																
Baked, piecrust made with unenriched flour (9-in. diam., 28.3-in. cir.):																
Apple: Sector, 3½-in. arc; ⅙ of pie—1 sector	118	47.6	302	2.6	13.1	45.0	9	26	.4	355	94	40	.02	.02	.5	1
Banana custard—1 sector.	114	54.4	252	5.1	10.6	35.0	75	93	.6	221	231	290	.05	.15	.3	1
Blueberry—1 sector.	118	51.0	286	2.8	12.7	41.2	13	27	.7	316	77	40	.02	.02	.4	4
Cherry—1 sector.	118	46.6	308	3.1	13.3	45.3	17	30	.4	359	124	520	.02	.02	.6	Trace
Chocolate chiffon—1 sector.	81	33.0	266	5.5	12.4	35.4	19	79	1.0	204	89	250	.02	.08	.2	0
Custard—1 sector.	114	58.1	249	7.0	12.7	26.7	109	129	.7	327	156	260	.06	.18	.3	0
Lemon chiffon—1 sector.	81	35.6	254	5.7	10.2	35.5	19	67	.7	211	66	140	.02	.06	.2	2
Lemon meringue—1 sector.	105	47.4	268	3.9	10.7	39.6	15	51	.5	296	53	180	.03	.08	.2	3
Mince—1 sector.	118	43.0	320	3.0	13.6	48.6	33	45	1.2	529	210	Trace	.08	.05	.5	1
Peach—1 sector.	118	47.5	301	3.0	12.6	45.1	12	34	.6	316	176	860	.02	.05	.8	4
Pecan—1 sector.	103	19.5	431	5.3	23.6	52.8	48	106	2.9	228	127	160	.16	.07	.3	Trace
Pumpkin—1 sector.	114	59.2	241	4.6	12.8	27.9	58	79	.6	244	182	2,810	.03	.11	.3	Trace
Rhubarb—1 sector.	118	47.4	299	3.0	12.6	45.1	76	31	.8	319	188	60	.02	.05	.4	4
Piecrust or plain pastry, made with																
Enriched flour—1 pie shell	180	14.9	900	11.0	60.1	78.8	25	90	3.1	1,100	89	0	.36	.25	3.2	0

Food	Weight (g)	Water (%)	Calories	Protein (g)	Fat (g)	Carbohydrate (g)	Calcium (mg)	Phosphorus (mg)	Iron (mg)	Sodium (mg)	Potassium (mg)	Vitamin A (I.U.)	Thiamine (mg)	Riboflavin (mg)	Niacin (mg)	Ascorbic Acid (mg)
Pigs' feet: Pickled—2 oz	57	66.9	113	9.5	8.4	0	—	—	—	—	—	—	—	—	—	—
Pimientos, canned, solids and liquid: 4 oz.—1 can or jar	113	92.4	31	1.0	.6	6.6	8	19	1.7	—	226	1,600	.02	.07	.5	107
Pineapple: Raw—1 cup	155	85.3	81	.6	.3	21.2	26	12	.8	2	226	110	.14	.05	.3	26
Canned, solids and liquid: Water pack, without artificial sweetener—1 cup	246	89.1	96	.7	.2	25.1	30	12	.7	2	244	120	0.20	0.05	0.5	17
Sirup pack: Heavy—1 cup	255	79.9	189	.8	.3	49.5	28	13	.8	3	245	130	.20	.05	.5	18
Extra heavy—1 cup	260	75.9	234	.8	.3	60.8	29	13	.8	3	244	100	.21	.05	.5	16
Frozen chunks, sweetened with nutritive sweetener—1 cup	245	77.1	208	1.0	.2	54.4	22	10	1.0	5	245	70	.25	.07	.7	20
Pineapple juice: Canned, unsweetened—1 cup	250	85.6	138	1.0	.3	33.8	38	23	.8	3	373	130	.13	.05	.5	23
Frozen concentrate, unsweetened: Diluted with 3 parts water by volume—1 glass	187	86.5	97	.7	.1	23.9	21	15	.6	2	254	20	.13	.04	.4	22
Pineapple juice and grapefruit juice drink: Canned (approx. 50% fruit juices)—1 cup	250	86.0	135	.5	.1	34.0	13	13	.5	Trace	155	30	.05	.03	.3	(¹)
Pineapple juice and orange juice drink: Canned (approx. 40% fruit juices)—1 cup	250	86.0	135	.5	.3	33.8	13	15	.5	Trace	175	130	.05	.03	.3	(¹)
Pinenuts: Pignolias, shelled—1 oz	28	5.6	156	8.8	13.4	3.3	—	—	—	—	—	—	.18	—	—	—
Pistachionuts: 1 lb	454	5.3	2,694	87.5	243.6	86.2	594	2,268	33.1	—	4,409	1,040	3.04	—	6.4	—
Pizza: From home recipe, baked (in 14-in. diam. pan): With cheese topping: Sector, 5½-in. arc: ⅛ of pizza—1 sector	65	48.3	153	7.8	5.4	18.4	144	127	.7	456	85	410	.04	.13	.7	5
With sausage topping—1 sector	67	50.6	157	5.2	6.2	19.8	11	62	.8	488	113	380	.06	.08	1.0	6
Chilled, with cheese, commercial: Baked—1 sector	60	45.1	147	5.5	4.1	21.9	86	89	.5	380	67	230	.04	.10	.6	4

APPENDIX A—Nutritive values for household measures and market units of foods—Continued

[Item numbers correspond to those in table 1 of Handbook No. 8, revised 1963. Values in parentheses denote imputed values usually from another form of the food or from a similar food. Zeros in parentheses indicate that amount of a constituent, if present, is probably too small to be measured. Dashes (—) denote lack of reliable data for a constituent believed to be present in a measurable amount. Calculated values, as those based on a recipe, are not in parentheses]

(B) Food, approximate measures, units and weight (edible part unless footnotes indicate otherwise)	Grams	(C) Water Percent	(D) Food energy Calories	(E) Protein Grams	(F) Fat Grams	(G) Carbohydrate Grams	(H) Calcium Milligrams	(I) Phosphorus Milligrams	(J) Iron Milligrams	(K) Sodium Milligrams	(L) Potassium Milligrams	(M) Vitamin A value International units	(N) Thiamin Milligrams	(O) Riboflavin Milligrams	(P) Niacin Milligrams	(Q) Ascorbic Milligrams
Frozen, with cheese, commercial:																
Baked—1 sector	57	45.3	139	5.4	4.0	20.1	89	89	0.5	367	65	250	0.03	0.10	0.6	3
Plantain (baking banana), raw:																
1 banana	365	66.4	313	2.9	1.1	82.0	18	79	1.8	13	1,012	—	.16	.11	1.6	37
Plums:																
Raw: Damson—1 cup	145	81.1	87	.7	Trace	23.5	24	22	.7	3	395	(400)	.11	.04	.7	—
Japanese and hybrid: Pitted—1 cup	185	86.8	89	.9	.4	22.8	22	33	.9	2	315	460	.06	.06	.9	11
Prune type: Pitted—1 cup	165	78.7	124	1.3	.3	32.5	20	30	.8	2	281	500	.05	.05	.8	7
Canned, solids and liquid: purple (Italian prunes), whole, unpitted style: Water pack, without artificial sweetener—1 cup	262	86.6	114	1.0	.5	29.6	22	25	2.5	5	368	3,110	.05	.05	1.0	5
Sirup pack, heavy—1 cup	272	77.4	214	1.0	.3	55.8	23	26	2.3	3	367	3,130	.05	0.05	1.0	5
Pollock:																
Cooked, creamed—1 cup	250	74.7	320	34.8	14.8	10.0	—	—	—	278	595	—	.08	.33	1.8	Trace
Pomegranate, raw:																
3¾-in. diam., 2¾ in. high—1 pomegranate	275	82.3	97	.8	.5	25.3	5	12	.5	5	399	Trace	.05	.05	.5	6
Popcorn:																
Popped, plain, large kernel—1 cup	6	4.0	23	.8	.3	4.6	[1]	[17]	[2]	[Trace]	—	—	—	[.01]	[.1]	[0]
Oil and salt added, large kernel—1 cup	9	3.1	41	.9	2.0	5.3	1	19	.2	175	—	—	—	.01	.2	0
Popovers:																
Baked (home recipe with enriched flour)—1 popover	40	54.9	90	3.5	3.7	10.3	38	56	.6	88	60	130	.06	.10	.4	Trace

Pork, fresh, retail cuts:															
Ham: Cooked (baked or roasted):															
Lean with fat (74% lean, 26% fat);															
Yield from 1 lb., raw ham with bone and skin—9.2 oz	262	45.5	980	60.3	80.2	0	26	618	7.9	148	675	(0)	1.34	.60	12.1	—
Baked or roasted loin roast. Yield from 1 lb., raw loin with bone—8.6 oz	244	45.8	883	59.8	69.5	0	27	625	7.8	147	670	(0)	2.24	.63	13.7	—
Shoulder cuts (Boston butt and picnic); Boston butt: Cooked (roasted): Lean with fat (79% lean, 21% fat); Yield from 1 lb., raw meat with bone and skin—10.2 oz	290	48.1	1,024	65.3	82.7	0	29	664	8.4	160	731	(0)	1.45	.67	12.8	—
Picnic: Cooked (simmered); Lean with fat (74% lean, 26% fat]; Yield from 1 lb. raw meat without bone and skin—10.2 oz	290	45.7	1,085	67.3	88.5	0	29	403	8.7	118	538	(0)	1.57	.73	13.9	—
Spareribs: Cooked: Yield from 1 lb. raw spareribs—6.3 oz	180	39.7	792	37.4	70.0	0	16	218	4.7	65	299	(0)	.77	.38	6.1	—
Pork, cured:															
Ham: Baked or roasted: Yield from 1 lb., unbaked ham without bone and skin—13.1 oz	372	53.6	1,075	77.7	82.2	0	33	640	9.7	2,782	870	(0)	1.75	.67	13.4	—
Boston butt: Baked or roasted: Lean with fat (83% lean, 17% fat]; Yield from 1 lb. unbaked meat without bone and skin—11.8 oz	336	47.7	1,109	76.9	86.4	0	34	622	10.1	2,753	861	(0)	1.78	.71	13.8	—
Picnic: baked or roasted: Yield from 1 lb., unbaked meat without bone and skin—11.8 oz	336	48.8	1,085	75.3	84.7	0	34	612	9.7	2,696	843	(0)	1.75	.67	13.4	—
Potatoes:															
Baked in skin: 2⅓-in. diam., 4¾-in. long—1 potato	202	75.1	145	4.0	.2	32.8	14	101	1.1	6	782	Trace	.15	.07	2.7	31
Boiled in skin—1 potato	250	79.8	173	4.8	.2	38.9	16	121	1.4	7	926	Trace	.20	.09	3.4	36

APPENDIX A—Nutrititive values for household measures and market units of foods—Continued

[Item numbers correspond to those in table 1 of Handbook No. 8, revised 1963. Values in parentheses denote imputed values usually from another form of the food or from a similar food. Zeros in parentheses indicate that amount of a constituent, if present, is probably too small to be measured. Dashes (—) denote lack of reliable data for a constituent believed to be present in a measurable amount. Calculated values, as those based on a recipe, are not in parentheses]

Food, approximate measures, units and weight (edible part unless footnotes indicate otherwise) (B)	Grams	Water (C) Percent	Food energy (D) Calories	Protein (E) Grams	Fat (F) Grams	Carbohydrate (G) Grams	Calcium (H) Milligrams	Phosphorus (I) Milligrams	Iron (J) Milligrams	Sodium (K) Milligrams	Potassium (L) Milligrams	Vitamin A value (M) International units	Thiamin (N) Milligrams	Riboflavin (O) Milligrams	Niacin (P) Milligrams	Ascorbic (Q) Milligrams
Boiled, pared before cooking:—1 potato	188	82.8	122	3.6	.2	27.3	11	79	.9	4	536	Trace	.17	.07	2.3	30
French fried: Length, over 2 in. to 3½ in.—10 strips	50	44.7	137	2.2	6.6	18.0	8	56	.7	3	427	Trace	.07	.04	1.6	11
Fried from raw—1 cup	170	46.9	456	6.8	24.1	55.4	26	172	1.9	379	1,318	Trace	.20	.12	4.8	32
Mashed, milk added—1 cup	210	82.8	137	4.4	1.5	27.3	50	103	.8	632	548	40	.17	.11	2.1	21
Scalloped and au gratin: With cheese—1 cup	245	71.1	355	13.0	19.4	33.3	311	299	1.2	1,095	750	780	.15	.29	2.2	25
Dehydrated mashed: Granules with milk—1 cup	210	81.4	166	4.2	4.6	27.5	65	92	1.3	491	704	190	.06	.11	1.7	6
Frozen—1 cup	155	56.1	347	3.1	17.8	45.0	28	78	1.9	463	439	Trace	.11	.03	1.6	12
French fried: Ovenheated: Yield from—9 oz., frozen french-fried potatoes—7 oz.	198	52.9	434	7.1	16.6	66.6	18	171	3.6	8	1,290	Trace	.28	.04	5.1	42
Potato chips: 10 chips	20	1.8	114	1.1	8.0	10.0	8	28	.4	—	226	Trace	.04	.01	1.0	3
Potato salad: Cooked salad dressing. seasonings—1 cup	250	76.0	248	6.8	7.0	40.8	80	160	1.5	1,320	798	350	.20	.18	2.8	28
Mayonnaise and french dressing. hard-cooked eggs. seasonings—1 cup	250	72.4	363	7.5	23.0	33.5	48	158	2.0	1,200	740	450	.18	.15	2.3	28
Pretzels: Rings: [piece. 1½-in. diam. with 1-in.-diam. hole: cross section of ring. ¼-in.—10 pretzels.	20	4.5	78	2.0	.9	15.2	4	26	.3	336	26	(0)	Trace	.01	.1	(0)
Thins—10 pretzels	60	4.5	234	5.9	2.7	45.5	13	79	.9	1,008	78	(0)	.01	.02	.4	(0)

Food																
Prunes:																
Dried, uncooked, whole—1 cup	185	28.0	411	3.4	1.0	108.5	82	127	6.3	13	1,117	2,580	.14	.27	2.6	5
Cooked, fruit and liquid: Without added sugar—1 cup	250	66.4	253	2.1	.6	66.7	51	79	3.8	9	695	1,590	.07	.15	1.5	2
With added sugar—1 cup	280	53.2	409	1.9	.5	107.3	45	71	3.6	7	624	1,430	.06	.14	1.4	2
Prune juice:																
1 glass	192	80	148	.8	.2	36.5	27	38	7.9	4	451	—	.02	.02	.8	4
Prune whip:																
Baked—1 cup	90	57.3	140	4.0	.2	33.2	20	30	1.2	148	261	410	.02	.13	.5	2
Puddings:																
Chocolate—1 cup	260	65.8	385	8.1	12.2	66.8	250	255	1.3	146	445	390	0.05	0.36	0.3	1
Vanilla (blancmange)—1 cup	255	76.0	283	8.9	9.9	40.5	298	232	Trace	166	352	410	.08	.41	.3	2
Pumpkin:																
Canned—1 cup	245	90.2	81	2.5	.7	19.4	61	64	1.0	5	588	15,680	.07	.12	1.5	12
Rabbit, domesticated, flesh only, cooked: Yield from 1 lb. ready-to-cook rabbit—8.6 oz.	245	59.8	529	71.8	24.7	0	51	635	3.7	100	902	—	.12	.17	27.7	—
Radishes, common, raw: Medium (¾- to 1-in. diam.)—10 radishes	50	94.5	8	.5	Trace	1.6	14	14	.5	8	145	Trace	.01	.01	.1	12
Raisins, natural (unbleached) seedless type—1 cup	165	18.0	477	4.1	.3	127.7	102	167	5.8	45	1,259	30	.18	.13	.8	2
Cooked, fruit (seedless raisins) and liquid, added sugar—1 cup	295	41.4	628	3.5	.3	166.4	86	139	4.7	38	1,047	30	.12	.09	.6	Trace
Raspberries:																
Raw: Black—1 cup	134	80.8	98	2.0	1.9	21.0	40	29	1.2	1	267	Trace	(.04)	(.12)	(1.2)	24
Red—1 cup	123	84.2	70	1.5	.6	16.7	27	27	1.1	1	207	160	.04	.11	1.1	31
Canned, water pack, solids and liquid, without artificial sweetener: red—1 cup	243	90.1	85	1.7	.2	21.4	36	36	1.5	2	277	220	.02	.10	1.2	22
Frozen, red, sweetened with nutritive sweetener—1 cup	250	74.3	245	1.8	.5	61.5	33	43	1.5	3	250	(180)	.05	.15	1.5	53
Rennin products:																
Tablet (salts, starch, rennin enzyme)—1 tablet	.9	9.0	1	Trace	Trace	.2	32	2	—	201	—	0	0	0	0	0
Dessert, home-prepared with tablet: Yield from recipe—1 cup	255	81.1	227	7.9	8.9	29.6	283	212	Trace	209	321	360	.08	.38	.3	3
Dessert made with milk—1 cup	255	77.9	260	8.7	9.7	36.0	311	245	Trace	133	319	360	.08	.38	.3	3

APPENDIX A–Nutrititive values for household measures and market units of foods–Continued

[Item numbers correspond to those in table 1 of Handbook No. 8, revised 1963. Values in parentheses denote imputed values usually from another form of the food or from a similar food. Zeros in parentheses indicate that amount of a constituent, if present, is probably too small to be measured. Dashes (—) denote lack of reliable data for a constituent believed to be present in a measurable amount. Calculated values, as those based on a recipe, are not in parentheses]

							Values for edible part of foods									
Food, approximate measures, units and weight (edible part unless footnotes indicate otherwise) (B)	Grams	Water (C) Percent	Food energy (D) Calories	Protein (E) Grams	Fat (F) Grams	Carbo-hydrate (G) Grams	Cal-cium (H) Milli-grams	Phos-phorus (I) Milli-grams	Iron (J) Milli-grams	Sodium (K) Milli-grams	Potas-sium (L) Milli-grams	Vitamin A value (M) Interna-tional units	Thia-min (N) Milli-grams	Ribo-flavin (O) Milli-grams	Niacin (P) Milli-grams	Ascor-bic (Q) Milli-grams
Rhubarb:																
Cooked, added sugar—1 cup	270	62.8	381	1.4	.3	97.2	211	41	1.6	5	548	220	(.05)	(.14)	(.8)	16
Frozen, sweetened: cooked, added sugar: Yield from 10 oz., frozen rhubarb—1¼ cups (approx.)	340	62.6	486	1.7	.7	123.1	265	41	2.4	10	598	240	.07	.14	.7	20
Rice:																
Brown: Cooked, long grain—1 cup	195	70.3	232	4.9	1.2	49.7	23	142	1.0	550	137	(0)	.18	.04	2.7	(0)
White (fully milled or polished):																
Enriched: Cooked—1 cup	205	72.6	223	4.1	.2	49.6	21	57	1.8	767	57	(0)	.23	.02	2.1	(0)
Parboiled, long grain.																
regular: Cooked—1 cup	175	73.4	186	3.7	.2	40.8	33	100	1.4	627	75	(0)	.19	.02	2.1	(0)
Precooked (instant), long grain:																
ready-to-serve, fluffed—1 cup	165	72.9	180	3.6	Trace	39.9	5	31	1.3	450	—	(0)	.21	( )	1.7	(0)
Unenriched—1 cup	205	72.6	223	4.1	.2	49.6	21	57	.4	767	57	(0)	.04	.02	.8	(0)
Rice polish:																
Stirred, spooned into cup—1 cup	105	9.8	278	12.7	13.4	60.6	72	1,161	16.9	Trace	750	(0)	1.93	.19	29.6	(0)
Rice products used mainly as ready-to-eat breakfast cereals:																
Rice, ovenpopped, added sugar, salt, iron, vitamins—1 cup	30	3.2	117	1.8	.1	26.3	6	28	.8	283	29	1,410	.35	.42	3.5	11
Rice, puffed, without salt and sugar: added iron, thiamin, niacin—1 cup	15	3.7	60	.9	.1	13.4	3	14	.3	Trace	15	(0)	.07	.01	.7	(0)
Rice, presweetened: Puffed, added honey or cocoa, salt, fat, iron, vitamins—1 cup	35	2.4	140	1.6	1.4	30.3	7	29	1.2	148	33	1,650	.41	.49	4.1	12

Food																
Rice, with protein concentrate, mainly—Wheat gluten and casein; added sugar, salt, minerals, vitamins; minute flakes—1 cup	85	3.0	325	34.0	.2	46.6	135	270	15.0	332	90	1,800	1.50	1.79	15.0	45
Rice pudding: With raisins—1 cup	265	65.8	387	9.5	8.2	70.8	260	249	1.1	188	469	290	.08	.37	.5	Trace
Roe, herring, canned, solids and liquid, 8 oz.—1 can	227	72.4	268	48.8	6.4	.7	34	785	2.7	—	—	—	—	—	—	5
Rolls and buns: Baked from home recipe, made with milk and enriched flour: roll (cloverleaf)—1 roll	35	26.1	119	2.9	3.0	19.6	16	36	0.7	98	41	30	0.09	0.09	0.8	Trace
Commercial: ready-to-serve: Danish pastry (plain without fruit or nuts): Prepackaged ring: Rectangular piece, approx. 6½ in. long, 2¾ in. wide. ¾ in. high—1 pastry	75	22.0	317	5.6	17.6	34.2	38	82	.7	275	84	230	.05	.11	.6	Trace
Hard rolls: Enriched: (round, or kaiser, 3¾-in. diam., 2 in. high)	50	25.4	156	4.9	1.6	29.8	24	46	1.2	313	49	Trace	.13	.12	1.4	Trace
Unenriched: (round, or kaiser, 3¾-in. diam., 2 in. high)—1 roll	50	25.4	156	4.9	1.6	29.8	24	46	.4	313	49	Trace	.03	.05	.4	Trace
Partially baked: Enriched, unbrowned: Cloverleaf and pan—1 roll	28	33.0	84	2.2	1.9	14.2	20	23	.5	136	25	Trace	.07	.06	.6	Trace
Browned—1 roll	26	26.9	84	2.2	1.9	14.2	20	23	.5	136	25	Trace	.07	.06	.6	Trace
Unenriched, unbrowned: cloverleaf and pan—1 roll	28	33.0	84	2.2	1.9	14.2	20	23	.2	136	25	Trace	.02	.02	.2	Trace
Browned—1 roll	26	26.9	84	2.2	1.9	14.2	20	23	.2	136	25	Trace	.02	.02	.2	Trace
Rolls prepared with roll mix and water, baked: Roll, cloverleaf. 2½-in. diam., 2 in. high—1 roll.	35	30.6	105	3.2	1.6	19.1	20	34	.2	110	43	Trace	.02	.04	.2	Trace
Rusk: 3¾-in. diam., ½-in. thick—1 rusk	9	4.8	38	1.2	.8	6.4	2	11	.1	22	14	20	.01	.02	.1	Trace
Rutabagas: Cooked (boiled), drained—1 cup	170	90.2	60	1.5	.2	13.9	100	53	.5	7	284	940	.10	.10	1.4	44
Rye flours: Sifted, spooned into cup—1 cup	88	11	314	8.3	.9	68.6	19	163	1.0	[1]	137	[0]	.13	.06	.5	[0]

APPENDIX A—Nutrititive values for household measures and market units of foods—Continued

[Item numbers correspond to those in table 1 of Handbook No. 8, revised 1963. Values in parentheses denote imputed values usually from another form of the food or from a similar food. Zeros in parentheses indicate that amount of a constituent, if present, is probably too small to be measured. Dashes (—) denote lack of reliable data for a constituent believed to be present in a measurable amount. Calculated values, as those based on a recipe, are not in parentheses]

Food, approximate measures, units and weight (edible part unless footnotes indicate otherwise) (B)	Grams	Water (C) Percent	Food energy (D) Calories	Protein (E) Grams	Fat (F) Grams	Carbohydrate (G) Grams	Calcium (H) Milligrams	Phosphorus (I) Milligrams	Iron (J) Milligrams	Sodium (K) Milligrams	Potassium (L) Milligrams	Vitamin A value (M) International units	Thiamin (N) Milligrams	Riboflavin (O) Milligrams	Niacin (P) Milligrams	Ascorbic (Q) Milligrams
Salad dressings, commercial:																
Blue and Roquefort cheese—1 tbsp.	15	32.3	76	.7	7.8	1.1	12	11	Trace	164	6	30	Trace	.02	Trace	Trace
Special dietary (low calorie)—1 tbsp.	16	83.7	12	.5	.9	.7	10	8	Trace	177	5	30	Trace	.01	Trace	Trace
French: Regular—1 tbsp.	16	38.8	66	.1	6.2	2.8	2	2	.1	219	13	—	—	—	—	—
Special dietary (low calorie), low fat (approx. 5 Cal. per teaspoon)—1 tbsp.	16	77.3	15	.1	.7	2.5	2	2	.1	126	13	—	—	—	—	—
Italian: Regular—1 tbsp.	15	27.5	83	Trace	9.0	1.0	2	1	Trace	314	2	Trace	Trace	Trace	Trace	—
Special dietary (low calorie, approx. 2 Cal. per teaspoon)—1 tbsp.	15	90.1	8	Trace	.7	.4	Trace	1	Trace	118	2	Trace	Trace	Trace	Trace	—
Mayonnaise—1 tbsp.	14	15.1	101	.2	11.2	.3	3	4	.1	84	5	40	Trace	.01	Trace	—
Russian—1 tbsp.	15	34.5	74	.2	7.6	1.6	3	6	.1	130	24	100	.01	.01	.1	1
Thousand Island: Regular—1 tbsp.	16	32.0	80	.1	8.0	2.5	2	3	.1	112	18	50	Trace	Trace	Trace	Trace
Special dietary (low calorie, approx. 10 Cal. per teaspoon)—1 tbsp.	15	68.2	27	.1	2.1	2.3	2	3	.1	105	17	50	Trace	Trace	Trace	Trace
Salmon, canned, solids and liquid:																
Atlantic: can and approx. contents: net wt. 7¾ oz.: drained solids..																
6¾ oz. (approx. 1 cup)—1 can	220	64.2	447	47.7	26.8	0	—	—	—	—	—	—	—	—	—	—
Chinook (king)—1 can	220	64.4	462	43.1	30.8	0	339	636	2.0	—	805	510	0.07	0.31	16.1	—
Chum—1 can	220	70.8	306	47.3	11.4	0	548	774	1.5	—	739	130	.04	.35	15.6	—
Coho (silver)—1 can	220	69.3	337	45.8	15.6	0	537	634	2.0	772	746	180	.57	.40	16.3	—
Pink (humpback)—1 can	220	70.8	310	45.1	13.0	0	431	629	1.8	851	794	150	.07	.40	17.6	—
Sockeye (red)—1 can	220	67.2	376	44.7	20.5	0	570	757	2.6	1,148	757	510	.09	.35	16.1	—

Food															
Salmon, broiled or baked with butter or margarine: Piece, 6⅜-in. long, 2½-in. wide, 1-in. thick (dimensions of uncooked steak)—1 steak	145	63.4	232	34.5	9.4	0	—	528	1.5	148	565	200	.20	.08	12.5	—
Salmon, smoked: 1 oz	28	58.9	50	6.1	2.6	0	4	69	—	—	—	50	—	—	—	—
Sardines, Atlantic, canned in oil: Solids and liquid—1 oz	28	50.6	88	5.8	6.9	.2	100	123	1.0	145	159	—	.01	.06	.05	1.2
Drained solids: Can and approx. drained contents: Size, 405×301×014 (No. ¼ Oil): drained wt., 3¼ oz.; 5–20 sardines—1 can	92	61.8	187	22.1	10.2	—	402	459	2.7	757	543	200	.03	.18	5.0	—
Sauerkraut: Canned, solids and liquid—1 cup	235	92.8	42	2.4	.5	9.4	85	42	1.2	1,755	329	120	.07	.09	.5	33
Sausage, cold cuts, and luncheon meats:—Blood sausage—1 oz	28	46.4	112	4.0	10.5	.1	—	—	—	—	65	—	—	—	—	—
Bologna—1 slice or 1 oz	28	56.2	86	3.4	7.8	.3	2	36	.5	369	—	—	.05	.06	.7	—
Braunschweiger (smoked liverwurst): package, net wt., 6 oz.; 6 slices—1 pkg	170	52.6	542	25.2	46.6	3.9	17	417	10.0	—	—	11,100	.29	2.45	13.9	—
Brown-and-serve sausage: Yield from 1 link—1 link	17	39.9	72	2.8	6.4	.5	—	—	—	—	—	—	—	—	—	—
Country-style sausage—1 oz	28	50.5	100	3.9	9.2	0	2	26	.6	—	—	(0)	.04	.03	.5	—
Frankfurters: Size, approx. 5 in. long, ⅞-in. diam.: wt., 2 oz.—1 frankfurter	57	55.6	176	7.1	15.7	1.0	4	76	1.1	627	125	—	.09	.11	1.5	—
Headcheese—1 slice or 1 oz	28	58.8	76	4.4	4.4	6.2	3	49	.7	—	—	(0)	.01	.03	.3	—
Knockwurst—1 link	68	57.6	189	9.6	15.8	1.5	5	105	1.4	—	—	—	[.12]	[.14]	[1.8]	—
Luncheon meat: Boiled ham—1 slice or 1 oz	28	59.1	66	5.4	4.8	0	3	47	.8	—	—	(0)	.12	.04	.7	—
Pork, cured ham or shoulder, chopped, spiced or unspiced, canned—1 oz	28	54.9	83	4.3	7.1	.4	3	31	.6	350	63	(0)	.09	.06	—	—
Meat loaf—1 lb	454	64.1	907	72.1	59.9	15.0	41	807	8.2	—	—	(0)	.59	1.00	11.3	—
Meat, potted (includes potted beef, chicken, turkey)—1 oz	28	60.7	70	5.0	5.4	0	—	—	—	—	—	—	.01	.06	.3	—
Polish sausage: approx. 5⅜-in. long, 1-in. diam.—1 sausage	76	53.7	231	11.9	19.6	.9	7	134	1.8	—	—	(0)	.26	.14	2.4	—
Pork sausage—1 patty	27	34.8	129	4.9	11.9	Trace	2	44	.6	259	73	(0)	.21	.09	1.0	—

APPENDIX A—*Nutritive values for household measures and market units of foods*—Continued

[Item numbers correspond to those in table 1 of Handbook No. 8, revised 1963. Values in parentheses denote imputed values usually from another form of the food or from a similar food. Zeros in parentheses indicate that amount of a constituent, if present, is probably too small to be measured. Dashes (—) denote lack of reliable data for a constituent believed to be present in a measurable amount. Calculated values, as those based on a recipe, are not in parentheses]

Food, approximate measures, units and weight (edible part unless footnotes indicate otherwise) (B)		Water (C) Percent	Food energy (D) Calories	Pro-tein (E) Grams	Fat (F) Grams	Carbo-hydrate (G) Grams	Cal-cium (H) Milli-grams	Phos-phorus (I) Milli-grams	Iron (J) Milli-grams	Sodium (K) Milli-grams	Potas-sium (L) Milli-grams	Vitamin A value (M) Inter-national units	Thia-min (N) Milli-grams	Ribo-flavin (O) Milli-grams	Niacin (P) Milli-grams	Ascor-bic (Q) Milli-grams
	Grams															
1 link	13	34.8	62	2.4	5.7	Trace	1	21	.3	125	35	(0)	.10	.04	.5	—
Salami: Dry—1 oz	28	29.8	128	6.7	10.8	.3	4	80	1.0	—	—	—	.10	.07	1.5	—
Cooked—1 slice or 1 oz	28	51.0	88	5.0	7.3	.4	3	57	.7	—	—	—	.07	.07	1.2	—
Scrapple—1 oz	28	61.3	61	2.5	3.9	4.1	1	18	.3	—	—	—	.05	.03	.5	—
Thuringer cervelat (summer sausage)—1 slice or 1 oz	28	48.5	87	5.3	6.9	.5	3	61	.8	—	—	—	.03	.07	1.2	—
Vienna sausage, canned: approx. 2 in. long, ⅞-in. diam—1 sausage	16	63.0	38	2.2	3.2	Trace	1	24	.3	—	—	—	.01	.02	.4	—
Scallops, bay and sea: Frozen, breaded, fried, reheated (sea scallops)—6⅔ oz	189	60.2	367	34.0	15.9	19.8	—	—	—	—	—	—	—	—	—	—
Sesame seeds: Dry, hulled, decorticated—1 tbsp	8	5.5	47	1.5	4.3	1.4	9	47	.2	—	—	—	.01	.01	.4	0
Shad: Baked—12⅔ oz	365	64.0	734	84.7	41.2	0	88	1,142	2.2	288	1,376	110	.47	.95	31.4	—
Shallot: Bulbs, raw, chopped—1 tbsp	10	79.8	7	.3	Trace	1.7	4	6	.1	1	33	Trace	.01	Trace	Trace	1
Sherbet: Orange—1 cup	193	67.0	259	1.7	2.3	59.4	31	25	Trace	19	42	120	.02	.06	Trace	4
Shrimp: Cooked (french fried)—1 oz	28	56.9	64	5.8	3.1	2.8	20	54	.6	53	65	—	.01	.02	.8	—
Canned—1 oz	28	70.4	33	6.9	.3	.2	33	75	.9	53	35	20	Trace	.01	.5	—
Shrimp or lobster paste: Canned—1 oz	7	61.3	13	1.5	.7	.1	—	—	—	—	—	—	—	.02	—	—

Sirups:																
Maple—1 tbsp	19.7	33	50	—	—	12.8	20	2	.2	2	35	—	—	—	—	0
Sorghum—1 tbsp	20.6	23	53	—	—	14.0	35	5	2.6	—	—	—	—	.02	Trace	—
Cane and maple—1 tbsp	19.7	33	50	0	0	12.8	3	Trace	Trace	Trace	5	0	0	0	0	0
Soups, commercial:																
Asparagus, cream of: 10½ oz.—1 can	298	85.8	161	6.0	4.2	25.0	66	92	1.8	2,444	298	750	.09	.21	1.8	—
Bean with pork: 11½ oz.—1 can	326	68.9	437	20.9	15.0	56.4	163	329	5.9	2,628	1,030	1,700	.36	.20	2.6	7
Beef broth, bouillon,																
consomme: 10½ oz.—1 can	298	91.6	77	12.5	0	6.6	Trace	77	1.2	1,943	322	Trace	Trace	.06	3.0	—
Beef noodle: 10½ oz.—1 can	298	86.4	170	9.5	6.6	17.3	18	119	2.1	2,277	191	150	0.12	.15	2.7	3
Celery, cream of: 10½ oz.—1 can	298	84.6	215	4.2	12.5	22.1	119	89	1.5	2,372	268	510	.03	.12	1.2	3
Chicken consomme:10½ oz.—1 can	298	93.7	54	8.3	.3	4.5	30	176	3.0	1,794	—	—	—	—	—	—
Chicken, cream of: 10½ oz.—1 can	298	83.8	235	7.2	14.3	20.0	57	86	1.2	2,411	197	1,040	.03	.12	1.5	Trace
Chicken gumbo: 10½ oz.—1 can	298	87.6	137	7.7	3.9	18.2	48	63	1.5	2,360	265	540	.06	.09	3.3	12
Chicken noodle: 10½ oz.—1 can	298	86.6	158	8.3	4.8	19.7	21	89	1.2	2,432	137	90	0.30	0.06	2.1	Trace
Chicken with rice: 10½ oz.—1 can	298	89.6	116	7.7	3.0	14.0	21	63	.9	2,277	244	390	Trace	.06	1.8	—
Clam chowder, Manhattan																
type: 10¾ oz.—1 can	305	83.7	201	5.5	6.4	30.5	88	116	2.7	2,336	458	2,170	.06	.06	2.7	—
Minestrone: 10¾ oz.—1 can	305	79.0	265	12.2	8.5	35.4	92	149	2.1	2,480	778	5,800	.18	.15	2.7	—
Mushroom, cream of: 10½ oz.—1 can	298	79.3	331	5.7	23.8	25.0	101	128	.9	2,369	244	180	.03	.30	1.8	Trace
Onion: 10½ oz.—1 can	298	86.9	161	13.1	6.3	12.8	69	69	1.2	2,608	256	Trace	Trace	.06	Trace	—
Pea, green: 11–11¼ oz.—1 can	316	72.8	335	14.5	5.7	58.1	114	288	2.2	2,319	506	880	0.13	0.16	2.8	19
Pea, split: 11¼ oz.—1 can	319	70.7	376	22.3	8.3	54.2	80	389	3.5	2,447	702	1,150	.64	.38	3.5	3
Tomato: 10¾ oz.—1 can	305	81.0	220	4.9	6.4	38.7	34	82	1.8	2,416	573	2,470	.15	.09	2.7	31
Vegetable beef: 10¾ oz.—1 can	305	83.8	198	12.8	5.5	24.1	31	119	1.8	2,605	400	6,710	.09	.12	2.4	—
Vegetarian vegetable: 10¾ oz.—1 can	305	83.7	195	5.5	5.2	32.3	49	98	2.4	2,086	427	7,020	.09	.09	2.1	—
Dehydrated: Onion (1½-oz. pkg.)—1 pkg	43	2.8	150	6.0	4.6	23.2	42	49	.6	2,871	238	30	.05	.03	.3	6
Pea, green (4-oz. pkg.)—1 pkg	113	3.1	409	25.3	4.6	69.6	68	354	6.1	2,667	988	140	.50	.52	4.6	1
Soybeans:																
Mature seeds, dry: Cooked—1 cup	180	71.0	234	19.8	10.3	19.4	131	322	4.9	4	972	50	.38	.16	1.1	0
Sprouted seeds: Cooked—1 cup	125	89.0	48	6.6	1.8	4.6	54	63	.9	—	—	100	.20	.19	.9	5
Soybean curd (tofu):																
(2½×2¾×1 in.)—1 piece	120	84.8	86	9.4	5.0	2.9	154	151	2.3	8	50	0	.07	.04	.1	0
Soybean flours:'																
Full fat, cup, stirred—1 cup	70	8.0	295	25.7	14.2	21.3	139	391	5.9	1	1,162	80	.60	.22	1.5	0
Low fat, cup, stirred—1 cup	88	8.0	313	38.2	5.9	32.2	231	558	8.0	1	1,636	70	.73	.32	2.3	0

APPENDIX A—Nutrititive values for household measures and market units of foods—Continued

[Item numbers correspond to those in table 1 of Handbook No. 8, revised 1963. Values in parentheses denote imputed values usually from another form of the food or from a similar food. Zeros in parentheses indicate that amount of a constituent, if present, is probably too small to be measured. Dashes (—) denote lack of reliable data for a constituent believed to be present in a measurable amount. Calculated values, as those based on a recipe, are not in parentheses]

(B) Food, approximate measures, units and weight (edible part unless footnotes indicate otherwise)	Grams	(C) Water Percent	(D) Food energy Calories	(E) Protein Grams	(F) Fat Grams	(G) Carbohydrate Grams	Values for edible part of foods									
							(H) Calcium Milligrams	(I) Phosphorus Milligrams	(J) Iron Milligrams	(K) Sodium Milligrams	(L) Potassium Milligrams	(M) Vitamin A value International units	(N) Thiamin Milligrams	(O) Riboflavin Milligrams	(P) Niacin Milligrams	(Q) Ascorbic Milligrams
Defatted, cup, stirred—1 cup	100	8.0	326	47.0	0.9	38.1	265	655	11.1	1	1,820	40	1.09	0.34	2.6	0
Soy sauce:																
1 tbsp	18	62.8	12	1.0	.2	1.7	15	19	.9	1,319	66	0	Trace	.05	.1	0
Spaghetti:																
Regular, thin, vermicelli, cooked—1 cup	140	73.0	155	4.8	.6	32.2	11	70	1.3	1	85	(0)	.20	.11	1.5	(0)
Spaghetti (enriched) in tomato sauce with cheese:																
1 cup	250	77.0	260	8.8	8.8	37.0	80	135	2.3	(955)	408	1,080	.25	.18	2.3	13
Canned—1 cup	250	80.1	190	5.5	1.5	38.5	40	88	2.8	955	303	930	.35	.28	4.5	10
Spaghetti (enriched) with meatballs and tomato sauce:																
1 cup	248	70.0	332	18.6	11.7	38.7	124	236	3.7	1,009	665	1,590	.25	.30	4.0	22
Spanish rice:																
Cooked from home recipe—1 cup	245	78.5	213	4.4	4.2	40.7	34	96	1.5	774	566	1,620	.10	.07	1.7	37
Spinach:																
Raw (chopped spinach)—1 cup	55	90.7	14	1.8	.2	2.4	51	28	1.7	39	259	4,460	.06	.11	.3	28
Cooked (boiled), drained—1 cup	180	92.0	41	5.4	.5	6.5	167	68	4.0	90	583	14,580	.13	.25	.9	50
Canned, whole leaf, cut leaf or sliced, chopped—1 cup	205	91.4	49	5.5	1.2	7.4	242	53	5.3	484	513	16,400	.04	.25	.6	29
Frozen: Chopped—1 cup	205	91.9	47	6.2	.6	7.6	232	90	4.3	109	683	16,200	.14	.31	.8	39
Leaf—1 cup	190	91.8	46	5.5	.6	7.4	200	84	4.8	93	688	15,390	.15	.27	1.0	53
Squash:																
Summer: Raw—1 cup	130	94.0	25	1.4	.1	5.5	36	38	.5	1	263	530	.07	.12	1.3	29

Food															
Cooked (boiled), drained—1 cup	180	95.5	25	1.6	.2	5.6	45	45	.7	2	254	700	.09	.14	1.4	18
Zucchini and Cocozelle: Raw—1 cup	130	94.6	22	1.6	.1	4.7	36	38	.5	1	263	420	.07	.12	1.3	25
Cooked —1 cup	180	96.0	22	1.8	.2	4.5	45	45	.7	2	254	540	.09	.14	1.4	16
Winter: Baked—1 cup	205	81.4	129	3.7	.8	31.6	57	98	1.6	2	945	8,610	.10	.27	1.4	27
Boiled—1 cup	245	88.8	93	2.7	.7	22.5	49	78	1.2	2	632	8,580	.10	.25	1.0	20
Acorn: Raw: Whole, 4-in. diam.. 4½-in. high: wt., 1¼ lb.—1 squash.	567	86.3	190	6.5	.4	48.3	134	99	3.9	4	1,655	5,170	.22	.47	2.6	60
Cooked: Baked—1 cup	205	82.9	113	3.9	.2	28.7	80	59	2.3	2	984	2,870	.10	.27	1.4	27
Boiled—1 cup	245	89.7	83	2.9	.2	20.6	69	49	2.0	2	659	2,700	.10	.25	1.0	20
Butternut, cooked: baked—1 cup	205	79.6	139	3.7	0.2	35.9	82	148	2.1	2	1,248	13,120	0.10	0.27	1.4	16
Boiled—1 cup	245	87.8	100	2.7	.2	22.5	71	120	1.7	2	835	13,230	.10	.25	1.0	12
Squash, winter, frozen: 1 cup	240	88.8	91	2.9	.7	22.1	60	77	2.4	2	497	9,360	.07	.17	1.2	19
Strawberries: Raw—1 cup	149	89.9	55	1.0	.7	12.5	31	31	1.5	1	244	90	.04	.10	.9	88
Canned, water pack, solids and liquid, without artificial sweetener—1 cup	242	93.7	53	1.0	.2	13.6	34	34	1.7	2	269	100	.02	.07	1.0	48
Frozen, sweetened—1 cup	255	71.3	278	1.3	.5	70.9	36	43	1.8	3	286	80	.05	.15	1.3	135
Whole—1 cup	255	75.7	235	1.0	.5	59.9	33	41	1.5	3	265	80	.05	.15	1.3	140
Sturgeon: Cooked, steamed—1 oz	28	67.5	45	7.2	1.6	0	11	75	.6	31	67	—	—	—	—	—
Smoked—1 oz	28	63.7	42	8.8	.5	0	—	—	—	—	—	—	—	—	—	—
Succotash (corn and lima beans), frozen: Not thawed: Cooked—1 cup	170	74.1	158	7.1	.7	34.9	22	145	1.7	65	418	(510)	.15	.09	2.2	10
Sugars: Beet or cane: Brown, spooned into cup—1 cup	220	2.1	821	0	0	212.1	187	42	7.5	66	757	0	.02	.07	.4	0
Granulated—1 cup	200	.5	770	0	0	199.0	0	0	.2	2	6	0	0	0	0	0
Powdered—1 cup	120	.5	462	0	0	119.4	0	0	.1	1	4	0	0	0	0	0
Maple—1 piece or 1 oz	28	8	99	—	—	25.5	41	3	.4	4	69	—	—	—	—	—
Sunflower seed kernels, dry: 1 cup	85	4.8	257	11.0	21.7	9.1	55	384	3.3	14	422	20	.90	.11	2.5	—
Sweetbreads: Calf—3 oz	85	62.7	143	27.7	2.7	0	—	—	—	—	—	—	.05	.14	2.5	—

APPENDIX A—Nutrititive values for household measures and market units of foods—Continued

[Item numbers correspond to those in table 1 of Handbook No. 8, revised 1963. Values in parentheses denote imputed values usually from another form of the food or from a similar food. Zeros in parentheses indicate that amount of a constituent, if present, is probably too small to be measured. Dashes (—) denote lack of reliable data for a constituent believed to be present in a measurable amount. Calculated values, as those based on a recipe, are not in parentheses]

							Values for edible part of foods									
Food, approximate measures, units and weight (edible part unless footnotes indicate otherwise) (B)	Grams	Water (C) Percent	Food energy (D) Calories	Protein (E) Grams	Fat (F) Grams	Carbohydrate (G) Grams	Calcium (H) Milligrams	Phosphorus (I) Milligrams	Iron (J) Milligrams	Sodium (K) Milligrams	Potassium (L) Milligrams	Vitamin A value (M) International units	Thiamin (N) Milligrams	Riboflavin (O) Milligrams	Niacin (P) Milligrams	Ascorbic (Q) Milligrams
Sweetpotatoes:																
Cooked, all: Baked in skin [refuse: skin, 22%]; Potato, 5 in. long, 2-in. diam.—1 potato.	146	63.7	161	2.4	.6	37.0	46	66	1.0	14	342	9,230	.10	.08	.8	25
Candied Piece, 2½-in. long, 2-in. diam.—1 piece.	85	60.0	143	1.1	2.8	29.1	31	37	.8	36	162	5,360	.05	.03	.3	9
Canned: 22 oz.—1 can.	638	70.7	727	6.4	1.3	175.5	83	185	4.5	306	(766)	31,900	.19	.19	3.8	51
Swordfish, broiled with butter or margarine [refuse: skin, 6%]: Yield from 1 lb., raw—10.1 oz.	305	64.6	499	80.3	17.2	0	77	788	3.7	—	—	5,880	.11	.14	31.3	—
Tangelo juice, raw, and tangelos used for juice—1 cup.	247	89.4	101	1.2	[.2]	24.0	—	—	—	—	—	—	—	—	—	67
Tangerines, raw: 2⅜-in. diam., size 176—1 tangerine.	116	87	39	.7	.2	10.0	34	15	.3	2	108	360	.05	.02	.1	27
Tapioca, dry: 1 tbsp.	8.4	12.6	30	.1	Trace	7.3	1	2	Trace	Trace	2	(0)	(0)	(0)	(0)	(0)
Tapioca cream pudding—1 cup.	165	71.8	221	8.3	8.4	28.2	173	180	.7	257	223	480	.07	.30	0.2	2
Tartar sauce: 1 tbsp.	14	34.4	74	.2	8.1	.6	3	4	.1	99	11	30	Trace	Trace	Trace	Trace
Tomatoes: Green, raw—1 lb.	454	93.0	99	5.0	.8	21.1	54	111	2.1	12	1,007	1,110	.25	.17	2.1	83
Tomatoes, ripe: Raw: Size, approx.2 3/5-in. diam.—1 tomato	135	93.5	26	1.3	.2	5.6	15	32	.6	4	290	1,070	.07	.05	.8	27
Cooked (boiled)—1 cup	241	92.4	63	3.1	.5	13.3	36	77	1.4	10	692	2,410	.17	.12	1.9	58
Canned, solids and liquid: Regular pack: 16 oz.—1 can or 1 lb	454	93.7	95	4.5	.9	19.5	27	86	2.3	590	984	4,080	.23	.14	3.2	77

Food															
Special dietary pack [low sodium]: 16 oz.—1 can or 1 lb	454	94.1	91	4.5	.9	19.1	27	86	2.3	14	984	4,080	.23	.14	3.2	77
Tomato catsup: Canned or bottled—1 tbsp.	15	68.6	16	.3	.1	3.8	3	8	.1	156	54	210	.01	.01	.2	2
Tomato chili sauce: Bottled—1 tbsp.	15	68.0	16	.4	Trace	3.7	3	8	[.1]	201	[56]	[210]	[.01]	[.01]	[.2]	[2]
Tomato juice: Canned or bottled: Regular pack—1 glass.	182	93.6	35	1.6	.2	7.8	13	33	1.6	364	413	1,460	.09	.05	1.5	29
Special dietary pack (low sodium)—1 glass.	182	94.2	35	1.5	.2	7.8	13	33	1.6	5	413	1,460	.09	.05	1.3	29
Tomato juice cocktail: Canned or bottled—1 glass.	182	93.0	38	1.3	.2	9.1	18	33	1.6	364	402	1,460	.09	.04	1.1	29
Tomato paste: Canned—1 can	170	75.0	139	5.8	.7	31.6	46	119	6.0	65	1,510	5,610	.34	.20	5.3	83
Tomato puree: Canned: Regular pack, 29 oz.—1 can.	822	87.0	321	14.0	1.6	73.2	107	279	14.0	3,280	3,502	13,150	0.74	0.41	11.5	271
Tongue: Beef, medium-fat, cooked (braised): Slice, approx. 3-in. long, 2-in. wide, ⅛-in. thick—1 slice.	20	60.8	49	4.3	3.3	.1	1	23	.4	12	33	—	.01	.06	.7	—
Tuna: Canned: In oil: Drained solids, 6 oz.—1 can	169	60.6	333	48.7	13.9	0	[14]	395	3.2	—	—	140	.08	.20	20.1	—
In water: 6½ oz.—1 can.	184	70.0	234	51.5	1.5	0	29	350	2.9	75	513	—	—	.18	24.5	—
Tuna salad: 1 cup	205	69.8	349	29.9	21.5	7.2	41	291	2.7	—	—	590	0.08	.23	10.3	2
Turkey: Cooked—8.6 oz.	245	55.4	644	66.2	40.2	0	—	—	—	—	—	—	—	—	—	—
Light meat without skin: Piece, approx. 4 in. long, 2 in. wide, ¼ in. thick: wt., 1½ oz.—2 pieces or 3 oz.	85	62.1	150	28.0	3.3	0	—	—	1.0	70	349	—	.04	.12	9.4	—
Dark meat without skin: approx. 2½ in. long, 1 5/8 in. wide, ¼ in. thick: wt., ⅞ oz.—4 pieces or 3 oz.	85	60.5	173	25.5	7.1	0	—	—	2.0	84	338	—	.03	.20	3.6	—
Turkey potpie: Home prepared, baked: Pie, whole (9-in. diam.)—1 pie.	698	56.2	1,654	72.6	94.2	129.1	188	705	9.8	1,906	1,382	9,280	.77	.91	17.5	14

APPENDIX A—Nutrititive values for household measures and market units of foods—Continued

[Item numbers correspond to those in table 1 of Handbook No. 8, revised 1963. Values in parentheses denote imputed values usually from another form of the food or from a similar food. Zeros in parentheses indicate that amount of a constituent, if present, is probably too small to be measured. Dashes (—) denote lack of reliable data for a constituent believed to be present in a measurable amount. Calculated values, as those based on a recipe, are not in parentheses]

Food, approximate measures, units and weight (edible part unless footnotes indicate otherwise) (B)	Grams	Water (C) Percent	Food energy (D) Calories	Protein (E) Grams	Fat (F) Grams	Carbohydrate (G) Grams	Calcium (H) Milligrams	Phosphorus (I) Milligrams	Iron (J) Milligrams	Sodium (K) Milligrams	Potassium (L) Milligrams	Vitamin A value (M) International units	Thiamin (N) Milligrams	Riboflavin (O) Milligrams	Niacin (P) Milligrams	Ascorbic (Q) Milligrams
Turnips:																
Raw, cubed or sliced—1 cup	130	91.5	39	1.3	0.3	8.6	51	39	0.7	64	348	Trace	0.05	0.09	0.8	47
Turnip greens, leaves including stems:																
Cooked (boiled), drained—1 cup	145	93.2	29	3.2	.3	5.2	267	54	1.6	—	—	9,140	.22	.35	.9	100
Frozen, chopped: Yield from 10 oz. frozen turnip greens—1½ cups	220	92.7	51	5.5	.7	8.6	260	86	3.5	37	328	15,180	.11	.20	.9	42
Veal:																
Chuck cuts and boneless veal for stew: Yield from 1 lb., raw veal with bone—8.4 oz.	240	58.5	564	67.0	30.7	0	29	362	8.4	117	536	—	.22	.70	15.4	—
Loin cuts: Yield from 1 lb. raw loin without bone—11.4 oz.	324	58.9	758	85.5	43.4	0	36	729	10.4	209	958	—	.23	.81	17.5	—
Vegetable juice cocktail:																
Canned—1 cup	242	94.1	41	2.2	.2	8.7	29	53	1.2	(484)	(535)	1,690	.12	.07	1.9	22
Vegetables, mixed:																
Cooked (boiled). drained: Yield from 10 oz. frozen vegetables—1½ cups	275	82.6	176	8.8	.8	36.9	69	173	3.6	146	525	13,610	.33	.19	3.0	22
Venison:																
Lean meat only, raw—3 oz.	85	74	107	17.9	3.4	0	9	212	—	—	—	—	.20	.41	5.4	—
Vinegar:																
Cider—1 tbsp.	15	93.8	2	Trace	(0)	.9	(1)	(1)	[.1]	Trace	15	—	—	—	—	—
Distilled—1 tbsp.	15	95	2	—	—	.8	(1)	(1)	—	Trace	2	—	—	—	—	—
Waffles:																
Baked from home recipe, made with Enriched flour-1 waffle.	200	41.4	558	18.6	19.6	75.0	226	346	3.4	950	290	660	.34	.50	2.6	1
Frozen, prebaked, waffle, 4⅝×3⅞×⅝ in.—1 waffle.	34	42.1	86	2.4	2.1	14.3	41	71	.6	219	54	40	.06	.05	.4	Trace

Food																
Walnuts:																
Shelled: Chopped or broken kernels—1 tbsp.	8	3.1	50	1.6	4.7	1.2	Trace	46	.5	Trace	37	20	.02	.01	.1	—
Persian or English: Chopped pieces or chips—1 tbsp.	8	3.5	52	1.2	5.1	1.3	8	30	.2	Trace	36	Trace	.03	.01	.1	Trace
Waterchestnut:																
1 lb.	454	78.3	276	4.9	.7	66.4	14	227	2.1	70	1,747	0	.49	.70	3.5	14
Watercress:																
Leaves including stems, raw: Whole. 1 cup (approx. 10 sprigs)—1 cup.	35	93.3	7	.8	.1	1.1	53	19	.6	18	99	1,720	.03	.06	.3	28
Watermelon, raw:																
piece, 1/16 of melon-1 piece.	926	92.6	111	2.1	.9	27.3	30	43	2.1	4	426	2,510	.13	.13	.9	30
Welsh rarebit:																
1 cup.	232	70.2	415	18.8	31.6	14.6	582	432	.7	770	320	1,230	.09	.53	.2	Trace
Wheat flour:																
Whole (from hard wheats)—1 cup.	120	12	400	16.0	2.4	85.2	49	446	4.0	4	444	(0)	.66	.14	5.2	(0)
All-purpose or family flour:																
Enriched—1 cup.	137	12	499	14.4	1.4	104.3	22	119	4.0	3	130	(0)	.60	.36	4.8	(0)
Cake or pastry flour—1 cup.	96	12	349	7.2	.8	76.2	16	70	.5	2	91	(0)	.03	.03	.7	(0)
Self-rising flour, enriched-1 cup.	115	11.5	405	10.7	1.2	85.3	305	536	3.3	1,241	—	(0)	.51	.30	4.0	(0)
Wheat products used mainly as hot breakfast cereals:																
Wheat, rolled: Cooked—1 cup.	240	79.7	180	5.3	1.0	40.6	19	182	1.7	708	202	(0)	.17	.07	2.2	(0)
Wheat, whole-meal, cooked—1 cup.	245	87.7	110	4.4	.7	23.0	17	127	1.2	519	118	(0)	.15	.05	1.5	(0)
Instant cooking (about 1 min. cooking time): Cooked—1 cup.	245	80.0	196	7.4	.7	39.4	22	201	2.2	250	Trace	(0)	.17	.05	—	(0)
Wheat products used mainly as ready-to-eat breakfast cereals:																
Wheat flakes, added sugar, salt, iron, vitamins—1 cup.	30	3.5	106	3.1	.5	24.2	12	83	4.5	310	81	1,410	.35	.42	3.5	11
Wheat, puffed: Without salt and sugar: added iron, thiamin, niacin—1 cup.	15	3.4	54	2.3	.2	11.8	4	48	.6	1	51	(0)	.08	.03	1.2	(0)
With sugar or sugar and honey, and salt: added iron and vitamins—1 cup.	35	2.8	132	2.1	0.7	30.9	7	53	1.2	56	61	1,650	0.41	0.49	4.1	12
Wheat, shredded: Without sugar, salt, or other added ingredients: Oblong biscuit (3¾×2¼×1 in. or 2½×2×1¼ in.)—1 biscuit.	25	6.6	89	2.5	.5	20.0	11	97	.9	1	87	(0)	.06	.03	1.1	(0)

APPENDIX A–Nutritive values for household measures and market units of foods—Continued

[Item numbers correspond to those in table 1 of Handbook No. 8, revised 1963. Values in parentheses denote imputed values usually from another form of the food or from a similar food. Zeros in parentheses indicate that amount of a constituent, if present, is probably too small to be measured. Dashes (—) denote lack of reliable data for a constituent believed to be present in a measurable amount. Calculated values, as those based on a recipe, are not in parentheses]

Food, approximate measures, units and weight (edible part unless footnotes indicate otherwise) (B)	Grams	Water (C) Percent	Food energy (D) Calories	Protein (E) Grams	Fat (F) Grams	Carbohydrate (G) Grams	Calcium (H) Milligrams	Phosphorus (I) Milligrams	Iron (J) Milligrams	Sodium (K) Milligrams	Potassium (L) Milligrams	Vitamin A value (M) International units	Thiamin (N) Milligrams	Riboflavin (O) Milligrams	Niacin (P) Milligrams	Ascorbic (Q) Milligrams
With malt, salt, sugar: iron and vitamins added: Bite-size squares—1 cup	55	3.2	201	5.0	1.6	44.9	21	176	19.4	383	99	2,590	.64	.78	6.4	19
Whey: Fluid—1 cup	246	93.1	64	2.2	.7	12.5	125	130	.2	—	—	20	.07	.34	.2	—
Whitefish, lake: Cooked (baked), stuffed—1 oz	28	63.2	61	4.3	4.0	1.6	—	70	.1	55	82	570	.03	.03	.7	Trace
White sauce: medium—1 cup	250	73.3	405	9.8	31.3	22.0	288	233	.5	948	348	1,150	.10	.43	.5	2
Wildrice, raw: 1 cup	160	8.5	565	22.6	1.1	120.5	30	542	6.7	11	352	(0)	.72	1.01	9.9	(0)
Yam: Tuber, raw—1 lb	454	73.5	394	8.2	.8	90.5	78	269	2.3	—	2,341	Trace	.39	.16	2.0	35
Yeast: Bakers: Compressed—1 oz	28	71.0	24	(3.4)	.1	3.1	4	112	1.4	5	173	Trace	.20	.47	3.2	Trace
Brewer's, debittered—1 oz	28	5.0	80	(11.0)	.3	10.9	60	497	4.9	34	537	Trace	4.43	1.21	10.7	Trace
Yogurt: Made from partially skimmed milk—1 cup	245	89.0	123	8.3	4.2	12.7	294	230	.1	125	350	170	.10	.44	.2	2
Made from whole milk—1 cup	245	88.0	152	7.4	8.3	12.0	272	213	.1	115	323	340	.07	.39	.2	2
Zwieback: Piece, approx. 3½ × 1½ × ½ in.—1 piece	7	5.0	30	.7	.6	5.2	1	5	Trace	18	11	Trace	Trace	Trace	.1	(0)

Appendix B
U.S. Recommended Daily Allowance

	Adults and Children Over 4 yrs. (U.S. RDA)	Children Under 4 yrs.	Infants Under 13 months	Pregnant or Lactating Women
Protein	65 g*	28 g*	25 g*	65 g*
Vitamin A	5,000 IU	2,500 IU	2,500 IU	8,000 IU
Vitamin C	60 mg	40 mg	40 mg	60 mg
Thiamin	1.5 mg	0.7 mg	0.7 mg	1.7 mg
Riboflavin	1.7 mg	0.8 mg	0.8 mg	2.0 mg
Niacin	20 mg	9.0 mg	9.0 mg	20 mg
Calcium	1.0 g	0.8 g	0.8 g	1.3 g
Iron	18 mg	10 mg	10 mg	18 mg
Vitamin D	400 IU	400 IU	400 IU	400 IU
Vitamin E	30 IU	10 IU	10 IU	30 IU
Vitamin B6	2.0 mg	0.7 mg	0.7 mg	2.5 mg
Folacin	0.4 mg	0.2 mg	0.2 mg	0.8 mg
Vitamin B12	6 mcg	3 mcg	3 mcg	8 mcg
Phosphorus	1.0 g	0.8 g	0.8 g	1.3 g
Iodine	150 mcg	70 mcg	70 mcg	150 mcg
Magnesium	400 mg	200 mg	200 mg	450 mg
Zinc	15 mg	8 mg	8 mg	15 mg
Copper	2 mg	1 mg	1 mg	2 mg
Biotin	0.3 mg	0.15 mg	0.15 mg	0.3 mg
Pantothenic acid	10 mg	5 mg	5 mg	10 mg

*If protein efficiency ratio of protein is equal to or better than that of casein, U.S. RDA is 45g for adults and pregnant or lactating women, 20g for children under 4 years of age and 18g for infants.

Appendix C
Nutrients Which Must Be on the Label

	Age (yr.)	Weight (lbs.)	Height (in.)	Protein RDA	Protein % of U.S. RDA which = RDA	Vitamin A 5000 I.U. RDA	Vitamin A % of U.S. RDA which = RDA	Vitamin C 60 mg RDA	Vitamin C % of U.S. RDA which = RDA	Thiamin 1.5 mg RDA	Thiamin % of U.S. RDA which = RDA	Riboflavin 1.7 mg RDA	Riboflavin % of U.S. RDA which = RDA	Niacin 20 mg RDA	Niacin % of U.S. RDA which = RDA	Calcium 1000 mg RDA	Calcium % of U.S. RDA which = RDA	Iron 18 mg RDA	Iron % of U.S. RDA which = RDA
Children	1-3*	28	35	23	35	2000	40	40	67	0.7	47	0.8	47	9	45	800	80	15	83
	4-6	44	44	30	50	2500	50	40	67	0.9	60	1.1	65	12	60	800	80	10	56
	7-10	66	54	36	55	3300	67	40	67	1.2	80	1.2	70	16	80	800	80	10	56
Males	11-14	97	63	44	70	5000	100	45	75	1.4	93	1.5	88	18	90	1200	120	18	100
	15-18	134	69	54	85	5000	100	45	75	1.5	100	1.8	106	20	100	1200	120	18	100
	19-22	147	69	55	85	5000	100	45	75	1.5	100	1.8	106	20	100	800	80	10	56
	23-50	154	69	56	90	5000	100	45	75	1.4	93	1.6	94	18	90	800	80	10	56
	51+	154	69	56	90	5000	100	45	75	1.2	80	1.5	88	16	80	800	80	10	56
Females	11-14	97	62	44	70	4000	80	45	75	1.2	80	1.3	77	16	80	1200	120	18	100
	15-18	119	65	48	75	4000	80	45	75	1.1	74	1.4	82	14	70	1200	120	18	100
	19-22	128	65	46	75	4000	80	45	75	1.1	74	1.4	82	14	70	800	80	18	100
	23-50	128	65	46	75	4000	80	45	75	1.0	67	1.2	70	13	65	800	80	18	100
	51+	128	65	46	75	4000	80	45	75	1.0	67	1.1	65	12	60	800	80	10	56
Pregnant*				+30	+50	5000	100	60	100	+0.3	+20	+0.3	+18	+2	+10	1200	120	18	100
Lactating*				+20	+35	6000	120	80	133	+0.3	+20	+0.5	+30	+4	+20	1200	120	18	100

*See Appendix B for U.S. RDA table for these groups.

U.S. RDA of 65 grams is used for this table. In labeling, a U.S. RDA of 45 grams is used for foods providing high-quality protein, such as milk, meat, and eggs.

Appendix D
Nutrients Which May Be on the Label

				Vitamin D 400 I.U.		Vitamin E 30 I.U.		Vitamin B$_6$ 2.0 mg		Folacin 400 mcg		Vitamin B$_{12}$ 6.0 mcg		Phosphorus 1000 mg		Iodine 150 mcg		Magnesium 400 mg		Zinc 15 mg	
Nutrient / U.S. RDA	Age (yr.)	Weight (lbs.)	Height (in.)	RDA	% of U.S. RDA which = RDA	RDA	%	RDA	%	RDA	%	RDA	%	RDA	%	RDA	%	RDA	%	RDA	%
Children 1–3*	1–3	28	34	400	100	7	23	0.6	30	100	25	1.0	17	800	80	60	40	150	38	10	67
Children 4–6	4–6	44	44	400	100	9	30	0.9	45	200	50	1.5	25	800	80	80	53	200	50	10	67
Children 7–10	7–10	66	54	400	100	10	33	1.2	60	300	75	2.0	33	800	80	110	73	250	63	10	67
Males 11–14	11–14	97	63	400	100	12	40	1.6	80	400	100	3.0	50	1200	120	130	86	350	87	15	100
Males 15–18	15–18	134	69	400	100	15	50	2.0	100	400	100	3.0	50	1200	120	150	100	400	100	15	100
Males 19–22	19–22	147	69	400	100	15	50	2.0	100	400	100	3.0	50	800	80	140	93	350	87	15	100
Males 23–50	23–50	154	69			15	50	2.0	100	400	100	3.0	50	800	80	130	87	350	87	15	100
Males 51+	51+	154	69			15	50	2.0	100	400	100	3.0	50	800	80	110	73	350	87	15	100
Females 11–14	11–14	97	62	400	100	12	40	1.6	80	400	100	3.0	50	1200	120	115	77	300	75	15	100
Females 15–18	15–18	119	65	400	100	12	40	2.0	100	400	100	3.0	50	1200	120	115	77	300	75	15	100
Females 19–22	19–22	128	65	400	100	12	40	2.0	100	400	100	3.0	50	800	80	100	67	300	75	15	100
Females 23–50	23–50	128	65			12	40	2.0	100	400	100	3.0	50	800	80	100	67	300	75	15	100
Females 51+	51+	128	65			12	40	2.0	100	400	100	3.0	50	800	80	80	53	300	75	15	100
Pregnant*				400	100	15	50	2.5	125	800	200	4.0	67	1200	120	125	83	450	113	20	133
Lactating*				400	100	15	50	2.5	125	600	150	4.0	67	1200	120	150	100	450	113	25	167

*See Appendix B for U.S. RDA table for these groups.

Appendix E
Food and Nutrition Board, National Academy of Sciences—National Council Research Recommended Daily Dietary Allowances,[a] Revised 1974

Designed for the maintenance of good nutrition of practically all healthy people in the U.S.A.

	Age (years)	Weight (lbs)	Height (in)	Energy (kcal)	Protein (g)	Fat Soluble Vitamins			Water-Soluble Vitamins							Minerals					
						Vitamin A Activity (IU)	Vitamin D (IU)	Vitamin E Activity (IU)	Ascorbic Acid (mg)	Folacin[b] (mg)	Niacin[b] (mg)	Riboflavin (mg)	Thiamin (mg)	Vitamin B6 (mg)	Vitamin B12 (µg)	Calcium (mg)	Phosphorous (mg)	Iodine (µg)	Iron (mg)	Magnesium (mg)	Zinc (mg)
Infants	0.0–0.5	14	24	kg × 117	kg × 2.2	1,400	400	4	35	50	5	0.4	0.3	0.3	0.3	360	240	35	10	60	3
	0.5–1.0	20	28	kg × 108	kg × 2.0	2,000	400	5	35	50	8	0.6	0.5	0.4	0.3	540	400	45	15	70	5
Children	1–3	28	34	1,300	23	2,000	400	7	40	100	9	0.8	0.7	0.6	1.0	800	800	60	15	150	10
	4–6	44	44	1,800	30	2,500	400	9	40	200	12	1.1	0.9	0.9	1.5	800	800	80	10	200	10
	7–10	66	54	2,400	36	3,300	400	10	40	300	16	1.2	1.2	1.2	2.0	800	800	110	10	250	10
Males	11–14	97	63	2,800	44	5,000	400	12	45	400	18	1.5	1.4	1.6	3.0	1,200	1,200	130	18	350	15
	15–18	134	69	3,000	54	5,000	400	15	45	400	20	1.8	1.5	2.0	3.0	1,200	1,200	150	18	400	15
	19–22	147	69	3,000	54	5,000	400	15	45	400	20	1.8	1.5	2.0	3.0	800	800	140	10	350	15
	23–50	154	69	2,700	56	5,000		15	45	400	18	1.6	1.4	2.0	3.0	800	800	130	10	350	15
	51 +	154	69	2,400	56	5,000		15	45	400	16	1.5	1.2	2.0	3.0	800	800	110	10	350	15
Females	11–14	97	62	2,400	44	4,000	400	12	45	400	16	1.3	1.2	1.6	3.0	1,200	1,200	115	18	300	15
	15–18	119	65	2,100	48	4,000	400	12	45	400	14	1.4	1.1	2.0	3.0	1,200	1,200	115	18	300	15
	19–22	128	65	2,100	46	4,000	400	12	45	400	14	1.4	1.1	2.0	3.0	800	800	100	18	300	15
	23–50	128	65	2,000	46	4,000		12	45	400	13	1.2	1.0	2.0	3.0	800	800	80	18	300	15
	51 +	128	65	1,800	46	4,000		12	45	400	12	1.1	1.0	2.0	3.0	800	800	80	10	300	15
Pregnant				+300	+30	5,000	400	15	60	800	+2	+0.3	+0.3	2.5	4.0	1,200	1,200	125	18 +[c]	450	20
Lactating				+500	+20	6,000	400	15	80	600	+4	+0.5	+0.3	2.5	4.0	1,200	1,200	150	18	450	25

[a] The allowances are intended to provide for individual variations among most normal persons as they live in the United States under usual environmental stresses. Diets should be based on a variety of common foods in order to provide other nutrients for which human requirements have been less well defined.

[b] Although allowances are expressed as niacin, it is recognized that on the average 1 mg of niacin is derived from each 60 mg of dietary tryptophan.

[c] This increased requirement cannot be met by ordinary diets; therefore, the use of supplemental iron is recommended.

Appendix F

Energy Output per Activity and Relationship to Selected Foods.

Food	Calories	Walking[1]	Riding bicycle[2]	Swimming[3]	Running[4]	Reclining[5]
Apple, large	101	19	12	9	5	78
Bacon, 2 strips	96	18	12	9	5	74
Banana, small	88	17	11	8	4	68
Beans, green, 1 cup	27	5	3	2	1	21
Beer, 1 glass	114	22	14	10	6	88
Bread and butter	78	15	10	17	4	60
Cake, 2-layer, 1/12	356	68	43	32	18	274
Carbonated beverage, 1 glass	106	20	13	9	5	82
Carrot, raw	42	8	5	4	2	32
Cereal, dry, 1/2 cup with milk, sugar	200	38	24	18	10	154
Cheese, cottage, 1 tbsp	27	5	3	2	1	21
Cheese, cheddar, 1 oz.	111	21	14	10	6	85
Chicken, fried, 1/2 breast	232	45	28	21	12	178
Chicken, TV dinner	542	104	66	48	28	417
Cookie, plain	15	3	2	1	1	12
Cookie, chocolate chip	51	10	6	5	3	39
Doughnut	151	29	18	13	8	116
Egg, fried	110	21	13	10	6	85
Egg, boiled	77	15	9	7	4	59
French dressing, 1 tbsp	59	11	7	5	3	45
Halibut steak, 1/4 lb.	205	39	25	18	11	158
Ham, 2 slices	167	32	20	15	9	128
Ice cream, 1/6 qt.	193	37	24	17	10	148
Ice cream soda	255	49	31	23	13	196
Ice milk, 1/6 qt.	144	28	18	13	7	111
Gelatin, with cream	117	23	14	10	6	90
Malted milk shake	502	97	61	45	26	386
Mayonnaise, 1 tbsp	92	18	11	8	5	71
Milk, 1 glass	166	32	20	15	9	128
Milk, skim, 1 glass	81	16	10	7	4	62
Milk shake	421	81	51	38	22	324
Orange, medium	68	13	8	6	4	52
Orange juice, 1 glass	120	23	15	11	6	92
Pancake with syrup	124	24	15	11	6	95
Peach, medium	46	9	6	4	2	35
Peas, green, 1/2 cup	56	11	7	5	3	43
Pie, apple, 1/6	377	73	46	34	19	290
Pie, raisin, 1/6	437	84	53	39	23	336
Pizza, cheese, 1/8	180	35	22	16	9	138
Pork chop, loin	314	60	38	28	16	242
Potato chips, 1 serving	108	21	13	10	6	83
Sandwiches:						
club	590	113	72	53	30	454
hamburger	350	67	43	31	18	269
roast beef with gravy	430	83	52	38	22	331
tuna fish salad	278	53	34	25	14	214
Sherbet, 1/6 qt.	177	34	22	16	9	136
Shrimp, french fried	180	35	22	16	9	138
Spaghetti, 1 serving	396	76	48	35	20	305
Steak, T-bone	235	45	29	21	12	181
Strawberry shortcake	400	77	49	36	21	308

[1]Energy cost of walking for 150-lb. individual = 5.2 calories/min. at 3.5 mph.
[2]Energy cost of riding bicycle = 8.2 calories/min.
[3]Energy cost of swimming = 11.2 calories/min.
[4]Energy cost of running = 19.4 calories/min.
[5]Energy cost of reclining = 1.2 calories/min.

Appendix G

CHOLESTEROL CONTENT OF FOODS

(From Feeley, Criner, Watt.)

Food	Portion	Cholesterol in Mg.
Beef, composite cut, cooked	about 3 oz.	80
All fat trimmed	about 3 oz.	77
Brains	3.5 oz.	over 2,000
Butter	Tablespoon (1/2 oz.)	35
Buttermilk from nonfat milk	cup	5
Cake, choc. devil's food	1/16 of 9 in. cake	32
Cake, sponge	1/12 of 10 in. cake	162
Cake, angel, from mix	1/12 of 10 in. cake	0
Caviar	1 tablespoon	48
Cheese, blue	1 oz.	24
Cheese, camembert	1 oz.	25
Cheese, cheddar, mild or sharp	1 oz.	28
Cream cheese	1 tablespoon (1/2 oz.)	16
Cheese, pasteurized process cheese food	1 oz.	10
Chicken, flesh and skin	about 3.5 oz.	87
Chicken, breast meat only	about 3.5 oz.	79
Chicken, drumstick, from 3 lb. bird	about 2 oz.	47
Crab meat	3.5 oz.	100
Cream, half and half	1 Tablespoon	6
Sour cream	1 Tablespoon	8
	1 cup	152
Cream, whipped	1 Tablespoon	20
Eggs, whole, scrambled	1 large egg	263
Egg Yolk	1 large egg	252
Flounder, lean meat only	3.5 oz.	50
Halibut, meat only	3.5 oz.	50
Heart (beef) cooked	3.5 oz.	274
Ice cream, regular	1 cup	53
Ice cream, rich	1 cup	85
Ice cream (frozen custard)	1 cup	97
Lamb, composite of cuts, cooked, lean only	3.5 oz.	70
Liver, cooked beef, calf, pork	3 oz.	372
Liver, chicken	3 oz.	640
Lobster meat, cooked	3 oz.	85
Margarine (all vegetable fat)	1 Tablespoon	0
Milk, whole	1 cup	34
low fat (2%)	1 cup	22
skim	1 cup	5
Muffins, home baked	1 3 in. diameter	21
Noodles, egg, cooked	1 cup	50
Oysters, 6	about 3 oz. meat	60
Pancake, from mix	1 six-inch	54
Pie, apple	slice	0
Pie, lemon meringue	1/8 of 9 in. pie	98
Pie, pumpkin	1/8 of 9 in. pie	70
Pork composite of cuts, cooked meat only	3.5 oz.	89
Salad dressings		
Mayonnaise	1 Tablespoon	80
Commercial mayonnaise type	1 Tablespoon	42
Salmon, cooked steak	3.5 oz.	59
Sardines in oil	3.75 oz. can	127
Sausage, frankfurter, cooked	One, 8 per lb.	34
Scallops, steamed	3 oz.	80
Shrimp	3 oz.	139
Tuna, drained	No. 1/2 can	102
Turkey, light meat, cooked, no skin	3 oz.	65
Turkey, dark meat, cooked, no skin	3 oz.	86
Veal, composite of cuts, cooked, lean only	3 oz.	84
Yoghurt	1 cup (8 oz.)	17

index

This book may be kept

FOURTEEN DAYS

A fine will be charged for each day the book is kept overtime.

GAYLORD 142   PRINTED IN U.S.A.